Advanced Praise for *100 Is the New 30*

I've been working with Dr. Jeff Gladden and his Longevity Institute for almost a decade. I feel that what I've learned and what we have implemented have significantly changed my outlook on aging and my performance as I age. I've seen my biological age get younger, noticed it through significant energy level improvements, and (through competitive CrossFit) had others notice it in my physical performance. I will be 65 this year and am more fit that when I was 40. (When I was 40, I was working out intensely and regularly, so I've been committed to a healthy lifestyle throughout my past.)

In this book, you benefit from the summary of knowledge that Dr. Gladden and his Longevity Institute team have learned. It is a comprehensive approach, and while its title seems a stretch (*100 Is the New 30*), I am further coming to believe it is very possible.

—Kent Pilcher

After reading *100 Is the New 30*, you will know that reversing aging is a choice. Dr. Gladden introduces us to a model of longevity like no other. This is a MUST READ for everyone who wants to take their health to a new level and look and feel better than anyone their age. This book will be a huge disruptor in the healthcare arena.

—Dr. Fabrizio Mancini
America's #1 "Healthy Living" Media Expert,
International Bestselling Author & Speaker, and
President Emeritus of Parker University

The ultimate message in *100 Is the New 30* is one that really resonates with me—aging is a choice. With the right lifestyle strategies and mindset, as outlined in this book, you can fight aging and keep your brain and body young for a lifetime.

—Daniel Amen, MD
Founder, Amen Clinics and author of
Change Your Brain Every Day

I'm lucky to have found Gladden Longevity. Personalized medicine is an understatement for the services they provide. After my dad passed away, I wanted to prioritize health and longevity. Jeff and his team have provided a roadmap, tools, and accountability to get there. I always tell people that in tough times, I'll cut everything before I stop seeing Gladden and his team.

—Eric Barvin

This book is powerful and brings to light a whole new way to approach aging or NOT aging, I should say. I started working with Dr. Gladden and his team at Gladden Longevity 2 years ago after asking myself the questions Dr. Gladden discusses. How good can I feel? Is this really how I'm supposed to age? The human body is meant to work, so why isn't mine? I have learned so much but, more importantly, improved in so many areas of my life. If you read this with an open, curious mind, you will have a whole new approach and mindset around your health.

—Autumn Calabrese
Beach Body

Dr. Gladden's latest book, *100 Is the New 30*, is a comprehensive manual that considers the entire body, inside and out, and gives you a guide to follow to keep you strong both physically and mentally. It covers everything from physical health and aging to the importance of keeping our mind fit as well. As you begin to age, you can take steps to reverse or stop the aging process, *100 Is the New 30* is the manual that will enable you to age gracefully and to live your best life ever.

—Jeff Russell
Founder & Exec Director of the IAPAM (International Association for Physicians in Aesthetic Medicine) and the CEO of the Oakridge Financial Group of companies

Dr. Gladden addresses the topic of aging with poise and grace like no other! In this society so obsessed with youth, we often overlook the quality of life and empowerment that comes from practicing self-care at a cellular level. Aging and time are not correlated. There is a chronology in evolution, yes, but how it is calculated and experienced is very much up to us. *100 Is the New 30* is a manual on how to reach the fountain of youth and quality of life within ourselves—a MUST read!

—Anna Cabeca, DO, FACOG
The Girlfriend Doctor
DrAnnaCabeca.com

When I first met Dr. Jeffery Gladden, I knew he was different. It was obvious from his practice and the quality of his team he was doing something different, doing something better.

When you read *100 Is the New 30*, you get a look into not just why he's different but how he's different!

While traditional medicine looks at "what's wrong" with the patient, Dr. Gladden provides a guide that starts with unique views of "Life Energy, Longevity, Health, and Performance." Clearly a superior plan for anyone trying to get the most out of life.

100 Is the New 30 is an excellent guide for anyone interested in optimizing health and performance!

—Don Moxley, Exercise Physiologist/Sport Scientist
Director of Applied Science, Longevity Labs, USA

100 Is the New 30 is not just a catchy title—the concept is closer to reality than ever, thanks to the strategies detailed in this inspiring, actionable, and revolutionary exposé on longevity. Dr. Jeff Gladden is a pioneer in longevity, with an unmatched combination of clinical experience, client successes, personal journey, and research acumen. From cutting-edge supplement recommendations to emergent testing methodologies, from critical emotional and mental techniques to detailed scientific explanations of specific body systems, this book has something for everyone—even the health enthusiast has so much to learn from *100 Is the New 30*!

—Megan Lyons
Board Certified Holistic Nutritionist, Certified Clinical Nutritionist, and Owner of The Lyons' Share Wellness

As a neuroscientist deeply committed to exploring the infinite potentials of the human mind, I have always been fascinated by the myriad ways we can tap into our own natural abilities to enhance our lives. Dr. Gladden's innovative approach to longevity, as illustrated in his latest masterpiece, *100 Is the New 30*, resonates strongly with my own principles and research.

Dr. Gladden's groundbreaking LIFE RAFT trial is a paradigm shift in our understanding of aging. What struck me the most was the inclusivity of his approach, accepting adults across a wide age range, and his emphasis on the immediate need to claim one's youthfulness. The synergistic integration of Life Energy, Health, Longevity, and Performance is not merely theoretical; it's a practical, actionable strategy that aligns perfectly with my own vision for enhancing human potential.

The meticulous detail with which Dr. Gladden has addressed the fifteen hallmarks of aging, including genomic instability, telomere attrition, and cellular senescence, offers readers an insider's look into the scientific mechanisms that contribute to aging. His proprietary techniques and strategies resonate with the forward-thinking methodologies I embrace with BrainTap, and I firmly believe his work will contribute profoundly to the field of longevity.

Gladden's work in optimizing the human condition is akin to a well-conducted symphony, where every note, every instrument, and every musician plays a vital role. *100 Is the New 30* is more than a book; it's a manual, a guide, a mentor that leads you to the very essence of what it means to live young for a lifetime. It's not just about extending our years but enriching the quality of those years, making every moment count.

I wholeheartedly endorse this book and encourage anyone who wishes to invest in themselves, their health, and their future to delve into its insightful pages. Dr. Gladden has provided us with a remarkable tool that transcends traditional boundaries and offers a tangible pathway to an enriched, youthful life. His magnum opus, the LIFE RAFT trial, represents the future of anti-aging medicine and will, without doubt, mark a transformative moment in human health and well-being.

—Patrick K. Porter, Ph.D.
Inventor of BrainTap and Advocate for
Human Potential and Wellness

Dr. Gladden is a leading Longevity clinician. In this book, he covers all the pillars of Longevity and how to practically adopt those within our lifestyles. A must-read for anyone who wants to add more life to his/her life!

—Dr. Joseph Antoun, MD, Ph.D
CEO & Chairman at L-Nutra Inc.

100 IS THE NEW 30

How Playing the Symphony of Longevity Will
Enable Us to Live Young for a Lifetime

100 IS THE NEW 30

How Playing the Symphony of Longevity Will Enable Us to Live Young for a Lifetime

Jeffrey Gladden, M.D.

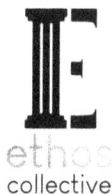

ethos
collective

Printed in the United States of America

Published by Ethos Collective™
PO Box 43, Powell, OH 43065
www.ethoscollective.vip

LCCN: 2023913993
Paperback ISBN: 978-1-63680-187-2
Hardcover ISBN: 978-1-63680-188-9
e-book ISBN: 978-1-63680-189-6

Available in paperback, hardcover, e-book, and audiobook

For bonus material, please visit GladdenLongevity.com/Book100 or scan the QR code below.

Dear Reader,

This book is dedicated to all of you. You who have wanted to find an answer to the aging problem and who want to continue to grow in your understanding of what it means to be truly alive. Learning to defy aging and understanding what it is to live well go hand in hand. My goal is to give you current, actionable scientific information but, more importantly, to give you a glimpse of what it can mean to have many more physically youthful years while simultaneously growing more wise, unencumbered, enlightened, and impactful. This is a life that combines a 300-year-old mind with a 30-year-old body. It is a life no one has yet to lead, and yet I believe we are the first to have this opportunity.

This book is also dedicated to my beloved family, all of whom have now passed. They instilled in me that it's hell to get old and admonished me to never get old. This book is a love letter to them.

Table of Contents

Foreword

From the moment I picked up *100 is the New 30*, I was captivated by the depth of knowledge Dr. Jeffrey Gladden was eager to share. His wisdom emanates from every page. His work resonated with me, touching the core of human experience and the intricacies of aging, resilience, and the pursuit of a life lived fully—a concept I have spent much of my career exploring with regenerative medicine.

100 is the New 30 has the potential to transform lives, inspire change, and provide peace to countless individuals who, like me, have pondered the complexities of aging and the relentless march of time. Through candid reflections, we journey through the challenges of maintaining vitality and question ideas we have often thought to be inevitable. I believe Dr. Gladden's insights will serve as a guide for those seeking to reclaim their vitality and zest for life.

In a world where time's passage is marked by decline and aging, we find ourselves at a crossroads. It is a narrative we've come to accept, a fate we've normalized. But what if we dared to question this narrative? What if we challenged the notion that aging is a linear journey into decline and instead embraced the possibility that it could be an exponential adventure into vibrancy and boundless potential? This is what Gladden does in his exploration.

As a practicing interventional cardiologist, Dr. Gladden has been a witness to the effects of time on the human body. He's seen the struggles, the challenges that often accompany the aging human body. But he's also seen something else—a spark of defiance, a glimmer of hope, and a yearning for something more. It was this refusal to accept the status quo that propelled him to question current conventions. It led him to explore the depths of Age Management Medicine, Functional Medicine, and Integrative Medicine—to seek out answers that would transform his own life and those of others.

Dr. Gladden shares his own transformation, his moments of realization, and the insights that emerged as he pieced together the puzzle of aging. He delves into the intricacies of the human body, unraveling the complex interplay of hormones, genetics, and environment that determine how we age. Dr. Gladden introduces us to the concept that our age is not singular but a collection of different biological markers. He discusses the exponential process that accelerates as we move through life and challenges us to imagine a future where we can shape the trajectory of our own aging.

In the pages of this book, Dr. Gladden confronts the conventional wisdom that aging is a graceless surrender. With a perspective that springs from both a medical career and a deeply personal transformation, Dr. Gladden takes us on a journey—a journey that unfolds in the corridors of science, genetics, and human experience. It's a journey that brings to light a new approach to aging—one that shatters the confines of accepted norms and charts a course toward a future that defies the limits of time.

This book invites the reader to be an active participant in their own longevity, to embrace the levers of health and performance. And in doing so, one can set forth a vision of a life that defies the confines of chronological age.

Welcome to a future where the question is not "How old are you?" but "How young can you be?"

—Anthony Atala, MD
G. Link Professor and Director Wake Forest
Institute for Regenerative Medicine
Winston-Salem, North Carolina
aatala@wakehealth.edu

Introduction

If you want to hear something that will create an existential crisis, think about the fact that you are getting older, and you have no effective strategy to meaningfully change the long road of steady decline that lies ahead. When we observe aging in those around us, we observe capable, vibrant, impactful people struggling to deal with daily loss and decline.

It is not an attractive future: Loss of energy, loss of stamina, loss of capability, loss of resilience, loss of independence, loss of appearance, loss of the ability to perform, loss of friends, loss of impact, and eventually, loss of relevance—even to those inside our own family.

We're told the ideal is to age gracefully. What does that even mean to make peace with loss? Do we smile as we struggle to do simple things and see ourselves drowning in the demise of our mind, body, and spirit? As a practicing interventional cardiologist for twenty-five years, I watched people age. I thought "age well" meant coming to grips with loss and learning to adapt to it. Aging gracefully, then, was an exercise in adapting to loss. What a terrible fate for all of us! I do not see anything graceful about it.

Since you picked up this book, I suspect you're unwilling to accept the traditional trappings of aging, and beyond that, you want a different outcome altogether.

Up to a certain point in my personal and professional life, aging had been an abstraction, not a reality . . . until it started happening to me. As I worked to crack my own code on aging, I noticed that one of the biggest problems we all face is the ubiquitous acceptance of the aging process. Our parents, peers, the medical profession, the government, companies, and even us as individuals have all normalized aging and, in doing so, acquiesced to it. Whenever I hear someone say, "Well, at my age . . . ," I always cringe; it means that both the speaker and the listener have bought into the idea that aging is inevitable, but it's not.

In life, I have discovered that we only get answers to the questions we ask. If we're asking questions like, *How do I retire? How do I adapt to my declining health? How do I find the right retirement community or nursing home?* then those are the answers that we'll find.

On the other hand, if we ask questions like, *How do I actually make 100 the new 30? How do I regain and maintain my youthfulness and vitality? How do I crack the code on this aging process, continue to be vital and relevant, and impact my family, work, and community for years and decades to come?* then *those* are the answers that we'll get. We are the luckiest generation of all time because we now understand how to accomplish what every other generation in every culture has wanted to do: maintain our youthfulness and live young for a lifetime.

Questions are the lifeblood of all progress. They provide the energy for transformation. Answers are resting places that protect the status quo. I wrote this book for those of you who are unwilling to acquiesce to the aging process and are asking the bigger, empowering, energizing questions that create a completely different future for you and every life you touch.

"It's Hell to Get Old!"

My quest to fight aging and stay young for a lifetime started at an unconscious level. I was very close to my maternal grandparents; when my family lived in Michigan, we saw them about every other Saturday. We moved to Philadelphia when I was seven, and they would come and stay with us for a week or two every few months. We spent holidays together, and each summer would take a two- or three-week-long family vacation. My mother was an only child, so my older sister and I got all their attention.

My grandfather was a character. He stood at five-foot, three inches due to scoliosis, had a great sense of humor, and was loved by everyone in his hometown of Marshall, Michigan. An avid golfer, fisherman, pheasant hunter, and mechanical whiz, he worked with my father in the insurance and estate-planning business, and they were the best of friends. When I turned twelve, we started doing "guy trips" together: initially, spin-fishing evolved into fly-fishing for trout, golf, and, occasionally, bird hunting. These were coming-of-age trips for me, and I loved them. I got to do things on those trips that Mom and Grandma would have frowned at, like driving them around New Brunswick, Canada, when I was fifteen and without a license.

My grandmother was sweet and loving, a great cook, and had a dry sense of humor when she wasn't upset about something. By the time she reached her sixties, she would complain about getting old. In her seventies, she periodically would tell me, "Jeff, you don't ever want to get old. It's hell to get old!" When she reached her eighties, this became her mantra; before she died, her bitter mantra about getting old became a daily one. When my grandfather passed away at ninety-seven, she lost her will to live and died six weeks later, at age ninety-six.

"Jeff, it's Hell to Get Old!!"

"You Don't Ever Want to Get Old"

-MY GRANDPARENTS AND PARENTS

I was still a child the first time I heard her say her aging mantra. I didn't understand what she meant, but she said it to me so many times, in so many ways, over so many years, that I started to think, *Okay, I don't think I ever want to get old.*

When my mother reached about seventy-five, she started to echo my grandmother's words: *Jeff, you don't want to get old. It's hell to get old!* At age ninety-three, she still told me this on a weekly basis: *Jeff, it's hell to get old!* She passed away just a few months ago following a fall and broken femur, from which she was too weak to recover.

As a medical student, I knew I wanted to help people recover from disease and sickness. After completing medical school at Temple University in Philadelphia and an Internal Medicine internship and residency at Case Western's University hospitals in Cleveland, I decided to become an interventional cardiologist. I moved to Denver to complete my training at the CU Health Science Center, where we worked at four different hospitals: The University Hospital, the VA, the city hospital, Denver General Hospital, and a private hospital, Rose Medical Center.

The spectrum of experience at those institutions, scattered across the country, prepared me very well for practicing cardiology. An interventional cardiologist conducts all the diagnostic treatments of a non-interventional cardiologist, but we also focus on performing procedures like cardiac catheterization, balloon angioplasty, and placing stents and pacemakers—in essence, trying to save people from needing open heart surgery.

TREATING A HEART ATTACK

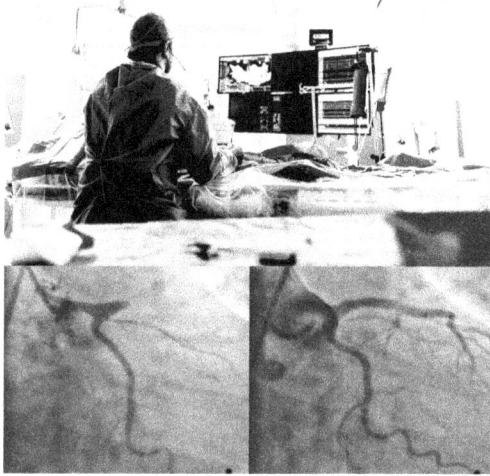

After completing my cardiology training, I moved to Dallas, thinking the chicken-fried-steak-eating, tobacco-chewing people in the great state of Texas might need my help. And I was right—it was a target-rich environment. I loved the work; it was a heady time to be in the field. We were seeing the sickest patients and doing amazing, innovative things; angioplasty was a cutting-edge technology when I left my training, stents became available soon thereafter, and intravascular ultrasound was just emerging, enabling me to achieve much greater precision in what I was doing. I jumped at the opportunity to learn and master each new technology and to train others. I ended up starting my own full-service cardiology group, growing to ten offices and twelve doctors serving Dallas and rural areas in northwest of Dallas and in east Texas. We also had a clinic in southeast Oklahoma. My mission was to make high-quality cardiology care accessible to those living far from the "big city."

For the first time, interventional cardiologists had a lot of new tools, and we developed a lot of new ways to help people. It was super-exciting to me, and I realized that my path forward would be to constantly investigate new technologies and methods to help patients—new medications, strategies, and approaches with more precision and better outcomes.

Quest for the Best

In time, I also satisfied my entrepreneurial spirit. As a college student, I started a summer house-painting business and was able to pay for one-third of my college tuition that way. I also put myself through medical school this way until my schedule would not allow it, and I had to resort to student loans. When the opportunity came for me to set up my own practice, I jumped at it. In the context of adding doctors and locations, we were able to pioneer many innovations for these outlying communities:

- I launched cardiac catheterization laboratories and cardiac rehabs in rural hospitals.
- I produced ST-elevation myocardial infarction programs, also known as STEMI programs, to care for people who had heart attacks, enabling us to respond quickly with treatment to open a closed artery within ninety minutes of EMS arriving at their home.

We continued to build, installing congestive heart failure and atrial fibrillation programs to systematize care. I worked with numerous hospital systems. We would bring more complex cases back to Dallas to perform more complex procedures and connect them with cardiothoracic surgeons if they required surgery. The problem with the large Dallas hospitals is that cardiology was only one of their "service lines." We could never get them to implement the changes we wanted to improve the experience of the cardiology patient and their family. After two years of meetings to do this in one large facility, they told us they were shelving the program for other more pressing needs.

I was dumbfounded, and my entrepreneurial instincts clicked in—which led me to explore other options and eventually reunite with a former partner of mine and Baylor University to co-found a heart hospital in the suburbs of Dallas, Texas. The Heart Hospital Baylor Scott and White Plano has become a shining example of traditional cardiology care and research. I'm very proud of what we did there, and it was all driven by asking different questions such as:

- How do we create the best patient and family experience?
- How do we provide the most cutting-edge technologies to patients with the best doctors?
- How do we make this care accessible to more people?

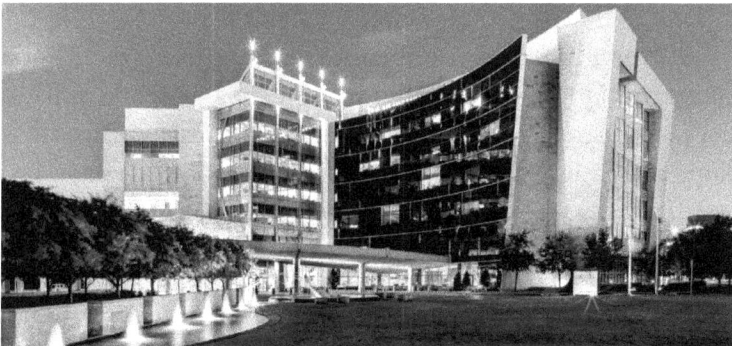

My quest for cutting-edge healthcare did not stop there. In an effort to improve upon the technologies we worked with, I began working with a few medical device companies. I spent time trying to put intravascular ultrasound onto a coronary artery guidewire, which ultimately failed. I also became involved with other kinds of guidewires and catheters, some of which are currently in sales and doing well. I also became part of a pharmaceutical start-up to improve an antiquated technology.

Currently, I sit on the board of two medical device companies that focus on interventional wires for cardiology and neurovascular procedures. I've learned a couple of foundational medical insights while practicing cardiology:

- Great technique cannot make up for poor protoplasm. If a patient has aged or deteriorated beyond a certain point, all the technology, skill, and care in the world would not be enough to overcome the fact that the tissues have aged and lost their resilience and regenerative capacity.
- If I had tools that enabled me to work with greater precision, I could always get a better outcome for a patient.

Leveraging these enabled me to start interventional programs at hospitals with no surgical backup and expand access to care. We utilized strategies and techniques that kept the patients safe. Our track record was excellent, and we did things in smaller communities that were as good or better than what I was doing in Dallas. When I began to focus on cracking the code on aging, I found those insights to be every bit as valuable.

My Confrontation with Aging
(and How I Initially Cracked the Code)

Having been athletic my entire life, I enjoyed running, playing soccer in high school and college, basketball, snow skiing, body surfing, water sports, motorsports, and so on. Medical school should be a sport unto itself, though I did manage to carve out time for physical activity in the first two years. After a day of classes and studying, weather permitting, I would run through the streets of Center City Philadelphia at 11:00 p.m. and ride my bike five miles to North Philly to med school.

As a practicing cardiologist, I was still physically active. I enjoyed snowboarding with my children and introducing them to soccer. I met a friend who introduced me to mountain biking, and I fell in love. I sold the dirt bikes and switched to mountain biking, which was more fun, accessible, and a better workout. Various members of my family excelled at these activities, and we loved spending time together doing them.

When I hit age forty, however, I had the first wave of feeling my age. I leveraged my health to attain my education, build my practice, and raise a family. This is not uncommon among medical professionals, professionals at large, or anyone getting started in life, for that matter. I was quite proud of my accomplishments in my chosen field. With a wife, two young daughters, and a son from a prior marriage, I no longer had the energy to do all the family-oriented activities I once enjoyed. Worse yet, I couldn't pop out of bed in the morning—it took all my effort just to do *that*.

As I mentioned, it was during this period that I also started putting on weight around the middle. I was twenty-five pounds up on my college weight. I thought, "Time to get back into shape—think I'll go for a run." It turns out I could run only two blocks before I had to stop. Wow, had I really, *really* gotten out of shape? I went from running all day in a soccer camp to barely making it two blocks.

I made a conscious decision to integrate exercise into my daily routine. I was super busy, so I alternated getting to work by riding a bike or jogging. Weekends usually included longer bike rides. Pretty soon, I was riding twenty-five miles at a faster and faster clip. I looked for other ways to exercise throughout the day, even if it was simply taking the stairs instead of an elevator. Sure enough, I could run three miles after a few months and felt pretty good.

From there, I started looking for novel ways to get in shape and discovered balance training with balance boards. I bought a Bongo Board® from FitterFirst and was surprised at how challenging it was. I put it in the bathroom to play with it while brushing my teeth and carried it to other places in the house to practice. I was stunned at how it improved my ability to run downstairs. If something fell off the table, like a ninja, I would simply reach out and grab it on pure reflex. My body was learning where it was in space (proprioception) and how to respond to the unexpected without being impacted.

I also *thought* I was making better decisions about my diet. Knowing what I know now, I could have eaten even better, but I cut back on drinking one or two beers two nights a week to two nights a month. What mattered was that I was intentional and committed to creating an environment that supported my mission, and I did things that were fun and challenging. It was exciting to see the results. This regimen worked well for the next ten years, and I staved off the exhaustion I'd felt in my early forties.

However, I started to feel poorly again when I reached my fifties. My "get-healthy" strategy—optimizing my diet and exercise—was no longer working. Yes, I was still involved in a good number of professional endeavors, but this was a different sort of tiredness. I would wake up tired and remain tired throughout the day. I would arrive home exhausted, and sleep—when it finally arrived—offered no relief. I would get up and repeat the cycle. My wife and kids started saying, "Dad's always tired!"

Here I was again: exhausted, putting on weight, and now with a new wrinkle, developing worse brain fog. The brain fog was very concerning because my father ultimately died with dementia. He had been a high-functioning financial planner and insurance professional who achieved national recognition as a general agent and sales leader at every company he ever worked for. Watching him slip away was not only upsetting for him but for me too. Thankfully, he always knew who I was, but to watch someone so capable become so incapable and for them to realize it's happening to them is tragic.

I Got Sick

Increased Weight

Tired and Exhausted

Stress = Anxiety and Depression

Brain Fog

My worst fear in life became that I would lose my mental capacities. This left me anxious and stressed, to the point I experienced bouts of depression. To underscore my mother's and grandmother's messages: "Jeff, It's hell to get old!" "You don't ever want to get old!"

I had some lab work done and met with an internal medicine physician. "Your results are fine," he said. "Everything checks out. You know you're just getting older. Why don't you take an antidepressant?"

"Your Results Are
Normal for Your Age"

"You're Just Getting Older"

Why Don't You Take
an Anti-Depressant"

There it was—the question that brought me one of the most existential moments in my life, the question that has brought so many of us to a poignant, existential moment. I felt like I was being told that I'd reached the full extent of my capabilities and that it was all downhill from there. To think that I could no longer keep up with the kids or perhaps with my younger colleagues was incredibly sobering.

That's when I had an obvious but powerful insight: traditional medicine, my medicine, was failing me.

From Sick Care to Health Care

At that point, I threw myself into integrative medicine, functional medicine, and age-management medicine. I attended conferences, read constantly, and acquired various certifications. Two-and-a-half years later, I cracked the code and understood what had been happening to me.

The reason that I was tired all the time is because I had subclinical hypothyroidism, which means low thyroid that didn't show up in the blood work. Everything indicated that my thyroid was within the "normal range." Remember, the only time we ever get the better answers is when we are willing to ask the better questions, and I wasn't satisfied with the answers I was getting.

I went beyond thyroid blood tests and completed biometric testing, where I tested my reflexes. The results indicated that my reflexes were significantly slower than they should be, which meant I was hypothyroid at a cellular level. Most hypothyroid patients are prescribed only inactive T4, Synthroid, or Levothyroxine, which the body is expected to convert to active T3. My genetics show that conversion from T4 to T3 was significantly compromised in my brain. Once I started taking a combination of both active T3 and inactive T4, I saw significant improvement. The lights came back on almost immediately. I could jump out of bed in the morning, ready to take on the day—and I had the energy to do it all day. I felt great!

My loss of strength and change in body composition—more fat, less muscle—was from a decrease in my testosterone and DHEA levels. Once I added them back into my system, I lost twenty pounds of fat and put on at least ten pounds of muscle. In six months, I was back to my college weight. Obviously, I was eating an even healthier diet by then, minus the beer, and still working out regularly, but my results were stunning.

From there, I looked at my genetics. I discovered that I have a predisposition for dementia and depression. This explained what happened to my father. I suspect Dad had untreated subclinical hypothyroidism and had a decrease in his ability to convert inactive T4 to active T3 in the brain. I am sure he was testosterone depleted. Additionally, I learned that I don't have the genes for Alzheimer's disease, but I do have genes that hinder my ability to make certain neurotransmitters efficiently. This lack of methylation capacity, coupled with a tendency to neuroinflammation, increases the risk of depression and dementia. I found this very useful to know *while I could still do something about it.*

Once I understood why I was feeling the way I was, I felt very empowered. I knew that if I adjusted my diet further to remove inflammatory foods and foods high in glutamate, and if I took certain supplements to decrease neuroinflammation and combined them with specific vitamins to optimize my methylation capacity, I could make the neurotransmitters I needed to make. Feeling razor-sharp is such a great feeling. And as long as I didn't waver from my routine, I was razor-sharp.

When I got myself on the correct hormone replacement strategy, with testosterone and DHEA, and managed my estrogen metabolites correctly, I could get my body composition back to where I wanted it to be.

If I'm on the proper thyroid medication, I can feel really good. I had been taught in medical school that all you need to do is look at TSH. If it's in a normal range, then simply prescribe T4, and there is no need to prescribe T3. I have learned from firsthand experience that nothing could be further from the truth.

That got me thinking . . . what *else* could I do to improve and optimize my health and performance? I wondered, *How good can I be?* How fit, how strong, how mentally sharp, and for how many years—and decades—can I carry this forward?

My mind was humming at this point, and my desire to help others moved to center stage: *If I can feel this good at this point in my life, I'm sure thousands of other people would like to benefit from this kind of approach.* Surely others resonate with the same questions I'm asking.

- *How good can I be?*
- *How fit, how strong, how mentally sharp can I be?*
- *How many decades can I carry that forward?*

Asking these bigger questions in general and this question, in particular, became my initial strategy and has remained my strategy to this today. While the strategy has remained the same, the questions, however, have expanded exponentially. I became fascinated, dedicated, and devoted to unraveling the knot of aging and finding actionable strategies to modulate our biology back into a youthful state.

So, in 2014, I created Apex, the precursor to Gladden Longevity, to focus on these and other questions. I was eventually able to conceptualize and encapsulate this strategy into a structure comprised of four circles and four levels. While the content held in each circle and on each level will change over time, the structure itself is proving to be durable. It is built around the Circles of Life Energy, Longevity, Health, and Human Performance. We begin by understanding all of the significant elements on each circle for each client. Then we address all of them with the proper sequence, appropriately weighted. By doing so, we create unexpected and exceptional results for our clients. Youthfulness can be achieved.

Gladden Longevity attracts people asking the same questions we are: How Good Can I Be? How Do I Make 100 the New 30? How do we live well Beyond 120? And How Do We Live Young for a Lifetime? I first listen to their stories, aspirations, and challenges. Then I build a program across all four circles to test, understand, and treat the drivers of aging as well as the root causes and symptoms of the problems they face. My staff and I also mentor them on optimizing their life energy as they organize their environment to support the implementation of their new behaviors and thought processes.

A New Toolkit

I had an epiphany: as an interventional cardiologist, I wasn't a healthcare provider, I was a sick care provider. In fact, I had spent my entire career practicing "sick care." People only came to see me when they were sick.

Medical professionals are trained at good institutions. They work hard, and well-intended, knowledgeable professors instruct them. When they finish their training, they have a toolkit that amounts to a set of answers built on a scientific model they believe to be gospel. The questions they have been taught are focused squarely on disease. For a cardiologist like myself, those questions include: *Are you short of breath? Do you have chest pain? Are you having palpitations? Are you dizzy? Are you lightheaded?* The toolkit contained the answers: medications and procedures like stents, bypass, valve replacement, etc.

I realized that getting married to a set of answers was a woefully inadequate way to address the needs of any patient. If my solutions didn't fit the patient, all I knew how to do was to send them down the hall to someone else. Maybe *their* answers would fit.

I Left
Sick Care
for
Health Care

Now that my entire focus is on optimizing health, longevity, performance, and life energy, I want to ask a different set of questions.

- *How good can we be?*
- *How do we make 100 the new 30?*
- *How do we live well beyond 120?*
- *How do we Live Young for a Lifetime*

This is the path forward.

The Questions We Ask Are Infinitely More Powerful Than the Answers We Currently Have

-JEFFREY R. GLADDEN, MD, FACC

Gladden Longevity literally has thousands of new answers, yet we are not married to any of them—we are only married to our empowering questions.

The other doctors in my cardiology group couldn't understand what happened to me, their group's founder and president was leaving the world as they knew it. Initially, they tolerated me staying in the group, but ultimately, we all agreed that we weren't aligned and decided to leave. The precursor to Gladden Longevity was born at that very moment, and I've never looked back.

An Exponential Process

You've probably noticed there are people in their thirties who are going on seventy and people who are seventies going on thirty. The difference between the two is their mindset. Our mindsets drive the questions we are asking, and those questions define both the present and the future. If we think about things differently, we also dramatically change our outcomes.

You see, not only have we normalized the aging process, we have mischaracterized it. We live our lives as if aging is a linear process when, in fact, it is an *exponential* process. We age much more between seventy and eighty than we do between thirty and forty. In 2013, "The Hallmarks of Aging," a paper by Carlos López-Otín et al., described nine specific features or characteristics of aging and has served as the catalyst for all longevity medicine and research. In fact, I believe it is the most cited paper in longevity literature. In 2022, another paper was published, expanding the number of hallmarks to fourteen. And later that same year, a fifteenth hallmark was added. Using these sixteen as a springboard, we will dive deeper into each one to demonstrate how they drive the aging process and how we can mitigate them.

Peter Diamandis, primarily known for his contributions to abundance and exponential thinking, describes humans as linear thinkers—yet many things humans deal with change at exponential rates. Applying this to the aging process, we think aging is linear. Every year we add another birthday; it's a linear process.

WE PERCEIVE AGING AS LINEAR

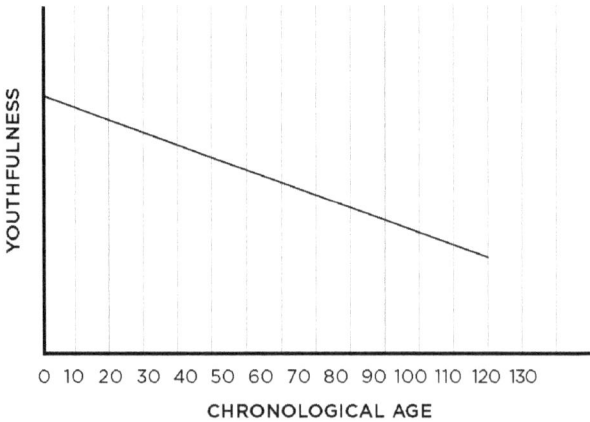

We formulate approaches and strategies based on this assumption, but we're wrong—dead wrong—because we don't realize we are playing an exponential game. If I were to ask you what you will be like ten or fifteen years from now, it is very difficult to imagine that you will be much different than we are today. We have a tough time relating to our inevitable, exponential decline.

AGING IS ACTUALLY EXPONENTIAL

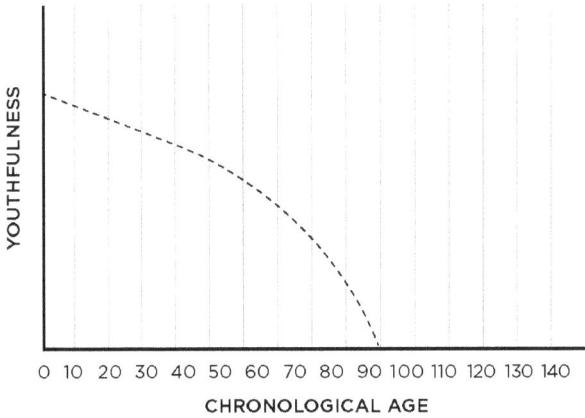

The evidence for exponential decline is right in front of us, and yet we live in denial of it ever happening to us . . . . until it does. An example would be running and skiing at age seventy, playing golf, or driving our own vehicle at eighty-three. By ninety-two, however, we can barely navigate inside our own homes. That is an exponential process!

EXPONENTIAL DROP IN IMPACT WITH AGING

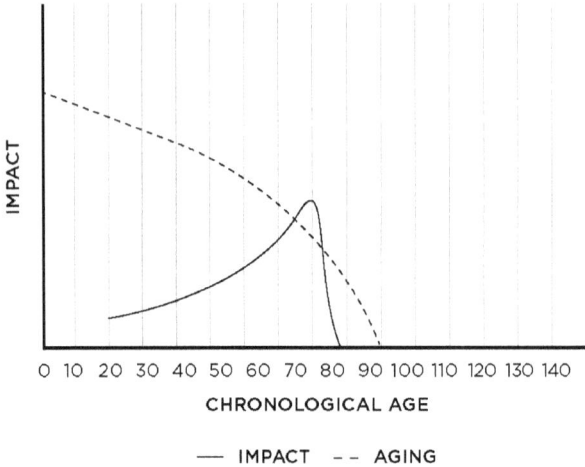

CHRONOLOGICAL AGE

— IMPACT   - - AGING

Wanting to fight against aging is not new; it is an integral part of human history. When we feel our mortality, one response (like mine was) is to get healthy. This applies a linear strategy to an exponential problem and will never work in the long term. A linear strategy may work for three, five, eight, perhaps even ten years, but the accelerating rate of aging will eventually rush past and sweep us up in its current.

I

Living Young Is the Currency of Exponential Impact!

How Young Am I?

What's My Status

The problem, then, is one of both mindset *and* strategy.

The Mosaic of Ages

One important misconception is that our chronological age is our actual age. Or that one biological measurement of our age accurately represents our age. In fact, we don't have one age; we are a mosaic of ages. Here are just a few:

- Telomere Length
- DNA Methylation Patterns
- Immune System
- Stem Cells
- Mitochondria
- DNA Damage
- Thyroid
- Hormonal
- Cardiovascular
- Bone, muscle, joints, ligaments, and tendons

The list goes on and on. As of this writing, we currently measure over sixty different ages for an individual, but we are in the process of expanding that to hundreds of ages by looking at the area of transcriptomics and proteomics. Transcriptomics and proteomics are the measure of DNA expression, which we'll talk more about later.

It's very important to understand your mosaic of ages because, looking at it through a risk lens, you are only as young as your oldest age: *Where is my Achilles heel? What is my weak link, and how can I identify and address it?*

Visualize the exponential strategy to combat aging as a series of four circles and four levels of these circles.

1. Life Energy
2. Longevity
3. Health
4. Performance

At the first level, foundational science informs each of the circles. On the second level, we have identified levers on each circle that need to be pulled or activated to optimize the status of the circles. When it comes to the longevity circle, we've learned that the key is not to pull all the levers simultaneously or randomly just because they are there. There is a timing, sequence, frequency, intensity, and duration with which they need to be pulled in order to experience the greatest effects. This symphonic strategy is a game-changer because so many approaches don't target all the critical levers, and never approach them as a symphony.

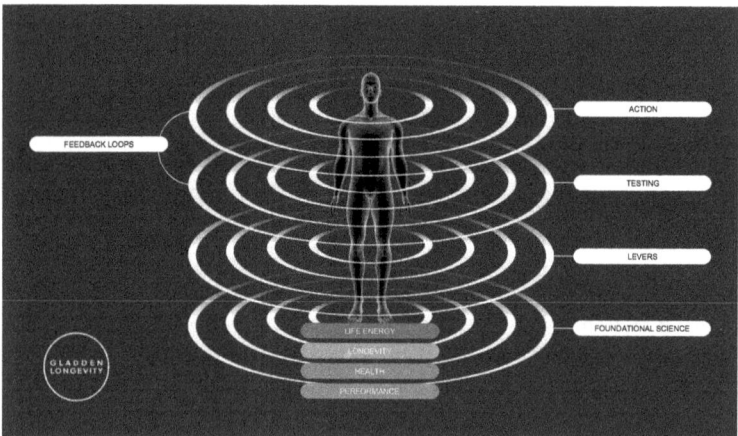

Through extensive testing, Gladden Longevity determines *the most important levers for the individual to have pulled.* A timed sequence of actions is prescribed, and repeat testing is employed to create feedback loops to optimize each circle. This becomes an exponential approach to the exponential problem and will enable an individual to optimize their Life Energy, Longevity, Health, and Performance.

As I mentioned above, I've likened it to a symphony. I call it The Symphony of Longevity™; there are sections, parts, sequences, timing, underlying rhythms, and harmony. This Symphony of Longevity™ approach reinforces that there will never be just one thing that solves the longevity problem—and it certainly won't be found in traditional medicine or an antidepressant. The response to aging must be a timed symphony composed of a number of individualized levers coupled with the underlying processes that drive aging, played in a particular and intentional manner. We believe this is the correct approach to cracking the code to make 100 the new 30 and Live Young for a Lifetime.

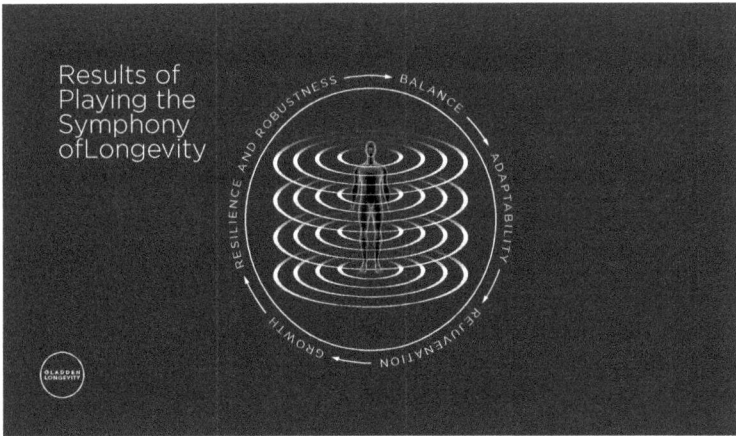

Results of Playing the Symphony of Longevity

Beyond the "Get Healthy" Answer

As you read this book, I think it's important to understand that I will present information to try and change your perspective on the aging process and how to understand, unravel, and approach it for yourself. The answer to your longevity is simply not to "get healthy"—a few notes do not comprise a symphony.

Disclaimer: It is beyond the scope of this book to give specific recommendations to an individual. In fact, that's one of the biggest problems in longevity medicine: linear thinkers, either practitioners or clients, are looking for a magic pill, a one-size-fits-all solution. While I described my own experience, your symphony will have a different melody, bass line, rhythm, tone, and time signature. Even in traditional medicine, what's great for one person is off-key for the next, and that couldn't be more true when it comes to optimizing health, longevity, performance, and life energy. This book will not directly recommend what to do, although I will outline things we do at Gladden Longevity.

One of the biggest mistakes people make is being seduced by doing what is referred to as "complete blood work." Some are conducted online, in a doctor's office, or even in a fashionable longevity clinic tied to a celebrity. What we have seen repeatedly is that comprehensive blood work is anything but.

Another mistake is believing that you have one biological age. An algorithm applied to simple blood tests or a more sophisticated DNA methylation age can calculate biological age. While both are useful, neither is adequate. Remember, we are only as young as our oldest age, so rather than asking, *what is my biological age?* using a single test, the question should be: *What are my oldest biological ages, and how do I address them?*

Many are seduced by a single test and high-five themselves if that single test suggests that they are four or five years younger than their chronological age. While it's a nice boost of confidence, it's also a false reassurance that everything is going well. Getting a comprehensive look at—and understanding of—your mosaic of biological ages is foundational. Understanding the genetic cards you've been dealt, coupled with other measurements and metrics, will help you play your hand optimally.

Can you imagine what Mozart's compositions would sound like without a woodwind section? Have you ever attended a junior-high band concert where one section's timing is off, and everyone gets confused? When you play the symphony of longevity with only partial information, you'll never be able to make good decisions, and ultimately, you will never enjoy the full experience of what your body is capable of becoming and doing.

The testing we do at Gladden Longevity is very comprehensive for a reason; it needs to be in order to define the entire mosaic of an individual's longevity, health, performance, and life-energy ages. The testing instructs us in what to do, when to do it, how to do it, and the sequence in which it needs to unfold for each client for them to achieve their best result. Our goal for each of them is that they lead their very best, most impactful life.

As you read, sometimes you'll notice I get into the weeds just a bit; do not be discouraged or intimidated by this. The goal is to provide you with a deeper understanding of the problem and the strategies currently in play to approach it. We have included a glossary of terms in the back and my contact information in the Afterword, should you want to contact me. We also discuss many topics on the *Gladden Longevity Podcast* at GladdenLongevityPodcast. com, formerly the *Living Beyond 120* podcast. My hope is that you will feel empowered to be your own advocate and, at the very least, have a strong foundation to ask the right questions as you move forward in playing the exponential game of aging, a game in which we are all playing for keeps.

Life on Mars

Making 100 to new 30 and living young for a lifetime is kind of like going to Mars—no one's ever done it before. If you embrace that, joining us means you will be an Age Hacker™ and age-onaut. With the associated questions, lifestyle, and approach, you will look, act, and feel different than your peers. They will wonder what you're doing, and you will likely get to a point where you don't even tell people what you're doing because they wouldn't believe or understand it. Worse yet, they may try to replicate something intricately designed just for you and dismiss it when it doesn't work for them. So it's important that you understand upfront that you will have to be willing to step outside of your social, cultural, and family norms if you intend to go down the path of making 100 the new 30 and living young for a lifetime.

An often-spoken paraphrasing of J.R.R. Tolkien's famous quote from *The Lord of the* Rings is "one ring that binds them all." In longevity, one circle also binds them all: the Life Energy circle. And that is where we'll begin.

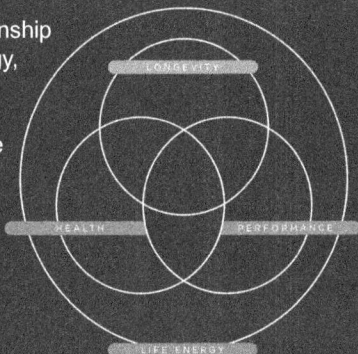

Inter-Relationship of Life Energy, Longevity, Health, and Performance

Introduction Notes

Carlos López-Otín et al., "The Hallmarks of Aging," *Cell* 153, no. 6 (June 6, 2013): 1194–1217, https://doi.org/10.1016/j.cell.2013.05.039.

Tomas Schmauck-Medina et al., "New Hallmarks of Ageing: A 2022 Copenhagen Ageing Meeting Summary," *Aging* 14, no. 16 (August 29, 2022): 6829–39, https://doi.org/10.18632/aging.204248.

Peter H. Diamandis, "How to End Your Linear Thinking," Peter Diamandis - Innovation & Entrepreneurship Community, February 6, 2022, https://www.diamandis.com/blog/how-to-end-your-linear-thinking#:~:text=Our%20brains%E2%80%94the%20100%20billion,world%20that%20is%20increasing%20exponentially.

For more references, please visit GladdenLongevity.com/Book100.

Part One

Life Energy

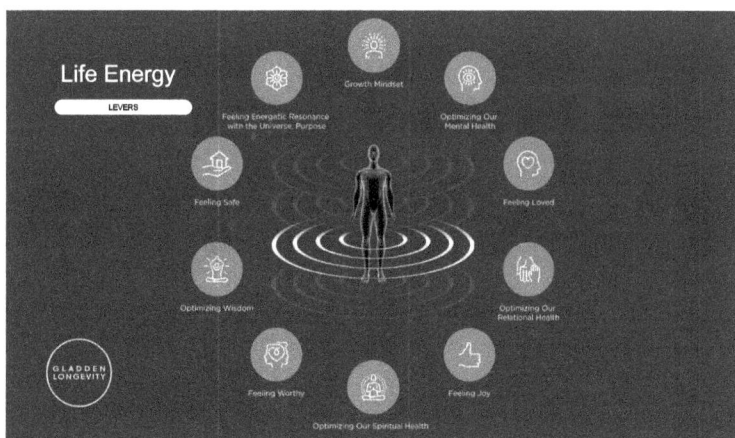

Empowering Questions:

How Good Can We Be?

How Good *Can* You Be?

I n the Introduction, you saw the Gladden Longevity Mosaic of Ages. Each of the Four Circles—Life Energy, Longevity, Health, and Performance—are composed of their own Mosaic of Ages, respective to that circle. For example, your muscle age contributes to your health age; your flexibility and balance ages contribute to your overall performance age; your immune system age contributes to your overall longevity age, and so forth. When we think about optimizing longevity, along with health and performance, it's easy for us to want to focus on the biochemistry of it all—how the muscles work, how the mitochondria work—in essence, how our cells age and how they stay young.

What I've discovered in my clinical practice and my own life experience, however, is that there is an energy foundation that runs beneath the "usual suspects" of biochemistry, diet, and exercise, a foundation that is far more critical to get the results we want: The Life Energy Mosaic of Ages.

While the mosaics of Longevity, Health, and Performance primarily involve tangible, measurable specifics, the Life Energy Mosaic is a bit more ethereal yet no less measurable. Think of it as the underlying rhythm section

3

in the Symphony of Longevity™. Without optimizing this deeper, rhythmic foundation, an organism cannot reclaim its optimal level of function.

Life Energy is the integration of a number of inter-related factors, but collectively, it's the bedrock on which everything else is built. If Life Energy isn't "dialed in," all the biochemistry, medicine, diet, exercise, and all the innovative, cutting-edge science we'll discuss in subsequent chapters will not optimize your quality of life, much less make you functionally age thirty as you approach age one hundred.

Life Energy, therefore, is the starting point in answering the question, *How good can you be?*

As seen in the Life Energies image at the beginning of Part One, we have currently identified ten life energies that are essential to making 100 the new 30 and living young for a lifetime:

- Growth Mindset
- Mental Health
- Feeling Loved
- Relational Health
- Feeling Joy
- Spiritual Health
- Feeling Worthy
- Wisdom
- Feeling Safe
- Feeling an Energetic Connection to the Universe, a Sense of Purpose

These ten should be considered central to you living your best life. As of this writing, these ten are the ones that I have found to be the most powerful, both in my own life and in the lives of my clients. Let's unpack each one and see why.

CHAPTER ONE

Growth Mindset

Perhaps the foundation of Life Energies is having a Growth Mindset, or better yet, an exponential growth mindset. In many respects, an exponential growth mindset is an optimization mindset. The two are almost synonymous. If you are asking questions like, *How do we do this better? How do I become better? How do we understand this to a greater degree?* then you have an optimization mindset. A fixed mindset already has answers and has stopped asking the bigger questions.

In her book, *Mindset: The New Psychology of Success,* psychologist Carol Dweck studied the effects of mindset on groups of schoolchildren. Some were told they were smart, while others were told they were hard workers and good at solving problems. When the "smart" children were presented with a new challenge, if they could not solve it immediately, they would shy away from it and would avoid trying it again.

The "hardworking, good problem-solvers," on the other hand, relished in the fact that they didn't know how to do this new challenge. They were excited that there was something to learn, their brain would get stretched, and their understanding and insight were about to grow. Essentially, they had the foundations of a growth mindset.

Reading Dr. Dweck's book had a profound impact on me as a physician and as a professional. Think about it; as professionals, we go to good schools, receive solid educations, and undergo immersive training in our respective disciplines . . . and we are basically taught a set of answers.

Someone has chest pain. Someone has palpitations. Someone has shortness of breath. Physicians know what to do. We know how to evaluate it. We know how to treat it. We have our answers.

And yet, when I confronted my health issues and found that these answers were inadequate, I started asking different questions.

When you have a growth mindset, you approach life with questions and an open mind. You stay married to the fundamental questions you're asking but not the current answers you have or are finding. When we get married to a set of answers and a new discovery appears, we are not open to it and, therefore, cannot embrace it. I see this frequently in the scientific community; Sir Isaac Newton was like this. He discovered fundamental principles about motion and gravity and became very skeptical and critical of others who were advancing thought in new directions. In essence, he got married to his answers instead of having an open mind and asking, *How do we understand this more deeply? How do we make sense of these findings that don't fit the model? What is the opportunity inside this "problem" to do this differently and better?*

If you are in the process of optimizing your health, longevity, and performance, you can't afford to be married to any of the answers you currently have; otherwise, you are sabotaging your opportunity to adopt appropriate new therapies and adapt to the new aging challenges time is serving up to you.

For example, I meet people who say, *Well, I know how to work out. I know how to eat. My hormones are good. I have my labs done yearly and know what they show.* They may have the right answers for now, but because they've stopped asking the right questions, they are being carried down an exponentially accelerating pathway of aging with no way to keep up. It's critical to understand that it will never be easier to be thirty than it is today, and it takes more than feeling good today to stay thirty. It takes preemptive thinking and actions fueled by ongoing questions to win.

You may have known how to exercise in your twenties, but that doesn't mean you know what's best in your forties, fifties, sixties, seventies, or eighties. A longevity growth mindset is empowered by many questions, like:

- *How do I become better than I am today?*
- *How do I play this symphony better?*
- *How do I understand this process to a greater degree?*
- *How do I orchestrate my environment to better support my aspirations?*

A growth mindset stays open to the idea that what is true today may change in the future, which means our answers must also change. When people are married to their answers, they get defensive and feel the need to dig in their heels on a particular topic. It puts them into a defensive posture and creates relational tension—just read today's headlines regarding discourse among religious groups, political parties, or countries. Look at conflict, perhaps even among your family members, and you will see that once someone is married to a point of view and can no longer entertain another point of view, it leads to conflict, tension, and resentment.

Within political or religious divisions, whenever someone sets aside their answers long enough to ask, *How can we collectively do this better?* growth and community can emerge. A growth mindset is empowering because you can receive new information you need to know at every point in your journey and lower the stress in your life. The benefit of stress decompression arrives when you release the need to be right or think you always have to have the right answer.

I think the entire educational system reinforces this mistaken way of thinking and is missing a huge opportunity to create a better future. It grades students on whether or not they have the correct answers instead of grading them on whether or not they are asking the right questions.

Measurement and Optimization

When we talk about measuring and assessing the Mosaic of Life Energies, there are some objective ways to accomplish this. However, I will continue to stress that due to the abstract nature of each one, the most helpful measurements are subjective. Nobody knows you better than you. You can feel when something is aligned, centered, and you are at peace; you also know when you're not.

Here are a few starter questions to help you assess your growth mindset:

1. *Do I see every event in my life as an opportunity or only a select few?*
2. *Am I becoming "antifragile"?* Author Nassim Nicholas Taleb's book, *Antifragile: Things That Gain from Disorder,* stems from the idea that there has never been a human language with a word that's the opposite of fragile. What does he mean by that? When something fragile meets an unexpected force, it's damaged. When we think about the opposite of fragile, we tend to think of strong, resilient, durable, tough, etc. Taleb would argue that those are good qualities, but when something strong or durable meets a challenge or force, it simply resists that force, and there is minimal impact on the system's integrity. That's not antifragile. His definition is that when something antifragile meets an unexpected force, it becomes stronger. Conceptualize your life energy, health, longevity, and performance as an opportunity to become antifragile. Reframe your challenges as opportunities and take action.
3. *How do I meet unexpected challenges and continue to grow stronger to become antifragile?* Reframe and take action.
4. *Is my resilience increasing?* Reframe and take action.
5. *Do I feel trapped in my current circumstances?* Reframe and take action.
6. *Do I feel like I'm a victim?* Reframe and take action.

I have often thought about my circumstances: *What if I lost everything?* I have gotten to a point in my life where I'm really not attached to things; I have a nice home that contains some nice things, but I'm not attached to them. My real assets are my growth mindset, spirituality, relationships, wisdom, connection to the higher vibration of the universe, love for myself and others, and the ability to give myself safety. If all my things were taken away tomorrow, including my health, my real assets—my life energies—would allow me to survive, reframe, learn, grow, take action, and rebuild.

So when optimizing a growth mindset, we should note that there is skepticism, and then there is *healthy* skepticism. What do I mean by that? Many people in general—and certainly, in the medical community—are skeptical when they hear new information, particularly if they are holding onto their current answers as a reference. They consider "intellectual rigor" to be their method of knowing, their epistemology: *This is not proven. We need to see results from double-blind, placebo-controlled trials before we'll believe it.* This is usually accompanied by a certain self-righteousness misconstrued as intellectual and even moral integrity.

A better approach might be to acknowledge that no one knows everything; therefore, let's look and see, try it, see if it works, understand how it works, and decide if it might contribute to our greater understanding. That's a healthy skepticism—or rather, how to approach new information with a growth mindset—with much more intellectual integrity than simply being skeptical and dismissing it because it's new information beyond your frame of reference.

However, there is a flip side to this, and that's quackery. In this space of longevity, health, and performance, some people have a quick, one-size-fits-all, this-is-all-you-need product or service equivalent to snake oil. These are easily sorted out, as excellent critical thinking skills are essential to a growth mindset. Because you are thinking critically, you will have a deeper understanding of what you are choosing to do and what not to do.

As I've mentioned, the most telling assessments of Life Energies cannot be measured and quantified by assigning a specific number to determine their level of existence or degree of success. So when we talk about optimization with our clients, there's no predetermined path to success, but there are success criteria.

Success is defined as:

- *Are they engaged?*
- *Do they enjoy healthy relationships?*
- *Does their behavior demonstrate self-love or self-destructive behavior?*
- *Do they feel safe, or are they anxious, worried, and angry?*
- *Do they feel worthy?*
- *Are they struggling with any mental health issues or addictions?*
- *What regular practices do they have in place to develop each area in the Life Energies Mosaic?*
- *What improvements are occurring in other areas of Health, Longevity, and Performance that these Life Energies practices have influenced?*

How do you optimize your growth mindset? You first need to determine if there are answers that you're married to or if you are willing to ask bigger questions.

In full transparency, the trickiest answers for many people involve religion and politics because they both hold up answers that are easy to get married to. We find that questions transcend any current answers in all areas, even religion and politics. *How can we do this better? How can we be more spiritually aligned? How can we find deeper meaning? How do we create a better community? How can we create more opportunities for others to thrive?* If you determine that you are, in fact, married to certain answers, you can hold certain positions. But those positions will be dramatically enhanced if you start asking optimization questions around them.

When you start asking the right questions, you invite other people to join you in solving the problem. When you cling to answers, you stand in judgment and, likewise, are being judged.

The more fixed your thinking, the more resistance you'll generate. Optimizing a growth mindset is about becoming married to the questions, not the current answers. Your brain automatically shifts into a growth mindset of looking for new answers and better solutions. It's very freeing, and you will love this creative process.

CHAPTER TWO

Mental Health

M any of us still think that mental health issues involve severe conditions like schizophrenia and the extremes of bipolar disorder. In fact, many of us are hindered by what I would call mild-to-moderate forms of mental health issues like anxiety, depression, post-traumatic stress disorder (PTSD), and attention-deficits. Everyone seems to have something going on, whether it's anxiety, depression, stress, etc. They cope as best they can but can't seem to resolve the underlying issues. Each of us has "run a gauntlet" of one sort or another. None of us had a perfect childhood, an atraumatic adolescence, or a smooth adult life.

The net effect of having run this gauntlet is that we end up living in reaction to the traumas we encountered along the way. We go through life "on tilt," not feeling safe, worthy, lovable, and not loving ourselves. Not only do these issues have a dramatic consequence on our health (and we'll go into that later in the book), but they also dramatically impact our decisions and actions. When we suffer from the echoes of these traumas, we inevitably make decisions and act in ways that are not in our best interest. Those decisions and actions sabotage our ability to thrive, reinforcing anxiety and depression, feelings of worthlessness, and self-loathing. It can become a downward spiral that is crippling, paralyzing, and begins to feel inescapable.

Many of us have genetic predispositions that exacerbate or protect us from mental health issues. Take, for example, the COMT and MAO gene configurations; it has been shown that those who have an optimal configuration of these two genes have greater resilience, even in the face of severe childhood trauma.

The cards you've been dealt are yours to play, but you need to know what cards you're holding so you can play them well and not be played by them instead. The Intellxx DNA genetic panels are a good place to discover the cards you're holding.

In genetics of this sort, almost everything is actionable. Meditation, reflective insight, energy work, Brain Frequency ™, and professional counseling are beneficial in bringing healing, or new and deeper understanding, which can be a catalyst for change. When you get your mental health right, you'll get to a place of equanimity and feel at peace in virtually all circumstances. Better decisions and actions reinforce feeling good about life and yourself, and the downward spiral becomes an upward spiral from which optimal health, performance, and longevity can grow. This is essential to living your best life.

In my own life, I've had some "bad things" happen to me; yet at this point, I have come to see that everything that has happened to me was teaching me what I needed to learn in order to enable me to become my best self, bring my best gifts forward, and allow me to make my greatest contribution and impact. Looking at my life from this perspective, there is no sorrow, pain, or regrets—only gratitude and love for the opportunities I have been afforded. It takes a concerted effort, time, attention, and resources to understand, heal, and ultimately transcend our traumas, but it is so worth it.

We tend to think of our genes as a blueprint that determines our destiny and that we have very little control of the genes or the destiny, but this couldn't be further from the truth. Genes are a set of possibilities, with a predilection for a certain outcome, but how they become expressed is a function of the environment they reside in.

Epigenetics is the interface between the environment and genetic expression. When we think about optimizing mental health—for example, the effects of post-traumatic stress disorder (PTSD)—consider the study conducted on pregnant women during the Nazi occupation of Holland during World War II. Expectant mothers were under tremendous psychological stress, with the uncertainty and ambiguity about what would happen to them and their unborn children on a day-to-day basis. That stress was transferred epigenetically to their offspring; when your mother is under a great deal of stress like that, it will have an impact on how your genes are expressed.

As they followed these children after they were born, they were noted to have significantly higher instances of anxiety, depression, mental illness, and chronic disease. In addition, they all died sooner than children carried by and born to mothers who were not exposed to that degree of stress.

In short, the stress you're feeling and your mental health are impacting your children, just like your parents and their parents had an impact on you. We are carrying three to five generations of epigenetic impact in our genomes. Understanding what your ancestors had to deal with can give you some insight into your own stress responses. Solving this mental health problem is not just for yourself but also for your children and the generations that follow you.

The world is, and always will be, an unpredictable place. The only thing that is guaranteed is change, and you can't guarantee what the change will be. Understanding that there are ways to make peace with that uncertainty and unpredictability—living in the present and being grateful for everything is a form of transcendence—can be very powerful and liberating.

We all live in reaction to things that have happened to us; in essence, they put us knowingly or unknowingly on tilt. Living on tilt in reaction to past traumas limits our ability to be our best selves and make our greatest impact. The goal, as I see it, is to reclaim our birthright to be unencumbered by past events so that we can actualize the full expression of ourselves, bring all our gifts to impact this world, and make it a better place.

Measurement and Optimization

When it comes to assessing mental health, we know there are some important genetic predispositions to understand. There are genes that predispose us to depression, and I have some of those genes myself. I struggled intermittently with depression in my twenties and thirties and became very depressed at other points in my life when my marriages failed. I've been through two divorces; when I went through the first one, I became so depressed at losing the dream of being a family that I became suicidal. It was the first time I'd felt such physical pain in relation to being depressed. Divine intervention and therapy helped me re-equilibrate and move on, but it wasn't until I later got on the right regimen of supplements to correct my genetic methylation cycle deficiencies that I came into a sustainable equilibrium.

Learning to meditate was also very helpful, and realizing if I began to feel depressed that taking a methyl donor SAMe, taking action in the areas I could control, and speaking with as many people as I could to increase my connection, sense of love, friendship, and wellbeing proved to be very helpful. My genetics haven't changed, but my life has dramatically changed because I kept asking how do I do this better and how do I avoid depression.

Food and alcohol can have an impact on our mental health genetics as well. Glutamate, for example, is an excretory neurotransmitter that, in excess, can cause brain fog and anxiety. Therefore, it makes sense that foods that are high in glutamate, or for that matter, histamine (or histamine-releasing foods), can trigger anxiety and depression. When I refrained from eating the wrong kinds of foods, I stopped getting anxious and depressed and had more mental clarity.

Alcohol or THC are used by many to self-medicate, but they never address the underlying issues. In many cases, based on genetic predispositions, drinking alcohol makes the anxiety better now . . . but *worse* tomorrow! We are fans of getting to the root cause, not masking the symptoms with prescription drugs or the use of alcohol or THC.

Hormones also play a role in mental health. If your thyroid levels are low, you may feel depressed. Women know premenstrual syndrome is very real, whether they are greatly affected by surging estrogen relative to progesterone or not. Men have hormonal changes that also affect their mental health; when they go through andropause (similar to menopause for women), testosterone drops, and their personalities can change from confident to insecure. Low testosterone not only affects libido but can cause men to be much less resilient in the face of stress.

So when we talk about mental health, it's fair to say that we are talking about a combination of genetics, epigenetics, biochemistry, our current life events, diet, and lifestyle choices. For example, for thirty years or more, those who exercise have been shown to have less anxiety and depression.

In addition to the influences I've outlined above, mental health has such a strong correlation to what we experienced growing up. Understanding your own history as well as your parents' and your grandparents', will help you unravel that knot and gain insight into how to take control of your mental health. There are many forms of therapy to help with this, but in general, they focus on resolving, making peace with, and forgiving the traumas and perpetrators we experienced. By resolving, I mean understanding and experiencing that whatever traumas we suffered do not reflect our lovableness, worthiness, or ability to feel safe. When we get back to our pristine, untainted self, say our toddler self, it is possible to rewrite our childhoods and, in so doing, claim and experience our birthrights to unconditional love, joy, and safety.

It is beyond the scope of this book to delineate all the useful therapeutic approaches, but everything from counseling to specific trauma work with EMDR (Eye Movement Desensitization and Reprocessing), Brain Frequency™, NeuroFeedback, Keatamine-assisted therapy, or Psilocybin-assisted therapy can be very helpful. If you want to optimize your life, addressing things that you are knowingly or unknowingly living in reaction to can have a massive impact on your health. When this psychological insight is coupled with genetic and biochemical insight, it can be life-changing.

A few questions to ask yourself:

- *Do I experience anxiety?*
  - *If so, how often?*
- *Is there a genetic component?*
- *Is there a food component?*
- *Does alcohol play a role?*
- *Is there a circumstantial component to this?*
- *Do I experience depression? (We found that depression is a function of inflammation in the brain.)*
  - *If so, how often?*
- *Do I feel stressed?*
- *Am I driven by stress?*
- *Do I have a family history of mental illness?*
  - *If so, what actions should I take to avoid going down those same pathways?*
- *Do I feel loved?*
- *Do I love myself unconditionally?*
- *Is there anything about myself that I hate?*
- *Do I criticize myself?*
- *Am I hard on myself?*
- *Am I living on tilt?*
- *Am I living in reaction to something?*

Be honest with yourself in your responses because everything that we will discuss in subsequent chapters has actionable steps. The more honest you are, the better the outcomes. This should give you hope. While we will address some of those life-energy questions in detail later in the chapter, these are all key signs that point to the current state of your mental health.

As mentioned above, there are some interesting, effective therapies available to help reprogram the brain. In fact, one of my working theories is that mental health optimization is a function of reprogramming the brain. And the reason I say that is because we tend to think of the brain as what's in between our ears, right?

I've moved beyond that concept. The way I think about it is that our entire body is, in fact, the brain. When I was a first-year medical student, I was studying for my final exam in anatomy, and it dawned on me. If I knew where all the nerves in the body were running and what structures they ran past, I would know anatomy extremely well and ace the exam. I ended up with the third-highest score in a class of 185 students.

The nervous system runs everywhere, so it is the key to everything in the body. If we can reprogram our brains using therapies, as I mentioned, and increase our neuroplasticity by boosting Brain-Derived Neurotrophic Factor (BDNF) with the right high-fiber foods or by using certain peptides like Semax, Selank, or Dihexa, we can effectively reprogram our brains to optimal mental health and function.

Understanding your genetics and biochemistry plays a big part in assessing your mental health, but reprogramming your brain and taking the right supplements will help you optimize it. Reintegrating your brain and neural pathways with things like neurofeedback and Brain Frequency™ can be massively helpful so that you think and feel about things differently, and they no longer stress you out.

If you are already on the path and have done the "shadow work" that brought you to be at peace with yourself, you know how to give yourself love and safety. You also accept your flaws, understand you are not perfect, and therefore, do not hate anything about yourself. Instead of beating yourself up when something happens, you ask, *What can I learn from this? I realize I made a mistake. I have apologized and made amends, and I will grow from this.* That is an optimization mindset for mental health.

Most of us already know that managing stress is one of the biggest things that we can do to improve our health and longevity. We know that chronic stress will lower the immune systems, therefore decreasing our ability to fight off diseases like COVID. Stress will raise blood sugars and put us into a state of high cortisol and high insulin. High-insulin levels drive the aging process, which we will cover in greater detail in Part Three. For now, make note that learning effective ways to manage stress—or better yet, having a sense of equanimity going into a situation where stress does not impact you—goes a long way toward slowing down the aging process.

You will not feel that equanimity, however, unless you feel loved and safe.

CHAPTER THREE

Feeling Loved

The next Life Energy area that I think is absolutely critical is feeling loved, including self-love, and there are sort of two facets to feeling loved. Imagine yourself when you're two or three years old. When you see that little person, how much love do you have for them? Do you want to just scoop them up in your arms and nurture them, celebrate them, love them, laugh with them, and encourage them to do great things? Do you want to share your joy and love with them? Is that your approach to yourself? Or do you beat yourself up, judging yourself harshly?

The lack of self-love does a lot of psychological and biological damage. It places us in a very stressful position, and then we're going out into the world without the confidence of being loved or that we are even lovable. That underlying software program has an impact that expresses itself in all our relationships, the decisions we make, who we marry, who our friends are, what business we get involved in, and so on. Figuring out that you're lovable, *truly* lovable, and giving that gift to yourself is a critical birthright to reclaim.

I'm the first person in my family to go through four years of college, and I didn't have a lot of guidance there. Initially, I wasn't accepted into medical school; I majored in chemistry, which made the process more difficult. Had I majored in biology, I probably would have had a 4.0 GPA, but chemistry was more challenging for me. I loved organic chemistry and biochemistry, but the complex, math-related subjects, like physical chemistry and calculus, were much more challenging. I deduced that I wasn't that smart. I wished I was so much smarter and would beat myself up over it.

When I did get accepted into medical school, I did exceptionally well—graduating near the top of my class, being an honors graduate, being elected to the Alpha Omega Alpha honor society, and being accepted into a very well-respected internal medicine program at Case Western Reserve in Cleveland. At some point in the process of going through medical school, I realized that I'm not the smartest person on the planet nor, in some areas, the smartest person in my class, but I'm smart enough to do exceptionally well at anything I'm interested in doing. From then on, I never looked back; I *was* good enough. I have enough aptitude, insatiable curiosity, and drive. I realized I was blessed with enough and that my gifts would enable me to make a real impact. I suspect the same is true for you.

When I got to a place in my life where I was just grateful for the gifts that I have and had made peace with it all, it made a major contribution to self-love. When we seek love and approval from external sources—through our families, friends, and significant others—we will never arrive at the same level of peace that we achieve when we are able to give that love to ourselves.

Parents are not perfect. Having been a parent and a child, I understand that parents are not perfect (and my four children will back me up on this). As children, we expect that our parents will love us, but it rarely works out that way. Parents have their own issues with self-love, agendas, and stressors. It's unlikely they gave you all the love that you needed.

In my case, love became associated with a couple of different things. For starters, when I was young. I felt like I could never get my father's attention; he was always so busy and brusk I referred to him as the angry giant. In contrast, my mother always seemed to want more of a relationship with me. I learned later as a teenager that this was a response to my father being so emotionally distant. My older sister was mentally handicapped, and I was evolving enough emotional intelligence to understand what everyone in the family was going through.

At the end of the day, I found that I was living in reaction to those two parental influences: a distant father for whom I was not enough to get his attention and a mother who wanted to smother and manipulate me into taking care of her needs. I equated love from a female as smothering and needy and love from a father as being something that was almost unattainable. I ended up making the major decisions in my life—my friends, my spouses, my career, my work ethic—living in reaction to that gauntlet of things I'd run as a child.

When my son was born, I felt unconditional love for another human being for the first time in my life. It was dramatic and life-changing. It dawned on me that many of my relationships were not going as I wanted, so I started to do a deep dive into myself: *If I can feel this much love for my son, why don't I feel that much love for myself? And why didn't I get this sort of love when I was a kid?*

Through visualization exercises, I manifested a maternal energy seat and a paternal energy seat in my psyche. I went back and removed my mother's energy and replaced it with the unconditional love that I felt for my son and then directed it at little Jeff—at age three—and it felt really good. I felt loved, celebrated, nurtured, and encouraged. At the time, I was really focused on solving the maternal side of the equation and the way it was impacting the women I was choosing to be with. Living unconsciously in reaction to her, I chose to be with women who would not smother me. Unfortunately, they were not able to engage in the level of emotional intimacy I was looking for.

Some years later, I did the same exercise with my father. I removed his energy from my paternal psychic energy seat and replaced it with the same unconditional love for little Jeff I described above. Once I did that, another major breakthrough occurred.

All of a sudden, I had love coming from both parental energy seats and energy from my adult self, all scooping up little Jeff and showering him with unconditional love, encouragement, nurturing, and celebration. It was like a three-legged stool of loving energy that had a firm foundation—I felt liberated from any questions of being loved, being lovable, being enough, or being worthy. I was free to stop living in reaction to my parents. Feeling replete in love, I could look at them with empathy for the lives they'd led, the gauntlets they had run, and who they *really* were instead of who I needed them to be. This allowed me to have much more compassion and love for them and to build warm, loving relationships with each of them that previously seemed impossible. This breakthrough led me to intentionally choose other people in my personal relationships, also.

While that was a quick synopsis of my journey, you have your own journey. To feel truly, unconditionally loved, this is work that you will need to do as well, but it is remarkable how it will change your perspective on the people closest to you—not to mention the impact that it will have on your health, your longevity, and your performance. Those who are in loving relationships and feel love for themselves have healthier and longer lives. So feeling loved is a big, big deal.

CHAPTER FOUR

Healthy Relationships

W e seek many things in a relationship, but ultimately, we crave to know and be known, to love and be loved. As a physician, I show up as wanting to know my client and have them feel cared for and nurtured. In a close relationship with either family or friends, I want there to be reciprocal—knowing and being known, loving and being loved. In my life partner, I want the deepest knowing and being known, loving and being loved.

Understanding what comprises a great relationship took me a while to figure out and understand. This process of knowing and being known is built up what I call Courageous Conversations. A Courageous Conversation is built upon the idea that in many relationships, we find a level of rapport; the goal going forward is to maintain that level of rapport. Conversations tend to shy away from taking risks, from us revealing how we feel in a non-judgmental way for fear of rejection, damaging the relationship, or being judged. Yet it is when we take a deep gulp, ask a question or say something that we think is risky we open the door to much deeper understanding, much deeper knowing and being known, loving and being loved.

Without Courageous Conversations, relationships can grow stale, repetitive, and stifling. With Courageous Conversations, relationships can continue to grow and evolve to new depths of understanding and intimacy. Before launching into a Courageous Conversation, it's best to have a conversation about having Courageous Conversations. It has to be done in a bidirectional, non-judgmental way and in the spirit of really wanting to understand the other person. When done in that context, it is like actively gardening in the relationship, plucking out weeds and preconceptions or misconceptions that no longer serve anyone, and planting understanding, mutual respect, and love. The closeness you feel and the intimacy you share will explode in your relationship. It takes courage.

Another area that comes up in relationships is the idea of forgiveness. This was always a nebulous concept for me; if I said I forgave someone, or they said they forgave me, I wasn't quite sure what had just happened and what it meant going forward. Any significant relationship that is functioning well is characterized by the unrestricted, uninterrupted flow of love, or positive regard, between ourselves and the other person.

Therefore, when something happens—or is done by one party—we no longer feel safe in a relationship. It could be a lie, an unkept promise, an act of disregard, or feeling judged, but whatever the details are, it leads us to a place of not feeling safe. The unrestricted, bidirectional flow of love, or positive regard, between ourselves, stops, and we build a psychic wall that no longer permits us to send or receive, to feel love or positive regard from that person. The problem is, maintaining that wall requires a lot of psychic energy. It takes a toll on us and our health.

Let's say, for example, you're dating someone and break up. Typically, something was going on in the relationship, and you no longer felt safe, nor did you see a pathway to feeling safe again, so you ended the relationship. Putting up a psychic wall is the typical response that enables you to feel safe with the net effect of cutting off that free flow of affection you had shared.

I've come to understand forgiveness as taking down the barrier. Dropping the barrier to the free flow of love or positive regard, even if you have left the relationship, has a very healing effect. Many times, we hear of or experience being forgiven or forgiving, yet, we still hold a grudge or a resentment. This is not forgiveness. More Courageous Conversations have to happen if the relationship is to be repaired to the point where forgiveness can happen. Knowing what constitutes forgiveness and when forgiveness has occurred is critical to healing, having great relationships, and letting go of the ones that can't be repaired with equanimity and no hard feelings.

As an experiment, think about a past relationship that was going great. You felt love, you received love, and then all of a sudden, for whatever reason, it changed. Now there's a wall between you. Say to yourself, *Okay, I'm going to take down the barrier and allow love or positive regard to flow freely from me to this person, and if there is any positive regard coming my direction, I will receive it.* (It doesn't matter who did what to whom, who said what to whom . . . none of that matters anymore because fundamentally, love really does conquer all.) When you open yourself up and feel an open channel for loving energy or positive regard to flow from you to that other person and vice-versa, your stress level goes down, and you start to be at peace. Notice what that does for your psychic energy. All of a sudden, your whole psyche just settles into a peaceful calm, and it feels really good. There is no longer this sort of edge or grudge that you're carrying around. These negative feelings we haul around are baggage, and it only harms *us*—not the other person.

When you love yourself—your Little Self and your Big Self—and do the work necessary to achieve a free flow of love between yourself and everyone in your life, that's an incredibly healthy position to be in.

That is also a really big challenge. Be kind to yourself and walk through the experiment I suggested to create a practice. Find a place that quiets your mind (which likely means finding somewhere that is quiet and free from distractions). Take time to think about that other person; settle into that thought, then go back to when you did feel love. Allow that to be the dominant force. Let love flow back and forth, unobstructed. You will see that your whole psyche settles down. It will also change your perspective on the other person.

You no longer have to live on tilt, where you are trying to hold on to that grudge. Nor will you carry the risk of sabotaging the next opportunity for a relationship with the negative residue from this one.

Healthy relationships are characterized by being interdependent but not codependent. Interdependence is two healthy individuals creating a Venn diagram of life activity. In the middle is a very large maximal area of overlap of knowing and being known, loving and being loved. They have their needs met internally with themselves in the relationship and outside the relationship with friends and colleagues. Codependent relationships are formed by two needy individuals who are trying to get all their needs met within the relationship and through the other person. Great relationships depend on you having done the work or being in the process of doing the work to become your unencumbered self—where you are not living in reaction to prior experiences but living out of your true, liberated nature. Finding a partner to do this with is life-changing. It certainly has been for me.

When we talk about optimizing the feeling that we are loved, it begins by loving ourselves. At the beginning of our lives, we're cute, innocent, and cuddly—nothing but lovable. As we grow up, we're scolded, corrected . . . sometimes too harshly. Maybe you were bullied at school or by a sibling. Or perhaps you felt abandoned. We end up feeling, on some level, that we're not lovable.

If that external message—that we're not lovable—gets imprinted into our psyche, it sabotages our ability to love ourselves and others. We internalize the criticism and judgment and start beating ourselves up. Every perceived shortcoming reinforces what we think is true.

By becoming the loving, present parent to that younger version of yourself, you can give yourself the unconditional love you deserve. That is your birthright. Your hero's journey is to reclaim your birthright. It's incredibly powerful, removing all of that judgment and all of that misaligned energy that was directed at you. This practice of scooping yourself up as the loving parent overrides all that.

You can rewrite your history if you really focus on optimizing self-love. I suggest you work with a therapist, a trusted friend, a mentor, or even by yourself to reclaim this love. Then, you can begin the work to optimize the love you share with others, to attract and build the great relationship you deserve with family, friends, and a significant other.

Solving the self-love equation is definitely a necessity for a great relationship, but it's not sufficient to sustain a relationship. In how many close relationships have you thought, *I really love this person, but I'm not sure I want to marry them?* Or, *I love so many things about him or her, but they are still not the right person.* Love is necessary but not sufficient.

Many will tell you that communication is the problem in relationships, and I have to agree. Recently, I have drawn the conclusion that language is a very poor form of communication. George Bernard Shaw famously said, "The single biggest problem in communication is the illusion that it has taken place." So, what is the solution?

Mental telepathy would work much better, as we could instantly know and be known. We could know how the other person feels, what they think, and how it makes an impact on us, collectively. But telepathy is not yet readily available, so we are stuck, dribbling out words to try and describe and explain a complex internal world that sometimes feels ineffable and incomprehensible.

For me, understanding the limitations of language changes the way I listen. Instead of assuming I know what the other person is thinking when they say something, I will say or ask things like:

- *Tell me more.*
- *Are you saying this?*
- *Did I get that right?*
- *I'm not sure I fully understand what you meant.*
- *Can you explain that to me?*

This type of active listening is a strategy to compensate for the limitations of language. The ultimate goal is to be heard and understood, and vice-versa.

Practice with the people who are closest to you—your children, your spouse, your significant other . . . you get the idea. It needs to be someone with whom you can talk to about this. Ask them, *How can I be more loving? What would make you feel more loved? What would make me feel more loved?*

Another key thing I've learned is that many things can be true at once. What I mean by that is that we can hold what ostensibly are contradictory ideas, thoughts, or judgments, yet they all make sense in defining a nuanced whole. Being able to communicate courageously around the multifaceted feelings and thoughts that exist within each of us and be heard, known, loved, and not judged is next-level communication. When you get there, it increases closeness and intimacy tenfold!

Here is a practical step you can take: it's called turning *toward* someone when they make a bid for closeness or intimacy. In the book, *The Love Prescription: Seven Days to More Intimacy, Connection, and Joy*, renowned psychologists and therapists John and Julie Schwartz Gottman discuss the importance of turning toward a loved one when they make a bid for attention. Doing so builds trust and connection, whereas *not* turning toward it fosters distance and resentment. In successful relationships, the person whose attention is being sought turns toward the person bidding for attention over 80 percent of the time, whereas in failed relationships, this only happens 30 percent of the time.

We tend to take all this for granted and usually don't talk about it—but it's quite helpful to courageously put everything on the table and look at everything as an opportunity, particularly if you've run into a snag in a relationship where one party or the other isn't feeling loved. Any understanding as to why one of you feels that way is important—people experience love in different ways.

In addition to language, we read each other's energy, pay attention to intonation, and so on. Albert Mehrabian, a researcher on body language, was the first to break down the components of a face-to-face conversation. He found that communication is 55 percent nonverbal, 38 percent vocal, and 7 percent words only. Actions, of course, speak louder than words, but what do they say? They, too, arise from a complex milieu of feelings and presumptions where many things can be true simultaneously. Nonetheless, unpacking those words and the nonverbal energy behind them is critical in knowing and being known and in giving and receiving love.

Robin Williams once said, "I used to think that the worst thing in life was to end up alone. It's not. The worst thing in life is to end up with people who make you feel alone." Many studies suggest that married people live longer, particularly married men who live longer than unmarried men. Interestingly enough, however, those results are only true if it is a good relationship.

Relationships that are truly nurturing—where you have each other's back but also respectfully and courageously tell each other the truth and hear the other person's truth—build deep, abiding trust and intimacy. During a meditative experience several years ago, I developed a new concept of heaven. It was two o'clock in the morning, and I could not sleep. I wandered into my office and sat down in a chair. Opening my copy of Eckhart Tolle's *The Power of Now*, I began reading when suddenly, the words were just resonating with me in a way that my head just kind of rocked back. I just went into this very meditative state where I immediately understood that there was love flowing through everything. On the other side of this river of love stood "God," not in a human form, but as pure consciousness. I had this incredibly powerful and reciprocal sense of being known and loved—it was unforgettable. We are children of God, i.e., God-like, and these experiences revealed this to me in a profound way. Living our unencumbered lives is to step into our birthright of being God-like. Think about that for a minute, and watch your joy rise and your problems and worries melt away.

All of a sudden, there was this feeling of absolute peace and reciprocity. It was the culmination of everything that anybody has ever been looking for in a relationship, and it was right there. I remained in that state for some time, at least an hour. In time, I went back to sleep, but it profoundly impacted me and really changed my idea of heaven—it was not about pearly gates and streets paved with gold, both of which always seemed kind of useless. My definition of heaven has now become knowing and being known, loving and being loved, and feeling absolute safety. That's also become my template for having the healthiest relationships.

Measurement and Optimization

Think about your best friends. They know parts of you and may or may not love you unconditionally. You feel the same about them. Heaven on earth is available to us in this concept of knowing and being known, loving and being loved. Initially with God, and then in relationship with others. When you examine and evaluate your other relationships, you can compare it to this ideal scenario:

- *Where am I truly known?*
- *Can I be really open with this person?*
- *Do I have the courage to speak about what is really on my heart?* (The courage in a relationship comes in

us revealing ourselves and taking responsibility for how we feel, not blaming the other person.)

- *Do I actively listen to know and understand?*
- *Am I replete, or am I needy?*

And vice-versa: *Am I asking my partner or my friend the questions that allow me to get to know them?* When you arrive at a place where you feel like you really know and love them unconditionally, that's your relationship North Star.

So when you think about optimizing relational health, it's not just that you get along, don't fight, have things in common, enjoy the same activities, or have children together. It boils down to whether you know and are known, love and are loved, and you create a safe, soft space for each other. That is the key to having a great relationship. To the extent that you can find friends and a partner who will go on this journey with you, you're well on your way to optimizing your health and longevity because there is so much peace and joy that comes from great relationships.

As a reminder, measuring and optimizing the Life Energies are highly personal. We can't weigh or assign a numerical value to tell you whether you have hit a scientifically substantiated "normal" range. With this in mind, however, we can assess our relational health in several ways.

1. First, ask yourself: *How many people actually know me?* Many times we're hesitant to allow people to know us because we feel fearful. We don't feel safe; we don't feel lovable. Are there people in your life who know you well, with whom you freely communicate, and you feel you could trust them with anything? How many people do you have like that in your life?

2. Next, how many people do you have in your life who actually love you? If you were to ask them, "Do you love me?" they would reply, "Yes, I really love you." How many of those people are in your life? Usually, the list is larger than you think.

3. Third, make three lists. The first list is those for whom you currently feel love; the second is for those for whom you used to feel love; and finally, the third list is the list for whom you *wish* you felt loved. It could be a parent, a sibling, or even a business partner . . . anyone you wish you could feel love for. Once you see those lists, you'll start to get a handle on where you are in your relational health.

4. Now review all three lists again, and ask yourself: *If I could change one thing about the way I show up in these relationships, what would that be?* Typically, it comes down to us starting with forgiveness, taking down the barrier, followed by being courageous.

Looking at your relationships through the lens of forgiveness and courage, you will be able to identify where to put your energies and where you are best to let go. This exercise also gives you a good idea of the character of your relationships and perhaps an insight into where you've been living on tilt, where you need to do more work on yourself so you can show up as a better friend or partner.

Having conversations where you're really unpacking the *language* to get to the experience and not relying on the words alone becomes a really helpful insight into building healthy relationships. This becomes advanced communication that enables knowing, being known, and love to flourish. Dr. Harville Hendrix and Dr. Helen LaKelly Hunt developed a form of therapy called Imago therapy. Basically, you start the Imago session by giving three affirmations to each person. Then one person invites the other "over the bridge" to come into their world, so to speak. It gives credence to the idea that there is something much bigger, and that there is a whole world that needs to be understood to be appreciated.

From there, the person who issued the invitation talks about what they think and feel about a particular topic. The other person remains empathetic, listening and asking more questions—unpacking, if you will. In that process, they agree to withhold any judgment, no matter what the other person says or if the listener believes it to be inaccurate. This unpacking process is beneficial for the person who needs to be understood and the person who is trying to understand. It is a reciprocal process. In the end, both parties understand more about themselves and each other because they have both been unpacking and listening with empathy and without judgment.

I did this with someone for whom birthdays were very important; for me, birthdays are not a big deal. I'm okay to celebrate or not celebrate on the exact day. I couldn't quite wrap my head around their emphasis on celebrating on the exact day, but once I was "invited over their bridge," I had the opportunity to hear the back story and ask more questions.

All of a sudden, I started to learn why this was so important. As we unpacked the topic, my heart went out to this person, and a lightbulb turned on in my head. *Oh wow, I get it. This is super important, and this would be great if I could do this for you. In fact, I would love to do this for you.* By withholding judgment and "visiting" the other person's world, you can change your entire perspective on a topic.

One final thought on relationships is to highlight that they begin with the relationship you have with yourself. The

Indian philosopher and founder of the Rajneesh movement, Osho, said:

> The capacity to be alone is the capacity to love. It may look paradoxical to you, but it's not. It is an existential truth: only those people who are capable of being alone are capable of love, of sharing, of going into the deepest core of another person—without possessing the other, without becoming dependent on the other, without reducing the other to a thing, and without becoming addicted to the other. They allow the other absolute freedom because they know that if the other leaves, they will be as happy as they are now. Their happiness cannot be taken by the other because it is not given by the other.

The goal here is for us to know and love ourselves with no reservations or qualifications. Then we are able to experience being known and loved by another while also knowing and loving them. If you have free-flowing, unencumbered energy in this space, this is where you optimize your psychology, spirituality, and energy. It will have a profound impact not only on your relationships and joy in life but your biology—via epigenetic inputs in the expression of your DNA.

CHAPTER FIVE

Spiritual Health

I t has been proven over and over again that individuals who are spiritually connected and have a spiritual belief system do better in life. In fact, according to a recent Harvard University study, ICU patients who have family members praying for them have a higher recovery rate. Those who believe in something, as opposed to nothing, have a sense of connection to something bigger than themselves. When we think about life and where we are on this speck of dust tumbling through space, circulating around a small star, in a small galaxy somewhere off in the corner of the universe, we can easily question the meaning of life and its purpose.

A lot of people equate spirituality with religion, primarily because religion deals with matters of the spirit and soul. If you are religious, I would encourage you to take a step back from the trappings of formalized religion and make space for spiritual health from a place unencumbered by the accepted dogma and doctrine. If you do, you'll find it renews, refreshes, and re-energizes your religious beliefs.

I grew up in a traditional Christian household and attended Christian schools from kindergarten through high school. I then attended Wheaton College, a conservative Christian college outside of Chicago. Before starting medical school, I attended Fuller Theological Seminary for six months as a special student to decide whether to go into ministry or attend medical school. It's fair to say that I have always had a spiritual bent. Even as a child, I was intrigued by spiritual topics such as meaning, purpose, enlightenment, and wisdom.

Today, I categorize myself as spiritual but not religious. I have moved away from organized religion because, much like today's healthcare, organized religion gets married to a set of answers and sits in judgment of everyone who doesn't have the same answers. It becomes the dogma of "We're right, you're wrong," "We're going to heaven, and you're going to hell," etc. Wars are fought, people die, and it's counterproductive to my vision of spirituality.

Voltaire's quote, "Cherish those who seek the truth, but beware of those who find it," rings true for me. The "We're right, you're wrong" mindset of organized religion never sat well with me; I found myself resonating more with people asking spiritual *questions* than I did with those who had spiritual *answers*. I have moved into a place of identifying with something bigger but doing it in an unencumbered and more enlightened way—one that is inclusive and pulls everyone together. There is a deep-seated peace and satisfaction in having a spiritual life that is not divisive but full of inclusion, love, and forgiveness.

Spirituality is something that many people reach for when they are facing difficult times. If you already have an established spiritual practice, I would just encourage you to expand it to tap into "something bigger" and achieve a greater experience of it. Mindfulness, meditation, prayer, and visualization are all great portals to get there and will likely lead you to additional practices that will enhance your personal experience of God, Source, or Universal Consciousness.

Henry Ford's famous quote also holds true: "Whether you think you can or think you can't, you are probably right." If someone is sick and believes they'll get better, there is a higher likelihood they will. If someone believes they will be successful in business, they likely will be. If you believe you can do or create something, you likely can.

I'm not a minister or spiritual guru. I do know, however, that my spiritual life and experiences have become very important to me, and the sense of peace, connection, and equanimity that I reside in melts away stress, anxiety, and fear. This impacts not only my mental health but my health and longevity, along with my effectiveness in every area of my life.

Measurement and Optimization

As one of the Life Energies, spiritual health is self-assessed and optimized the same way. These are a few questions you can ask to assess your spiritual status:

- *Do I have any spiritual practices?*
- *Do I take time out to think about spiritual matters and resonate with spiritual energies?*
- *Do I feel spiritually aligned in my soul, or do I feel out of sync?*

- *Is there a sense that I'm out of sync with this whole spiritual thing, or do I feel aligned with my spirituality and this greater good, greater purpose?*
- *Do I have a sense of purpose?*
- *Do I have a definition of wealth beyond tangible assets?*
- *What does wealth mean to me?*
- *How would I describe what wealth looks like now?*
- *How would I like to describe what wealth looks like going forward?*
- *Is it something in the spiritual realm? Is it something related to Health? Relationships? Impact?*
- Take a few minutes and be very specific. Ask yourself, *Is this what I really want to define me and my life, or is there more?*

My personal definition of wealth does not involve acquiring things; it's about curating the capabilities, resources, and relationships to create new ways of empowering people to get what they really need and want. In short, it's about making a positive impact.

This is where you should distinguish between what you're passionate about and finding your purpose. They can be two different things. You can be passionate about playing golf, but that doesn't mean it's your purpose. When you realize what you're passionate about, you discover something you love and enjoy. Your purpose, on the other hand, is what resonates with you so deeply that you would do it even if you weren't compensated and were ridiculed for doing it. You fundamentally do it because you *have* to, as much as you *want* to.

Passion and purpose can be synchronized. What you're passionate about might indeed become your purpose, and when you identify it, you certainly will be passionate about your purpose.

Find a spiritual practice that you can resonate with. There are lots of guided meditations, spiritual leaders, and practices out there; don't be afraid to try several until you find one that fits. I personally enjoy reading a paragraph or a few pages of Eckhart Tolle's, *The Power of Now*, but there are other spiritual books to consider. Commit to exploring this area of your life each day, even for just a few minutes; experiment with practices, the time of day you undertake them, and so on.

I try to meditate for five minutes twice a day—early morning and before bed at night. Book-ending my day with meditations like this has transformed my sense of peace and tranquility. I usually sit until my whole "being" is still and open; then, I read something and meditate on what I've just read. How you approach it makes a difference, so find your entry point.

Whether it's a guided meditation, attending a church or synagogue service, talking to someone you deem as a spiritual mentor or colleague, or somebody who simply has wisdom that you would like to tap into, optimizing your spiritual health involves exploration to find what resonates for you, and then turning it into a daily practice.

CHAPTER SIX

Wisdom

Many people say they don't remember their childhoods; for some reason, I have many memories from mine. For example, I remember attending Sunday school from a young age and asking questions about the teachings. When I was three, there was a pond I often visited, trying to catch polliwogs, frogs, skip rocks, and climb trees. One day, while walking home from the pond, I distinctly remember debating the existence of God and deciding that when I grew up, I wanted to become wise.

I've come to understand that wisdom is a perpetual state of learning and discerning. It is the process of creating a deeper understanding—of ourselves, the people around us, and the situations and experiences we encounter. Seeking wisdom over time enables us to have discernment, to understand things and see them for what they are . . . and what they aren't. Wisdom allows us to cut through the BS and hype and get to the heart of the matter and make the best decisions for everyone involved.

When coupled with emotional intelligence, wisdom gives us the ability to read people and situations where we understand what is being said, what is not being said, and what needs to be said. Our lives are much, much better if we aspire to be wise and practice it, as it enables us to have a better, more enduring impact.

Becoming wise is a journey. It requires us to not be married to our current answers but instead ask the bigger questions. In my own journey, I have learned that *no one can hear the wisdom you have to contribute until they feel heard themselves.* Therefore, all wisdom begins with listening and exploring the other person's thoughts, feelings, and positions.

Today, I feel wiser than ever; but if I'm going to live to be 120 years old, I know that I have space to become much wiser still. Wisdom never goes out of style or relevance. Technology and AI will disrupt our world, but wisdom will always be in demand.

Seeking wisdom requires an optimization mindset, which is a subset of a growth mindset. Wisdom really asks: *How do we understand this better? How do we do it better? How do we make it better? How do we make this the best? How can I bring my best self to bear on the situation? How do I want to make my best contribution?* Wisdom fuels our purpose because it invites expansion and abundance.

An additional key component of wisdom is that many things can be true at once, something I mentioned earlier. Many times, we feel we must reduce our thoughts and feelings down to one unified view, one statement, or one position; wisdom understands, however, that many things may be true simultaneously. The breadth of what is true simultaneously may even include thoughts, beliefs, or positions that are ostensibly contradictory to each other, yet all of them are true for the individual or group. For example, you may want to do something, and yet a part of you does not want to do it, or you may love someone but simultaneously have feelings of resentment toward them.

A good analogy for understanding that many things can be true at once is the difference between binary computing and quantum computing. In binary computing, a bit is either one or zero. In quantum computing, a qubit can simultaneously be all values between -1 and +1. I have observed that the human psyche is much more like a quantum system than a binary one, with many things being true simultaneously. Wisdom wants to understand all those truths and incorporate solutions that account for all of them. My assessment is that a great deal of conflict arises between humans when we fail to understand the full extent of what is true for a person and try to reduce a complex quantum system of thought and feelings into a binary one.

There is a certain joy in knowing that I have an expansive future in front of me, one of learning—not only academic and scientific knowledge, but relational knowledge, self-love, the meaning of my life, spiritual enlightenment, and, in order to do this, it is important to embrace the quantum nature of our reality. It's super fun for me to think about getting wiser and wiser in the process.

Measurement and Optimization

If wisdom is the ability to see a situation in its entirety and the circumstances, feelings, thoughts, and energies of the parties involved. Only then can we discern how to unravel the knot and tie it into a bow. Wisdom is expressed as loving discernment that simultaneously enables us to dodge bullets, disarm tense situations, and create beautiful solutions.

Passion and purpose without wisdom are prey to greed and placing self-interest first. Our endeavors have more staying power when they are guided by wisdom. So how do we become wise? We acquire wisdom through courageously stepping into experiences and actively working to understand all the thoughts, feelings, energies, and agendas in play. Courageously engaging with diverse experiences is a prerequisite for, but not a guarantee of, becoming wise. Wisdom requires reflection and commitment.

When assessing your own wisdom, think about whether wisdom is important to you and why.

- What is your definition of wisdom?
- What are you doing to become wise?
- How do you go about expanding your wisdom?
- Do you understand that many seemingly contradictory things can be true simultaneously?
- Are you developing skills to unravel the knot of someone else's reality?

I can't overemphasize the need for personal reflection on your experiences. These could be internal experiences or experiences that involve others. When you go into a situation, learn some things along the way. Reflect on what went well and what did not, what felt like progress, and what was impeding progress.

When things result in win-win-win solutions, think about why it went so well:

- *What sort of energy did you bring to it?*

- *How did you listen to understand others and allow them to feel heard?*
- *Do you see the many things that are simultaneously true in these circumstances?*
- *Did you discuss with compassion and non-judgment in a way that people responded favorably?*
- *How did this impact others and enable everyone in the room to move forward?*
- *If you had approached this differently, would there have been a better outcome if you had had a deeper understanding?*

Turn it over, look at all facets, and apply or modify your approach based on what you've learned.

For me to show up in a place where I can be at my wisest, it is critical that I not show up living in reaction to traumas I've experienced in the past. If I show up with those old programs running, I inherently don't feel safe, which will put me on tilt, which will impede my understanding of myself, the situation, and the others involved. When we feel resistance from anyone including ourselves, we know there is more to unpack. The knot has to be fully unraveled before wise solutions can emerge.

On the other hand, if I go into a situation in a state of equilibrium, with a solid sense of safety, I am in a much better position to be inquisitive, to learn to understand all the facets of what is true for each of those involved, and we will all end up making wiser decisions. I have discovered that wisdom grows when I stop judging and focus more on understanding.

I saw how judgment sabotaged progress and relationships while practicing sick-care. If a patient wasn't doing well in traditional medicine, the physicians or staff would blame the patient: "Well, they just don't blah, blah, blah . . ." or "It's all in their head," and that was simply not the case. When I talked to the patient, many things would be simultaneously true, some of which were impeding their progress. Once they were heard and understood, they began to feel safe. The knowledge could then be unraveled and progress could be made.

At the same time, the professionals had their own unresolved issues that caused them to struggle with the patient's reactions. They believed that they were well-trained and that *they* were the experts; therefore, the patient couldn't possibly be right. This led them to be dismissive as a kind of self-defense to protect the image and beliefs they had about themselves.

The more you find yourself judging other people, the more you are pulling yourself away from the opportunity to grow in wisdom. The more you find yourself considering, *I wonder why this is happening. I wonder what is true for them,* the more you open the door to wisdom.

Think about all the things and people you judge throughout the day. The next time you catch yourself doing this, or even just feeling agitated by someone's mere presence, ask yourself, *What could be causing me to feel this way? Is there something going on with this person that's making them feel unsafe that I don't yet understand? Is there something in my own life that I'm projecting onto them?* Many times, when we judge, it is because we also don't feel safe on some level. Exploring those questions will help you grow in wisdom. Ask yourself:

- *What am I doing to become wise?*
- *Do others see me as wise?*

- *Am I taking time to reflect on my experiences, good and bad, to pull valuable lessons from them?*
- *What do I intend to do with this new knowledge?*
- *What kind of situations will I put myself in to enable and encourage me to gain more wisdom?*
- *Am I developing the skill to see that many things may be true at once?*
- *What assumptions am I making about the other parties that preclude my understanding of who they are and what they want and need to feel safe?*

Finally, which resources are you consulting to gain more wisdom? Reading this book may be part of that, but you need a larger sphere of influence than any one book or person. You need wise counsel, mentoring from others, and time to reflect on your life's events.

When people come up to me, as they do now, and say, "You know, you're really wise," I smile, but the smile goes much deeper than the implied thank you; it goes into my heart and my soul because it's an indication that I'm making progress and three-year-old little Jeff is smiling.

CHAPTER SEVEN

Feeling Safe

W e hear it all the time: Love is the answer. All you need is love.

For a long time, I believed it. As I've grown wiser, however, I have come to a different understanding. Love—as we've talked about it up to this point—is absolutely necessary, but it's not sufficient. What I mean by that is there is another Life Energy that can be connected to love but isn't the same as love; it's feeling safe.

My only sibling was my older sister. She suffered brain damage during her birth. Her brain was without oxygen for some minutes as they waited for the obstetrician to arrive; she was otherwise normal, and her mental deficits were not fully appreciated until she started kindergarten. She was athletic, musical, sweet, funny, and extroverted, and we were very close; but with an IQ of fifty and unable to live independently, she required ongoing care and supervision. When she was five, the doctors advised my parents to put her in an institution and forget about her. To their credit, as a twenty-nine-year-old father and twenty-five-year-old mother, they said, "We will never abandon her," and undertook taking great care of her and, ultimately, gave her a great life.

Growing up in a family with a special-needs child is a challenge for everyone; books have been written on the topic of how it affects the members of the family, and it shaped me in several important ways. It was a driver for me to go to medical school and figure out how to better help those who have tragic events happen to them.

Another way it impacted me happened when I was about twenty-seven. I remember getting a phone call from my father.

"Jeff, you're in medical school," he began. "You're doing really well, and you're going to do great in life. I just wanted to let you know I had a life insurance policy with you as the beneficiary, but I canceled it. Your mother and I have been thinking about this a lot, and we've decided to modify our wills to leave everything to your sister."

It was jaw-dropping, quite honestly, like a punch to the solar plexus. I didn't know what to say; I certainly didn't want to feel like I was trying to take anything away from my sister or her care, but I also felt like, *Wow, I am really on my own. There's nobody out there who has my back. I'm absolutely on my own.*

Suddenly, I didn't feel like I had any real safety net and wasn't safe. It had a real impact on my life, to the point that I lived on tilt, in reaction to this feeling of not being safe, for a long, long time even after I had plenty of money. It left an imprint on me, both consciously and subconsciously.

If you've ever seen a poker player lose a big hand or a series of hands, many times they'll go on-tilt, which essentially means that they're now playing in reaction to the recent losses and are prone to play poorly. Similarly, we can live on tilt following a traumatic event, loss, or perceived loss. Many times, others around us see or sense that we are on tilt; but we have so integrated the events into our psyche, thinking, and emotional responses that we no longer see it in ourselves. This manner of living in reaction is so ingrained it becomes part of our DNA and impacts our epigenetics. At that point, it is very hard to change because we don't see it; we have normalized its integration into how we see and approach the world.

Many of us feel loved but, on some level, still don't feel safe. Likely, this has to do with things that happen early in our lives, often related to our families or close relationships. Regardless of the specifics, these are important issues to examine because they create ongoing stress in the body and sabotage our relationships and success, all of which affect how we age.

Solving this puzzle requires deep work because we are often unaware the problem exists, let alone understand its root causes. Once you are courageous enough to ask, *Am I living on tilt,* others will tell you what you can't see. They have likely seen it all along. You can then revisit the incidents that put you on tilt and begin to understand the ways in which you don't feel safe.

From there, you can determine how to provide yourself with safety. One major insight I learned is that nothing external to us can ever make us safe—no amount of money, education, accolades, family, or relationships. Safety, like self-love, is an inside job.

It took a long time to get here, but with others helping me see what I couldn't, I've been able to give myself safety the same way I gave myself unconditional love—by scooping up my small, three-year-old self and giving him safety. When I did this in early 2022, I felt safe for the first time in a long time.

I also realized I feel safe from a spiritual perspective. Realizing that I'm an eternal being living out a divine purpose who ultimately can't be harmed by things that go on in this life gave me a deep sense of peace and safety.

Utilizing those two approaches, I now do "safety checks" when I enter a room. Do I feel safe? If not, I consciously give myself safety. When I feel safe, I'm liberated to bring my best self into the situation. Try it for yourself.

It's important to understand that every time you feel stressed or anxious, it is because, on some level, you don't feel safe. When you have love and safety, it enables you to live in a world of abundance. Without love and safety, we live in a world of scarcity—where nothing we do or accumulate will ever be enough.

Confidence is also a direct result of feeling safe. Giving yourself safety can transform you from anxious to confident in an instant. Feeling safe and unconditionally loved is our birthright. When we claim and give both of them to ourselves, it frees us up to live an unencumbered life. Being unencumbered means, we are no longer knowingly or unknowingly living in reaction to past traumas. It liberates us and enables parts of ourselves that we have kept repressed to shine. We can then bring our best, most creative, generous, and generative gifts forward. When you do this, you will have a life lived in equilibrium, with little-to-no stress and loads of opportunity and joy.

Measurement and Optimization

Is it possible to feel safe and not feel loved? I think so. They typically go hand-in-hand, but there are nuances. Perhaps you feel safe and not loved. Or maybe you are still holding energetic resistance to the flow of love between yourself and someone else.

When you feel loved, however, I think you have a better chance of resolving whether you feel safe. And when you feel safe, you have a better chance of resolving whether you feel loved.

Before we can take steps to feel safe or safer, we need to assess our current state. Ask yourself the following questions:

- *I feel loved, but why don't I feel safe?*
- *I don't feel loved, and I don't feel safe. Why?*
- *Am I making selfish decisions because I'm trying to feel safe?*
- *How do I reclaim my birthright of feeling loved and safe?*
- *How does not feeling safe put me on tilt?* In other words, look at your relationships: *What's going right about them; what's going wrong; what vulnerabilities you are feeling—financial, emotional, physical—that are impacting how you show up?*
- *If I feel safe, do I feel confident, or do I have to fabricate confidence?* If you're wearing confidence like a cloak, you probably don't feel safe.
- *Does confidence flow out of you effortlessly?* If it does, it comes from feeling safe.
- *How do I do my own safety checks?*
- *How can I give myself safety?*

These are questions for internal reflection, but you may need additional resources to crack this code, like a therapist, a spiritual confidant, a close friend, or a significant other.

Ultimately, it takes time with yourself to reflect on these foundational pieces. It is vital work, however, because it impacts not only you but everyone and everything you care about in your life.

Many people are waiting for confidence before they start something. Feeling safe encompasses a lot more than feeling confident. Confidence is a byproduct that occurs at the very end of the process, not the beginning.

Dan Sullivan, the founder of Strategic Coach®, created a tool that he calls the The Four C's Formula®, which I have expanded to the five:

- Make a **Commitment** to what you want.
- **Courage** is required in order to move forward, even though you don't yet know how you're going to do it.
- Building on the first two **Cs** enables you to develop the **Capabilities** required to make good on your commitment.
- Then, and only then, will you develop **Confidence**.

My addition is **Clarity:** Become *clear* on what you want. I think this is important to add with *Commitment* and *Courage* to help you develop *Capabilities*.

This becomes a repeating cycle and moves us forward. Your acquired confidence gives you refined clarity, enabling you to make an even bigger commitment, which takes more courage, which adds more capabilities, which leads to greater confidence, and so on.

Those loops can start small, and starting small is one way to attain confidence. The other way to augment confidence is by feeling safe. When you think about it, no matter how much money, resources, and people surround them, many people simply don't feel safe.

I have four daily affirmations that put me into a confident, safe, and loving space.

1. I'm 27 years old. I wake up 27 every day.
2. I have access to unlimited resources.
3. I am on the path to enlightenment.
4. I live in an energetic fabric of mutual love and support with everyone I come in contact with.

These affirmations set me up each day to feel loved and safe.

Feeling safe is fundamental to our decision-making and can explain why many people's actions are fear-based and irrational. When people feel safe, it gives them tremendous confidence to walk into any situation, friendly or hostile, and not be on tilt. Instead, they arrive with their gifts, abilities, and imagination, ready to make their contribution in a much more powerful and effective way.

Likewise, if they are walking into a situation preoccupied, either consciously or unconsciously, with their lack of safety, people will definitely take notice. We read each other's energies very, very well, whether we realize it or not. In fact, these energies are contagious.

Dr. Drew Pearson, a doctor of Chinese medicine and a savant at reading EEGs and setting up neurofeedback programs likens the contagiousness of our energy to the sympathy of two clocks effect. As he explained, if you place a number of clocks with pendulums in the same room, over time, the pendulums all start to swing in synchrony.

This is also true when it comes to the energy in the room, including feeling safe and confident.

If you walk into a room and you are exuding safety, it will change the energy of the room, and the other people in the room will also start to feel safe.

If feeling safe is much more valuable than money, how do we attain it? I reached a point in my personal deep dives where I was trying to figure out the things I couldn't see that were holding me back. Until then, I had solved a lot of the things that I could see, but wondered, *What am I missing?* Talking over some of this with a very insightful woman at a conference I was attending on optimizing brain function, I got my answer.

"Jeff, you think you have an issue with money because of what happened between you and your father when you were 27," she said. Exactly—I thought I had an issue with money because of that phone call from my father all those decades ago.

"In fact, it's not about money at all. It's about feeling safe," she determined. In her school of thought, she equated it to the first chakra, which has to do with safety and security.

All of a sudden, I had this epiphany: *If I could give little Jeff love both from the maternal and the paternal positions, can't I give him safety, too? I'm just going to surround little Jeff with safety. I'm going to take care of him. He is going to be okay.*

This did not come from a place of anger. In my mind, I was not snatching little Jeff away from my parents and gnashing my teeth while hissing, "I'm gonna make him safe." Not at all. This epiphany came from a very loving, nurturing place. Once I did that, I could suddenly feel things going back into alignment, as though some sort of chiropractor had realigned me and adjusted things back into place.

I was no longer on tilt. *I am safe. I'm actually safe.*

The process you go through may mirror mine or be completely different, but I encourage you to discover safety for yourself.

Why is this so important for longevity? Because when we start to align with our true birthright of feeling loved and safe, it dramatically decreases stress while increasing joy and the quality of our relationships. In subsequent chapters, I will illustrate the effects of stress in biochemical terms and how it is aging us through many different pathways. Being able to lower stress by feeling safe is huge if you are going to live young for a lifetime.

Now some of you may be thinking: *I'm driven by stress. I actually love stress. I live for stress.* You might live for stress, but you won't live as long. You're paying a very high price if you use stress to push or motivate you. If you come into that same situation feeling safe, I can guarantee you that you'll be able to bring more capabilities, more wisdom, and more expansive thinking to whatever situation you find yourself in. Your sense of safety will enable you to do much more than you could if you are only being driven by stress.

Think about final exams in college. If you waited until the last minute when you really felt the stress to start studying, did you learn as much as somebody who just enjoyed the material over time, felt safe in learning it, and walked into the test confident in their knowledge and capabilities? Who had the better learning experience? Who is in a better position to use the information?

One very important note: If you have been in an abusive relationship, feeling safe is challenging but imperative. Those who have been in abusive relationships will often look for an external source to provide their safety and mistake this for love. Ultimately, your path to feeling safe is up to you—you provide it to yourself. When we give ourselves safety and love, we suddenly don't go into a relationship on tilt, constantly asking, *Does this person love me?* Or, *Is this person making me feel safe?* If you find that you are constantly asking these questions about someone in your life, you are at risk of repeating the cycle of abuse.

Go back and look at the things that made you feel unsafe and unpack them. You will need to find a quiet, safe space to do this, as it will likely bring up some very painful memories. It takes work; those events and subsequent response patterns are imprinted into the brain, and your goal is to rewrite your software to provide the safety you should have been given long ago.

Consider looking into a number of therapeutic techniques and tools to help you. Neurofeedback, Brain Frequency™, EMDR, brainspotting, and others have yielded tremendous results in treating trauma. Understanding your genetic proclivities for anxiety, addiction, and depression with Intellxx DNA can be profoundly helpful. You can heal and reach a point where you feel safe, and it will dramatically change your world.

Remember, we read each other's energies; it's our sixth sense. People in your personal and business lives will take advantage of you once they know you are looking to feel safe. They will abuse the power that you give them. Giving yourself safety will not only transform those relationships, it will transform your life—and it will transform your health.

CHAPTER EIGHT

Energetic Resonance with the Universe, Having a Sense of Purpose

W e have talked about spiritual alignment, but being aligned and in resonance with the energy of the universe is different. Many times, we equate spirituality with religious practices, attending services, singing, and praying. Prayer typically has a petitionary quality to it; we are asking for something, holding up a situation with a desire for an answer, guidance, wisdom, or next steps.

There is certainly nothing wrong with the petitionary prayer, but being in resonance with universal energy or God's energy is different. It's more analogous to being in the presence of Source Energy, Consciousness, or God and experiencing knowing and being known, loving and being loved, being at peace, and feeling safe and aligned. It's an energy that starts to flow through your body, and when you are connected, you feel at one with everything. The environment begins nurturing you—the trees, the ocean, and the people around you.

It's a different sort of construct than just being spiritually aware. The key to accessing it is removing *I* from the equation. This may sound tricky; *How do I remove* I *from the equation?* It's doable if you remove *I* from the present moment. You see, *I* is the ego. Eckhart Tolle speaks to the ego needing time to exist—a past and a future. All pain comes from reliving the past or projecting the future. Being present is the first step, and removing *I* from the present and allowing yourself to merge with all this is the second step. In doing so, we can access the quantum realm of universal energy, i.e., *Being.* Try it. You'll like it!

Nikola Tesla said, "If you want to find the secrets of the Universe, think in terms of energy, frequency, and vibration." We now understand, in our current physics model, that on a quantum level, everything we see and touch, as well as what we *can't* see and touch, is composed of waves of quantum energy. *How* these waves coalesce and interface with the perceiver creates the raw data which our brain then uses to create the reality we each experience.

The 2022 Nobel Prize in Physics was awarded to Drs. Aspect, Zellinger, and Clauser for describing the quantum entanglement of photons. Entangled photons assume the same state synchronously without regard to the distance between them. This can happen instantaneously over great distances—billions of light years. The effect between the entangled particles is faster than the speed of light.

Another feature is that they do not take on a particular set of physical properties until they are observed or measured, that is until the energy of the observer is put into the system. The implication is that the universe does not exist *a priori* but only comes into existence when it is observed and can come into existence in many different ways, depending on who the observer is. What this means to me is that we live in a universe of possibilities, and our energetic input into the system can result in the creation of a reality that reflects our energy. Energetically speaking, we create not only our own reality based on how we think but our own physical universe based on the energy we bring to the system. This is what people are talking about when they speak of manifesting a great life, health, relationships, financial abundance, and so on.

When you understand that everything is vibration, energy, and frequency, coming to the point of present-moment awareness and removing the *I* enables a state of resonance with Being or Consciousness. Accessing this is life-changing. It has massive benefits in terms of how you feel, your equanimity, your ability to handle stress, your health, your relationships, and what you're capable of doing and accomplishing.

Before you think I'm getting too woo-woo here, I'd ask you to keep an open mind. You'll be impressed with what you find there if you are open to it. Working with different people who are gifted in this area—who have developed the gift of being in contact with this energy—has been very helpful to me as a pilgrim moving toward the same. When you walk into a room with them, you can *feel their energy* and connect to it. It's really quite fascinating. And highly therapeutic.

Sound is another energy that we can connect to and through. Many people find music calms them, amps them up, and helps them concentrate, or sleep. Certain frequencies can be very therapeutic. Jason Campbell has combined breathwork with music to help people access this universal energy. He also composed music to help people focus. Focus at Will™ is a source of music to help you focus at work or when you are on task. I'm listening to it right now. Frequencies like 432hz and 528hz can aid meditation and stress reduction. Tibetan monks rub the rims of bowls to create sounds that enhance their meditative state. Resonating with these musical energies feels great and is calming and healing.

Measurement and Optimization

There's been a long discord around how to integrate Einstein's theory of relativity with quantum mechanics. Relativity is a construct used to explain things on a macroscopic scale, while quantum mechanics is a construct used to describe things on a microscopic scale. In quantum mechanics, a particle is not a particle—it's both a wave *and* a particle. The famous double-slit experiment—where a photon functions as a wave—can be demonstrated by sending the photon through a partition with two slits that are side-by-side—goes through both slits. The photon as a wave goes through both slits. This is understood by observings the wave interference pattern created on the other side of the partition. However, when the photon is measured, it only goes through one slit and functions as a particle.

As I was listening to an Oxford professor talking about quantum reality as he described the underpinnings of everything, quantum waves of energy flowing through the universe, it dawned on me that the universe is not a fixed reality but a field of possibilities.

(Stay with me here because this does make an impact on longevity.)

Remember what Tesla said about everything that exists? That it comes down to frequency, energy, and vibration? When you look at things from a quantum perspective—a table, a chair, the room you're currently seated in, and so on—they are basically quantum waves. All of reality comes down to quantum energy waves that coalesce and combine with our perception to create the reality we experience. It's also true that our thoughts have energy, and we can influence reality with the energy of our thoughts. This allows the field of quantum energy to coalesce into a measured reality that's different than it might have been.

At first glance, this sounds very woo-woo, but it's well-grounded in physics and understanding that thoughts are the energetic waves. Our thoughts have a dramatic impact on the physical realm. Our thoughts impact our health, epigenetics, performance, and longevity.

Our thoughts create realities. Many of us tend to ignore this, opting for a worldview that's more binary and black-and-white—an external objective view of reality. The door opens, and the door closes. I studied, and I got an *A* on my test. I worked *x* number of hours, and I got a paycheck . . . . But by understanding the energetics of what's happening at the quantum level, we can create outcomes that would otherwise not have happened: I developed a new attitude at work and got a raise, and so on.

So now, let's consider how to measure and assess our energetic resonance with the universe:

- Do you feel things at an energetic level?
- Do you have a method for quieting your mind, letting go of the past and future, and creating present-moment awareness?
- Are you able to remove your *I* from the equation?
- Do you feel a resonance with the sense of possibility that exists inside the energetic of Being and Consciousness?
- Do certain sound frequencies impact your mood, concentration, and ability to meditate and focus?

For example, if you're in a relationship and bring a certain energy to it, it will shape that relationship. If you bring a lot of loving energy into a relationship, it becomes a loving relationship. If you bring a lot of judgment into a relationship, it becomes a resentful relationship. Your thoughts have the power to sculpt how things turn out.

Being energetically aligned with the universe, with this universal energy, is another way to view and experience your life in terms of all the possibilities that exist. Whatever looks like a hurdle or setback to you is also a possibility—an opportunity that has presented itself to you. It's the energy that you resonate with that determines whether it be an obstacle or an opportunity.

The idea of resonating with this universal energy becomes very important and profound. Nikolai Kardashev, a Russian astrophysicist and radio astronomer, devised a multi-level scale to grade the sophistication of civilizations that could be found in the universe. Now known as the Kardashev Scale, it grades a civilization's level of development by measuring its ability to master and utilize energy. Kardashex level 1, for example, would be a civilization that can master and utilize all of the energy of its home planet. For perspective, humans on Earth are believed to be a Kardashev 0.7 civilization. A level 2 Kardashev civilization would have the ability to control and utilize all of the energy in its entire solar system, including the sun(s), planets, moons, comets, and asteroids. A level 3 Kardashev civilization would be able to master and use their entire galaxy's energy. A level 4 Kardashev civilization would be able to master and utilize all the energy of the observable universe. There are levels beyond 4, of course, but it leads to abstractions in physics like parallel universes, the multiverse, the omniverse, etc.

The point is that when I feel overwhelmed by something, I will visualize myself as a citizen of a Kardashev-3 civilization. If such a civilization exists, and there are beings who can control all of that energy, I ask myself, *How much of that can I tap into?*

Whether a level 3 civilization exists or not doesn't matter since this is a construct in my mind. This exercise enables me to say, *Okay, I can control more energy than I think I can. Let me shape reality in the positive directions I want it to go.*

So how do you optimize energetic resonance with the universe? In my mind, I started by exploring the nature of the quantum realm. I took physics in college, but then I took a deeper dive and listened to a few Oxford University professors and other notable experts in the field, like the 2022 Nobel Laureates. This started shifting my thinking about the fact that reality is a set of *potential* realities, and we shape our reality based on the energy that we put into the system, along with the energy of the system that we resonate with.

From there, I gained a greater understanding by working directly with some individual experts, including Barry Morguelan. M.D., a UCLA Gastroenterologist and

Chinese-trained Energy Grand Master. Dr. Morguelan and others opened my eyes to the fact that there is a direct connection between my ability to connect to universal source energy and the reality I create in my own life.

If this is an area that you're interested in pursuing, I would encourage you to do so. It's a definitive "leveling-up" to your life that we often overlook or, if we pause long enough to consider it, we quickly shrug it off as not practical. When you tap into it, all of a sudden, you are *really* living. It's as though you are a visitor on this planet because you're experiencing this energetic space that enables you to move through every situation effortlessly. It's really cool, and guess what? Optimization goes through the roof, stress falls away, and health, longevity, performance, and life energy expand exponentially.

Building on those foundational energies of feeling safe and feeling loved prepares you to feel the resonance with this universal energy. This is how people start to manipulate their health; you hear stories about people healing themselves and "miracles" occurring, and it's happening at this level.

If you are super skeptical of this, then feel free to pass it by. But if you resonate with this, it can be very powerful in your life. Understand that what you're trying to build is *already built*—you just need to get out of the way and live into it. By doing so, we are accessing the most important things we need to thrive: Resilience and Adaptability.

We spend so much time stressing about building a business, writing a book, buying a home, or forming relationships, yet at a profound, energetic level, those things already exist. When we resonate with this universal energy, we are able to live in what already exists. Now, we're just leaning into it with our intentions. Stress dramatically decreases as we set aside the uncertainty of not feeling safe and simply *will* into existence the life we want, which already exists and is waiting for us.

> *Everything is energy and that's all there is to it. Match the frequency of the reality you want and you cannot help but get that reality. It can be no other way. This is not philosophy. This is physics.*

–Anonymous

Think about it: Why have over 99 percent of all species that have ever lived on this planet gone extinct? It's because they lacked resilience in the face of new challenges and the ability to adapt to new circumstances. If we want to make 100 the new 30, we need to prioritize resilience and adaptability. Learning to tap into and resonate with these energetics enables us to shape our reality, and restructuring our environment will have a major impact on how our DNA is expressed.

CHAPTER NINE

Finding Joy, My Personal North Star

What comes to mind when you think about *joy*? Do you equate it with happiness? Or does it guide you even on the darkest of days?

Joy is deeper and stronger than happiness. Happiness is superficial, contextual, and dependent on things going our way, happiness is always fleeting; therefore, it is always connected to pain when things go wrong. Pursuing happiness usually becomes a rollercoaster punctuated, if not characterized by, unhappiness.

Joy, however, is not contextual. It is aligned with our deeper sense of being. Joy can be present even in dire circumstances. Humans are social creatures; if we create joy for another person, it reverberates back to us. In fact, I'm not sure it's possible to create joy for another person and not experience joy in the process. As the joy resonates back and forth, it becomes amplified and only creates more joy.

Joy is also amplified when we feel safe and loved. This can be generated when we give ourselves the gift of unconditional love or safety, and it also reveals itself in our relationships. When you show up to bring joy, it will happen, and everyone will benefit.

Measurement and Optimization

In a sense, joy operates similarly to loving and being loved, knowing and being known. We cannot optimize joy if we do not feel love or feel safe, either in our relationships or with ourselves. As you assess your level of joy, ask yourself the following questions:

- *What is my North Star? What am I using to guide me on my path?*
- *In how many current situations do I feel joy?*
- *Am I creating joy in other people's lives?*
- *Do I feel joy when I create joy for others?*
- *Is joy a glue that holds my relationships together?*
- *Does my joy tend to grow and reverberate? If so, when?*
- *Would I like to have more joy in my life?*
- *If I don't currently have joy, what is the underlying reason?*

Discovering what guides you—your personal North Star—is important. If you walk into a situation and the energy is right, you bring your gifts and want to share them.

On the other hand, if you're not feeling joy, you are likely to question why you are doing this.

- *What is it about this situation that joy simply won't arise?*
- *Why am I not feeling joy here?*
- *What about me is impeding my ability to feel joy?*
- *Am I living on tilt to the extent that I am unable to experience joy here?*

Because joy has become my North Star in life, I know that if I feel joy, I am on the right track. If, for some reason, I'm not feeling joy, then I do a deep dive and look at how I'm thinking or feeling about the situation and make an adjustment. These deep dives enable me to deconstruct faulty preconceptions or understand the true underpinnings of joy with greater clarity. If I'm not feeling joy, then potentially, it's not an activity I should participate in. If something isn't joyous but is in a category I aspire to participate in, I work to get back to being joyful. This may sound selfish, but showing up with joy allows me to show up for others in a way that also optimizes their joy. A true win-win!

It's nice to find joy in a complex world with so many different things coming at us, competing for our attention. When joy serves as your North Star, you can rock back into a peaceful perspective and ask, *Is this really what I need to be doing right now?*

When we emphasize joy, we are also simultaneously emphasizing gratitude. I learned a lot about the power of gratitude from a dear friend of mine, Lee Brower, who was my original coach at Strategic Coach. Lee often said to begin by "going BIG"—*Begin In Gratitude*. That always resonated with me, but I found that adding joy to that makes it a bit more robust.

The next time you're headed to a meeting, headed to work out, have a relationship conversation, or any sort of activity, activate these statements: *I want this to be joyful, and I am going in here to experience joy. I'm here to give and receive joy.* This changes your whole mindset and ushers in a sense of gratitude. Suddenly, we are so grateful to have this opportunity, whatever it is, that it just changes everything. When joy serves as your personal North Star, you have the discernment to figure out that you should probably avoid that which does not bring you joy.

That's not to say that we shouldn't step out of our comfort zones. In fact, those events can be an opportunity to make what would otherwise be uncomfortable, comfortable. I have also found that the combination of joy and feeling safe is an incredibly powerful combination. For example, if I go into a meeting and, for some reason, I think there may be some antagonism, I can go in there kind of living in reaction to whatever that was before. As I drill down into it, I realize that joy is not present, and on some level, I don't feel safe. So if the meeting is not going to lend itself to joy, I focus instead on giving myself safety and affirming that I live in an energetic fabric of love and mutual support. I visualize my three-year-old self, scoop him up, and tell him he is safe. I am going to protect him. This reminds adult Jeff that he is safe, too. Now that I realize I'm safe, I don't have to live in reaction mode, which frees me up to be my best self, bringing and expecting love, mutual support, and joy.

As a healthcare professional, I have gone into many situations where I'm there to give; somebody's coming to see me with their very personal problem. That has always been a very sacred space for me. The door closes, and somebody pours out their heart to you in a way they wouldn't with anybody else. There is a great deal of trust and compassion, and that's a very sacred space.

Walking into that situation and feeling like I'm going to give them something has always been my default mode.

But I've learned that it's better if I walk into that situation feeling safe, with a sense of joy, and fully expecting to receive from this person. I know that I will make my contribution. I will definitely give what I'm supposed to, but actually receiving what they have to tell me changes everything. Now, they are validated, we're collaborating, we are on the same team, and we're getting things done. This whole mix of the conversation shifts into something that I think is very special, and I have expanded it to other areas like at the grocery store, in a restaurant, or when I bump into an old friend.

This approach has the propensity to create compounding joy in your life, which is the exact opposite of stress, anxiety, anger, fear, and living on tilt. Negative emotions undermine not only your health but your ability to perform, they prevent you from making the contributions that, in your heart, you want to make.

Find joy, give joy, and receive joy!

CHAPTER TEN

Feeling Worthy

I have found that many people—even successful people—on some level don't feel worthy. Usually, they don't feel worthy enough to achieve something great or worthy of something they have already received. I believe this is due to old software running in the background, making us feel like we aren't enough.

What I mean by *enough* is to be able to do, have, or achieve something wonderful. Many times, this software is written at a point where we are being judged by someone we respect or someone from whom we want respect. It's helpful to understand that many of these judgments have nothing to do with us but have everything with the baggage of the person judging us. It could be their belief system, their sense of who they are, and what they were taught is or isn't possible that gets ladled onto us at younger, more vulnerable ages and leaves us believing we are not worthy.

Feeling worthy means that you have no limits to what you can do or accomplish. There is no artificial ceiling. It is very energizing and enables us to dream big and then dream bigger.

Measurement and Optimization

Ask yourself these questions:

- *Do I feel worthy?*
- *Has someone told me, "You are not capable of this"?*
- *Am I still holding on to their belief?*
- *What would I do if I had no limitations?*

Joseph Campbell, in *The Hero's Journey*, speaks of us having to courageously leave behind what is familiar to explore and fight to reclaim our birthright to be our unencumbered selves and, in that liberation, dream as big as we want to. (We talk more about Joseph Campbell and *The Hero's Journey* in Chapter Thirty-One.) Getting to that point will likely require some reflective work and therapeutic intervention, but it is well worth it to wake up energized every day—knowing you're stepping into your dream life and completely worthy of it!

What Does "Live Young for a Lifetime" Look like?

A 30 Year Old Body with a 300 Year Old Mind

Final Thoughts on Life Energies

At Gladden Longevity, we are empowered by four questions:

- How do you make 100 the new 30?
- How do you live "well" beyond 120?
- How good can you be?
- How do you live young for a lifetime?

As you can see, these are global questions within the Life Energies Mosaic. It's not just how fit, how fast, how dense your bones can be, and how sharp your mind can be. It's actually about how good your life can be as an individual in order to make a global impact.

The state of your mind and outlook have a tremendous impact on aging. If you are making poor decisions and choices, living in reaction to old traumas, and engaging in self-destructive behavior, you are self-sabotaging—and consequently, short-changing—your health, longevity, performance, and impact.

When we think about optimizing these life energies to become the best iteration of ourselves, our unencumbered selves, we do so with the intent of making a larger contribution to our world. Once we gain clarity, we can do unbelievable things with our lives. We can not only optimize our lives but also help optimize the lives of those around us. Ultimately, that becomes our greatest joy.

Life Energies Notes

Carol S. Dweck, *Mindset the New Psychology of Success* (New York: Ballantine Books, 2016).

Nassim Nicholas Taleb, *Antifragile: Things That Gain from Disorder* (New York, NY: Random House, 2016).

Susanne R. De Rooij et al., "Lessons Learned from 25 Years of Research into Long Term Consequences of Prenatal Exposure to the Dutch Famine 1944–45: The Dutch Famine Birth Cohort," *International Journal of Environmental Health Research* 32, no. 7 (May 5, 2021): 1432–46, https://doi.org/10.1080/09603123.2021.1888894.

"Epigenetics & Inheritance," Learn.Genetics, accessed April 7, 2023, https://learn.genetics.utah.edu/content/epigenetics/inheritance.

Eva Jablonka and Gal Raz, "Transgenerational Epigenetic Inheritance: Prevalence, Mechanisms, and Implications for the Study of Heredity and Evolution," *The Quarterly Review of Biology* 84, no. 2 (June 2009): 131–76, https://doi.org/10.1086/598822.

A. Byrne and D.G. Byrne, "The Effect of Exercise on Depression, Anxiety and Other Mood States: A Review," *Journal of Psychosomatic Research* 37, no. 6 (September 1993): 565–74, https://doi.org/10.1016/0022-3999(93)90050-p.

John Gottman and Julie Schwartz Gottman, *The Love Prescription* (Random House USA, 2022).

"Mehrabian's 7-38-55 Communication Model: It's More than Words," The World of Work Project, July 26, 2021, https://worldofwork. io/2019/07/mehrabians-7-38-55-communication-model/.

Lee A Lillard and Constantijn (Stan) Panis, "Health, Marriage, and Longer Life for Men," RAND Corporation, January 1, 1998, https:// www.rand.org/pubs/research_briefs/RB5018.html.

"Imago Relationships Worldwide - Imago Relationships," Imago Relationships, October 3, 2021, https://imagorelationships.org/.

Tracy A. Balboni et al., "Spirituality in Serious Illness and Health," JAMA 328, no. 2 (July 12, 2022): 184, https://doi.org/10.1001/jama.2022.11086.

Michael Balboni and Tracy Balboni, "Do Spirituality and Medicine Go Together?," Bioethics, June 1, 2019, https://bioethics.hms.harvard.edu/ journal/spirituality-medicine.

Eckhart Tolle, *The Power of Now: A Guide to Spiritual Enlightenment* (Vancouver, BC: Namaste Pub., 2004).

"The Nobel Prize in Physics 2022," NobelPrize.org, accessed April 9, 2023, https://www.nobelprize.org/prizes/physics/2022/popular-information/.

"Double-Slit Experiment," Wikipedia, July 7, 2023, https://en.wikipedia. org/wiki/Double-slit_experiment.

"Kardashev Scale," Wikipedia, June 21, 2023, https://en.wikipedia.org/ wiki/Kardashev_scale.

Alex Hughes, "Kardashev Scale: What Is It and Where Is Earth Listed?," BBC Science Focus Magazine, May 18, 2022, https://www.sciencefocus. com/future-technology/kardashevs-scale/.

Hannah Ritchie, Fiona Spooner, and Max Roser, "Biodiversity," Our World in Data, December 19, 2022, https://ourworldindata.org/biodiversity.

Joseph Campbell, The Hero's Journey: Joseph Campbell on His Life and Work (Joseph Campbell Foundation, 2020).

Michael J Gonzalez et al., "Metabolic Correction and Physiologic Modulation as the Unifying Theory of the Healthy State: The Orthomolecular, Systemic and Functional Approach to Physiologic Optimization," *International Society for Orthomolecular Medicine* 38, no. 2 (2023), https://isom.ca/article/metabolic-correction-physiologic-modulation-unifying-theory-healthy-state/.

Khyatee, et al., "Impact of Cranial Electrical Stimulation Based Analysis of Heart Rate Variability in Insomnia," *Communications in Computer and Information Science*, November 24, 2019, 296–307, https://doi.org/10.1007/978-981-15-1718-1_25.

Khyatee et al., "Impact of Cranial Electrical Stimulation on Statistical Indices of Time Domain Parameters of Heart Rate Variability in Hypertensive Individuals," *Indian Journal of Public Health Research & Development* 11, no. 3 (March 23, 2020), https://doi.org/10.37506/ijphrd.v11i3.726.

Katie Daughters et al., "Salivary Oxytocin Concentrations in Males Following Intranasal Administration of Oxytocin: A Double-Blind, Cross-over Study," *PLOS ONE* 10, no. 12 (December 15, 2015), https://doi.org/10.1371/journal.pone.0145104.

Jennie R. Stevenson et al., "Oxytocin Administration Prevents Cellular Aging Caused by Social Isolation," *Psychoneuroendocrinology* 103 (May 2019): 52–60, https://doi.org/10.1016/j.psyneuen.2019.01.006.

Chiara Porro, Tarek Benameur, and MariaA Panaro, "The Antiaging Role of Oxytocin," *Neural Regeneration Research* 16, no. 12 (December 2021): 2413, https://doi.org/10.4103/1673-5374.313030.

Joseph A Boscarino et al., "Higher FKBP5, COMT, CHRNA5, and CRHR1 Allele Burdens Are Associated with PTSD and Interact with Trauma Exposure: Implications for Neuropsychiatric Research and Treatment," *Neuropsychiatric Disease and Treatment*, February 11, 2012, 131, https://doi.org/10.2147/ndt.s29508.

Arterosil and endocalyx fact sheet - microvascular, August 2022, https://microvascular.com/wp-content/uploads/2022/08/Arterosil-Endocalyx-Classic-FactSheet-Aug-2022.pdf.

For more references, please visit GladdenLongevity.com/Book100.

Part Two
Longevity

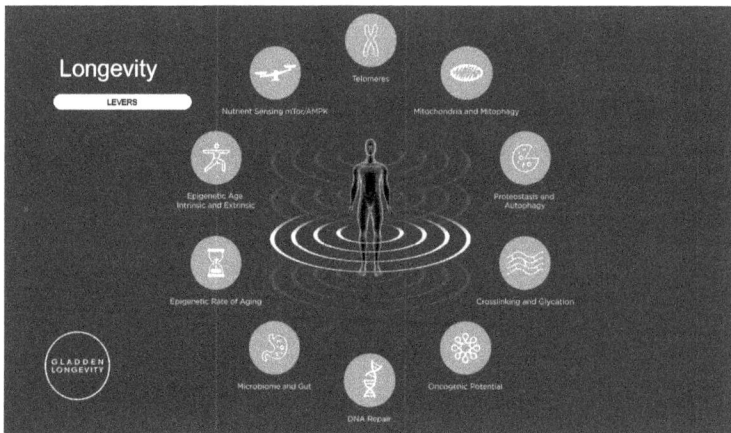

How Do We Live "Well" Beyond 120?

How Old Are You?

Most people would respond to that question with a single number, the number of years they have been on the planet. Gladden Longevity defines it differently. As of this writing, we measure sixty-three different "ages" to come up with a composite that identifies where an individual is in their aging process, and we are actively adding more. Your composite age consists of the elements identified in the Mosaic of Ages and includes the ages attached to the Life Energy, Longevity, Health, and Performance Circles. Some of the ages are obvious like heart age, brain age, or bone age. Others are more obscure like mRNA splicing dysregulation, DNA Methylation age, Mitochondrial Age, and Altered Nutrient Sensing.

While you may have forgotten most of these biological structures and functions after high school or college biology, they are extremely important to understanding aging and cracking the code of why and how we age. If you are depressed and suffer a cardiac event, for example, your chances of a full recovery increase if you have loving, supportive family and friends. We can have all the best biochemical solutions and answers in the world, but if we don't have our Life Energy in order, they won't have nearly the positive impact they could.

I have created an avatar that I use to help Gladden Longevity clients, prospective clients, and even prospective employees understand our process. The Avatar, as you've seen earlier, consists of four concentric circles, all represented on four ascending levels. The four circles are Life Energy, Longevity, Health, and Performance. The four ascending levels are referred to as information, levers, testing, and actions. When it comes to information, we are constantly utilizing several AIs: The Levers are things that need to be targeted, pulled, or activated to have an impact on an area of interest; Testing performed to evaluate the status and age of a system, process, or organ; and Actions are things we would ask you to do or not do, take or not take, and the coaching we provide to enable you to succeed. Actions can also include procedures we do for you, with you, or recommend you have done.

In addition, we have Feedback Loops between the Testing and Actions to continue to refine and adjust our interventions to bring the ecosystem into an equilibrium that optimizes all four circles. In essence, the Avatar explains how we think, conceptualize, take action, initiate research, and adapt our strategies. Although the specifics are always reflecting new information and insights, we have found the construct to be durable, and it helps tremendously getting your arms around aging and longevity. You realize it's not all about stem cells, DNA damage, or epigenetic age; you don't think saunas are the sole answer or whatever else is trending. It helps us to understand how the next shiny object may make a contribution, at which points, and in what manner.

That's not to say things like stem cells are not important, and saunas are not beneficial. Not at all. I want you to understand that there is *no single solution* that is going to make 100 the new 30. Biology is best addressed through a complex systems approach, much like the approach to an ecosystem. It is critical to understand that biology and ecosystems are an economy of balance. Thinking of ourselves as an ecosystem, i.e., a complex system with many feedback loops, checks, and balances, is very helpful. Ecosystems like us do not respond well to being forced into one state or another and held there; it thrives on rhythmic, circadian oscillations between states. For example, the idea that being "keto" all the time is good reveals a fundamental misunderstanding of the body and how it works. When we push the body into a corner, it will either find a way out or begin to break down. When we optimize its natural rhythms and oscillations between states, it thrives. Here are some simplified obvious examples to illustrate the point:

- Eating is good. Eating all the time is bad.
- Being awake is good. Being awake all the time is bad.
- Sleeping is good. Sleeping all the time is bad.
- Exercise is good. Too much or not enough exercise is bad.

Bio Hacking
+
"Getting Healthy"
=
A Linear Strategy to an Exponential Problem

Age Hacking™

Bio Hacking

+

Longevity Medicine

=

Live Young for a Lifetime

An Exponential Strategy for an Exponential Problem

It all comes down to balance. When an ecosystem is healthy and vibrant, it is youthful, and it is characterized by being robust and resilient. So what's the difference between being robust and resilient? If something is robust, it can encounter unexpected stress and be minimally affected. If something is resilient, it has the capacity to recover from the damage caused by an unexpected stress. Together, they are the underpinnings for being anti-fragile. When the ecosystem is anti-fragile, after it either resists or recovers from an unexpected stress, it grows stronger. This is a constellation of characteristics—being robust, resilient, and anti-fragile are, collectively, my definition of youthfulness. That is why we want to focus on staying thirty for a lifetime. If we stay young, longevity comes along as a byproduct of our youthfulness.

The real target in longevity medicine is youthfulness. The entire goal of this book is to show you how to be robust, resilient, and antifragile so you can Live Young for a Lifetime.

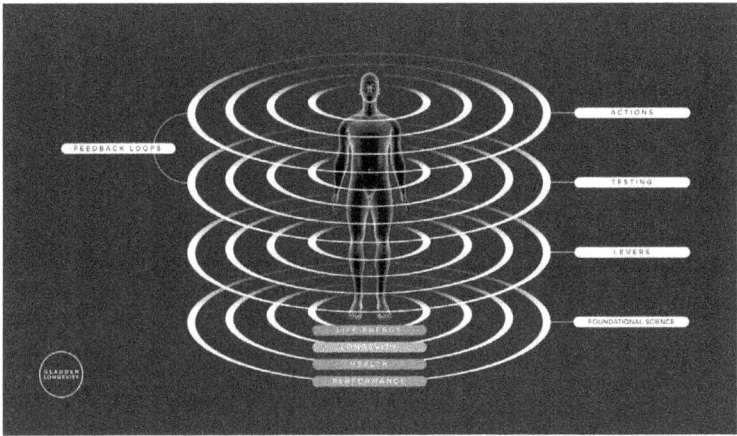

FEEDBACK LOOPS

ACTIONS

TESTING

LEVERS

FOUNDATIONAL SCIENCE

LIFE ENERGY
LONGEVITY
HEALTH
PERFORMANCE

GLADDEN
LONGEVITY

Let's return to the Avatar. What is true for all the circles, especially the Longevity Circle, is that there is a timing, sequence, frequency, intensity, and duration with which the levers need to be pulled in order to push our ecosystem back into a youthful state.

The four circles are also interrelated in this way:

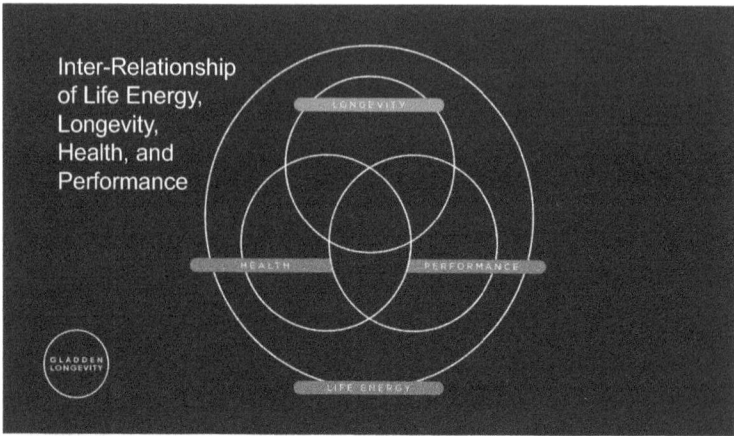

Inter-Relationship of Life Energy, Longevity, Health, and Performance

LONGEVITY

HEALTH   PERFORMANCE

GLADDEN LONGEVITY

LIFE ENERGY

Note that longevity, health, and performance form a Venn diagram, and life energy is the circle that encompasses those three.

As we move further into each section of the book, I hope you're seeing that the answer isn't just to "get healthy" by eating cleaner, prioritizing sleep, taking supplements, and exercising more. That strategy will work for a number of years, but in time, you will start to feel your "age" again. In time, the "get healthy" approach becomes more restrictive in what you can and cannot do; you have more days where you don't feel great or have great energy, and it gradually becomes an ineffective strategy.

If you are building or have built a business, career, or family, you are likely leveraging or have leveraged your health to do so. While diet and exercise will always play an essential role in the symphony of longevity, the complete musical score is much more intricate and nuanced.

"Getting healthy" is a linear strategy for an exponential problem. Human beings are linear thinkers. We find it hard to imagine exponential decline for ourselves. Ask yourself, *What will I be like in ten years?*

The answer I experience and hear from others is: *I don't know, I'll probably be about like I am now.* The reality of aging that we see all around us is difficult for us to personalize; we have difficulty imagining that aging is an exponential process, and that our decline will accelerate in an exponential way.

There was an article published recently from Stanford University that demonstrates the non-linear and exponential nature of aging. One thing that becomes clear is that youth typically ends around age twenty-six. There is an acceleration in the rate of aging in our late twenties that peaks at thirty-four. Another acceleration occurs in our late fifties, peaking at sixty, but the real story is that the fifteen years between sixty-three and seventy-eight represents a massively exponential increase in the aging process.

It is so important that you understand we are not playing a linear game. Do you have an exponential strategy?

We have also learned that aging occurs in bursts, superimposed on this timeline. For example, when you get COVID, it temporarily ages you more quickly. Women carrying a child to term ages them more quickly. The flu also ages us more quickly, and yet the body can recover youth after these insults and regain youthfulness provided there is enough underlying robustness to minimize the aging and resilience to recover youthfulness.

I have walked you through portions of my own journey and how I cracked the code for myself. For a while, it seemed like I was in a long-term game of whack-a-mole. In my forties, *whack*, I cleaned up my diet and exercised more until that no longer worked. In my fifties, *whack*, I figured out that my subclinical hypothyroidism was the reason I was tired all the time. Then *whack*, my testosterone levels were also going down, which decreased my muscle mass, energy, and libido, so I addressed that. Then another *whack*; I realized my anxiety, depression, and brain fog were related to my methylation genetics . . . and so *whack*, I corrected that. It was in this process that I realized optimization is not a one-time event but an ever-evolving and adapting strategy. I stopped believing the whack-a-mole approach was the way forward and began composing the symphony of longevity.

It wasn't that the "whacking" wasn't purposeful; I just realized it wasn't enough. It wasn't comprehensive enough, and the results weren't durable enough. I realized we needed an exponential strategy for an exponential problem and a symphonic strategy for optimizing our complex biological ecosystem.

As I composed my own symphony of longevity, I felt really good again, inside and out. Each day was better than the day before, and I realized I could be the conductor and compose symphonies for clients. That's when I left cardiology to ask the bigger questions:

- *How good can we be?*
- *How do we make 100 the new 30?*
- *How do we live "well" beyond 120?*
- *How do we live Young for a Lifetime?*

Let's digress, for a moment, on the symphonic nature of this. Have you ever heard an orchestra warming up? Each section, and each instrument, is playing independently, and it sounds like chaos. Finally, one player strikes a note, and everyone else follows to ensure they're collectively in tune. Once the conductor takes the podium, every player and every section awaits their cue to perform. They won't play all at once. They won't all play the same notes; neither will they play at the same decibel, and they don't have the same roles. But when they play the symphony with the right timing, sequence, frequency, intensity, and duration, the result is beautiful and transcendent.

Understanding our mosaic of ages and getting each one in tune is important…but the key to playing the symphony correctly involves the way the levers are played. Playing the levers correctly across all four circles becomes an exponential strategy, a strategy I believe can compete and win at the exponential game of aging!

The landmark article by Carlos Lopez-Otı'n et al. published in 2013 defined nine Hallmarks of Aging:

1. **Genomic instability**, meaning genes, DNA, or the proteins intertwined with DNA get damaged and are not adequately repaired.
2. **Cellular Senescence and Senescence Associated Secretory Phenotype (SASP)** ultimately leads to tissue dysfunction and increased cancer risk.
3. **Telomere attrition** is the end caps on the chromosomes that shorten with each cell division. When they get critically short, they accelerate the aging process.
4. **Epigenetic alterations**, DNA methylation patterns that evolve over time, and are a very good predictor of a mammal's biological age.

5. **Loss of proteostasis,** which addresses how the DNA is transcribed to make proteins and how the proteins fold, function, and are disposed of.
6. **Deregulated nutrient sensing** involves important mechanisms called mTOR and AMPK, which are responsible for the pacing of cell division, growth, repair, and rejuvenation.
7. **Mitochondrial dysfunction,** where the mitochondria are told to stop making energy in the form of ATP, typically due to damage by excessive oxidative stress or a dysfunctional immune system.
8. **Stem-cell exhaustion,** which affects the cells that are supposed to rejuvenate us. When we run out, it's over—but don't worry, we all have a secret supply.
9. **Altered intracellular communication,** which essentially boils down to a lot of excess inflammation and oxidative stress in the system due to miscommunication between cells.

In 2022, five more hallmarks were also added:

10. **Inflammation,** which accelerates aging by creating excess oxidative stress. Excess oxidative stress is causing the body to "rust" from the inside out.
11. **Compromised Autophagy,** the ability of cells to do "spring cleaning" and get rid of dysfunctional elements.
12. **Microbiome Disturbances** involve a different distribution of bacterial types that populate the intestinal tract as we age.
13. **Altered Mechanical Properties** occur when cell structures are damaged. Think the termites are eating the wood that holds your house up.

14. **mRNA Splicing Dysregulation** occurs when what the DNA wants to make and what is made are not aligned due to miscommunication between the blueprint and the factory where it is made.

And just recently in Nov of 2022, another hallmark was proposed, bringing the total to fifteen:

15. **Cell Size** because cells increase in size as they age.

In July 2023, another Hallmark was mentioned.

16. **Disrupted nucleocytoplasmic compartmentalization (NCC)** David Sinclaire's Group at Harvard recently published a paper stating that NCC is "one of the most well-conserved physiological hallmarks of aging. It can be understood as the deterioration of nucleocytoplasmic compartmentalization (NCC), it can be visualized as the leakage of nuclear proteins into the cytoplasm and failure of proteins to be imported into the nucleus from the cytoplasm." This leads to a loss of information transfer and is both an expression of and accelerates the aging process.

Let's discuss some of these hallmarks, which can be understood as both expressions and drivers of aging.

CHAPTER ELEVEN

Telomere Attrition

T elomeres are nucleic acid repeats located at the ends of our twenty-three chromosomes. Like the aglets on the tips of your shoe laces, they protect the integrity of the ends of the chromosomes. They are repeating sequences of nucleotides—TTAGGG—but they do not code for a protein. Instead, telomeres provide both protection for the ends of the chromosome and serve as timekeepers for the cell. Each time a cell divides, between thirty and two hundred base pairs are lost. Therefore, the telomeres are shortened each time a cell divides.

When we are conceived, let's say we may have 15,000 base pairs that comprise our telomeres. By the time we're born, we may have whittled that down to 10,000 base pairs in our white blood cells as we age, and as more cells divide, we lose more base pairs and the telomeres become shorter and shorter.

Telomeres are a finite resource unless they are re-lengthened. As we go through life, our cells divide at different rates, depending on the tissue type; for example, our immune cells divide much more frequently than our bone cells do. The telomeres in more rapidly dividing cells shorten more quickly. When they shorten to a critical point, they inform the cell that it is now old, and the cell's DNA is expressed differently, which can lead to either cellular senescence or cell suicide.

The Hallmarks of Aging are interrelated; for example, a decrease in telomere length leads to a reduction in mitochondrial ATP production. Think of telomere attrition as both an expression and driver of aging.

Even within a single tissue, there is a bell-shaped curve of telomere lengths. For example, it is routine to measure a bell-shaped curve of telomere lengths in our white blood cells. The report describes a median length which is the most frequently occurring length, and the mean is the average length; these are useful to know but can be misleading. Therefore, we also look at something called a "'20th percentile length," which is a measure of short telomeres. The shorter the 20 percent length is, the more the population of telomeres comprising the bell-shaped curve are shifted toward being short telomeres. This is the critical number, as it is the short telomeres that cause cells to become senescent or to undergo suicide. Conversely, the longer the 20 percent number is, the less prone our cells are to becoming senescent by this mechanism, and the younger and more resilient we are.

If you've had a telomere test done and all they are reporting is your median telomere length—and they're suggesting it's your "telomeric or biologic age age"—you can easily be misled. We like Life Length in Barcelona, Spain, as a high-quality, comprehensive telomere testing platform.

What lifestyle choices contribute to telomere shortening?

- Smoking
- High stress
- Lack of sleep
- Shift work
- Low Vitamin D level
- Lack of natural dietary antioxidants
- Lack of plant-based polyphenols and anti-inflammatories
- Lack of fish oil and plant-based Omega 3s

What are the effects of shortened telomeres? Telomeres are responsible for preventing DNA damage, so if telomeres are shortened, the DNA is more likely to be damaged. Having short telomeres can also lead to

- genetic mutations;
- chromosomal instability, which can cause a variety of problems with the DNA;
- cellular aging;
- decreased gene expression, which can lead to a decrease in the expression of important genes;
- a decrease in the ability of the cell to repair damaged DNA;
- increased susceptibility to diseases and cancer; and
- reduced energy production by the mitochondria.

And the above is just for starters. We know that COVID infections shorten telomeres and, upon recovery, decrease a patient's ability to regenerate damaged lung or heart tissue. Patients with shorter telomeres who get COVID also suffer more hospitalizations and complications and die more often. It appears that longer telomeres also confer more protection for those who choose to receive the vaccines. Interestingly, we are observing telomere shortening with vaccination.

Telomeres can be lengthened by the enzyme telomerase. It is found in all cells but typically is only active in stem cells and reproductive cells. Telomerase is also frequently turned on by cancer cells as part of their strategy to remain immortal. This raises the question: If we activate telomerase to re-lengthen telomeres, will it cause cancer? It is an important question.

We know that having short telomeres increases the risk of cancer. Senescent cells resulting from shortened telomeres that become secretory cells or undergo SASP also promote cancer. Short telomeres in immune cells weaken the immune system's surveillance and elimination of malignant cells and, therefore, make us more susceptible to cancer.

There is a "Goldilocks zone" for telomere lengths, as having telomeres that are too long may also be associated with cancer.

So what should we do—leave them short or re-lengthen them?

As far as the research tells us and what we've observed, the answer is *that humans do better with re-lengthening short telomeres but not over-lengthening longer telomeres.* Telomerase itself has not been shown to be responsible for making a cell malignant. Once a malignant cell has become malignant, turning on telomerase is a mechanism the cancer cell uses to maintain its immortality, but it is not the initiating event in cancer cell development.

On the other hand, genetic variants in telomerase cellular promoters that cause over-activity of telomerase have been linked to melanoma. To be safe, we do not recommend lengthening telomeres in patients with cancer or those with certain genetic predispositions to cancer. While it is possible that lengthening telomeres with telomerase would improve the immune system and help cure cancer—and there is anecdotal evidence to this effect—it has yet to be shown in a clinical trial, so we are being cautious.

If you are using a product to re-lengthen telomeres, we have seen repeatedly that it is the short telomeres that are preferentially lengthened. This is perfect because we are lengthening the telomeres that drive aging and not over-lengthening the ones that have a good length. This lack of further lengthening of telomeres that are at an optimal length is due to the fact that the telomeres are combined with shelterin proteins that serve to halt the re-lengthening process when the telomeres reach an optimal functional length. This built-in "governor" leads to an ideal outcome of lengthening the senescence-producing short telomeres without over-lengthening the longer normal telomeres. Despite this governor, controversy persists about whether re-lengthening telomeres is safe, and therefore, we test clients for malignant cells prior to initiating therapy. We also monitor the appearance of malignant cells during therapy.

Following my bout with COVID, I was in the twenty-sixth percentile for short telomeres. In other words, 74 percent of people my chronological age had a better telomere profile. Today, using a proprietary product, my percentile characterization is literally off the chart; my telomere age is in the seventy-fifth percentile for a thirty-year-old! While my median telomere length has also improved, the dramatic change has been in my short telomere lengths. This is exactly what I wanted to see happen.

With this proprietary product, we have conducted tests on cell cultures to see if we can transform cells from normal fibroblasts into cancer cells. It hasn't happened. We have also given telomerase to HeLa cells—known cancer cells—in tissue culture and have seen no increase in their malignant nature. We are also working on additional studies to do more testing in different models to ensure that there is no cause or effect with cancer-cell formation.

When looking at the drivers of aging, we find that genomic instability goes hand-in-hand with telomere length. Genomic instability refers to DNA damage that may result from DNA replication, endogenous oxidative stress, or from exogenous physical, chemical, or biological agents. These insults can lead to a lot of different disruptions in the DNA itself, which, if not repaired, will accelerate cellular dysfunction and aging.

There are many ways the genetic information can be damaged. DNA is not just composed of nucleic acids; the nucleic acids are entwined with proteins called *chromatin*. When the chromatin protein is damaged, it can also cause problems. Chromatin is the architectural structure of the DNA—think of chromatin as the structural backbone that holds the DNA in place. Damage to the backbone can also lead to genome instability and inappropriate gene transcription and expression.

Note that, by default, DNA will always be damaged. We live in a world where that is a given, so the issue is not whether DNA *will* be damaged but rather how well we *repair* the damage. Damage is not a problem if it can be repaired, but youth is lost when the repair mechanisms can no longer keep up with the rate of damage.

Measurement and Optimization

It is important to understand that telomere length is best correlated to biological age in the middle of life. After age eighty, telomere length is a less reliable "clock" because there are alternate mechanisms for telomere lengthening and shortening that come into play. This is in addition to the shortening that occurs with cell division.

That being said, telomere length is still very important, and having optimal lengths is necessary to be youthful. The first step in any process of optimization is to stop doing the things that are undermining our youthfulness. When our clients come to us and tell us they want to focus on getting healthy, getting their longevity and youthfulness on the right trajectory, and getting their performance levels back, we run them through a battery of tests and questionnaires that initially address one key point: What should they stop doing?

We don't start with what we can add—we start with what should be subtracted. What are you doing that's destroying your youthfulness? Maybe it's smoking, excess alcohol, excess stress, or lack of sleep . . . getting those lifestyle drivers of aging out of your life is the first big step. Below is a partial list of critical factors:

- Regular alcohol consumption (if you don't have a drinking problem, some alcohol is good, perhaps one drink on two different days of the week)
- Eating processed foods, vegetable oils, sugar, and calorie-rich/nutrient-poor foods
- Eating too much and too often and not fasting
- Poor quality sleep
- Too little or conversely, too much sun exposure
- Lack of daily exercise for cardiovascular fitness, strength, and balance
- Sitting vs. standing, or getting up and moving every twenty minutes
- Caffeine dependence, as an aid to wake up and for energy

- Mental health issues: anxiety, depression, PTSD, ADD, addictions, unresolved trauma, and excessive stress
- Not wearing sunglasses
- Tobacco use in any form
- Lack of close friendships and a romantic partner
- A closed mindset, being married to your current answers, and not your empowering questions

We have worked with people who ostensibly want optimal life energy, health, longevity, and performance, but are sabotaging themselves with anxiety, stress, lack of purpose, and addictive behaviors. When this is the case, we have found focusing on the Life Energy circle is the best place to start. Starting here does improve telomere attrition.

As mentioned, we use Life Length in Madrid, Spain, to measure our telomere lengths. By assessing the white blood cell median, average, and 20th percentile values, we are able to define your starting point. The more short telomeres are present, the more drive there is for cellular senescence. From there, we can make recommendations and interventions to improve your telomere lengths.

Optimizing lifestyle habits is key. Understanding that a great lifestyle comes from having an optimized life energy circle is a game-changer. Lifestyle will always be out of sync if life energy is not prioritized.

If you take only one thing away from this book, please understand that the most critical circle to address and the one you can take the most control over is life energy. You can't fix your boat if you're constantly drilling holes in it. The same is true with self-sabotaging thoughts and behaviors; you can't optimize your health and habits if your life energy is not addressed to support the mission.

Let's say you have taken steps to optimize your life energy and lifestyle. Your Vitamin D, fish oil, diet, sleep, and stress are under control, and you have quit using tobacco, drinking excessively, and started exercising, and your telomeres are still not getting any longer. There are some products that have been somewhat effective in activating telomerase:

- TA 65 is the middle of the road in terms of its ability to activate telomerase. Studies have shown that TA 65 works quite well at lengthening short telomeres, and we use it at Gladden Longevity.
- TAM 818 is more potent than TA 65 but more expensive. At Gladden Longevity, we have seen some good results of TAM 818 lengthening short telomeres.
- IsaGenis appears to affect telomeres by being a powerful blend of antioxidants to blunt telomere attrition, but as of writing, it has less data than TA65 or TAM 818 for actually re-lengthening telomeres.

Gladden Longevity is currently collaborating with an independent researcher and running an IRB-approved trial to test a proprietary telomerase product for safety and efficacy. As of writing this, our yet-to-be-published data is very encouraging in that short telomeres are re-lengthened, but longer telomeres are not over-lengthened. This is also what I used to take my telomeres from being five years older than my chronological age to being almost forty years younger than my chronological age. Stay tuned!

CHAPTER TWELVE

DNA Repair

As we discussed, telomere re-lengthening is a form of DNA repair. Our DNA is damaged all the time by internal processes like cell replication and oxidative stress and by external processes like radiation and toxin exposure. Fortunately, we have robust DNA repair mechanisms, but they don't always work. Some people are genetically gifted in their DNA repair capabilities, and this gift correlates with longevity. Others are genetically challenged in their ability to repair DNA, and this shortens life expectancy and increases the risk of cancer.

BRCA1 and BRCA2 are examples of a genetic variant that decreases the ability to correctly repair double-stranded DNA breaks. Women who have a BRCA1 or BRCA2 genetic mutation are at an increased risk of breast, ovarian, and pancreatic cancers. Men who have a BRCA1 or BRCA2 genetic mutation are at an increased risk of prostate, pancreatic, and breast cancers. We are currently looking at the status of DNA repair capabilities with sophisticated AI-enhanced transcriptomic and proteomic testing to better understand an individual's ability to perform DNA repair, identify where they are at risk, and create strategies to help protect them.

When it comes to DNA repair, there are at least 130 genes that code for proteins that contribute to the repair process. For example, when the gene known as BUBR1 is overexpressed, it increases protection from cancer. It does so by ensuring proper chromosome alignment and kinetochore-microtubule attachment in cell division. Mice genetically engineered to overexpress BUBR1 have extended healthy lifespans.

Effectively managing oxidative stress is a very important strategy for minimizing damaged DNA. Note that simply taking antioxidants has never been associated with improved longevity. For now, understand that the idea of taking high doses of Vitamin C, Vitamin E, etc., has never been shown to improve longevity. We became fans of molecular hydrogen in 2015 as a way to manage oxidative stress. Following *in silico* testing (computer-simulated testing), seeing all the benefits of hydrogen (H2) in oxidative stress and pain signal-balancing, we have developed H2 products that balance the redox system and can be used in higher doses as an adjunct to relieve pain.

Hydrogen is the perfect oxidative-stress modulator. It modulates oxidative stress by upregulating the genetic expression of three genes, SOD, GPX, and CAT, involved in turning oxygen-free radicals into water (H_2O). In addition, it down-regulates COX2 and inflammation genes associated with pain pathways.

Measurement and Optimization

Measuring levels of DNA damage and the extent of repair is difficult to do clinically. Our approach has been to develop transcriptomic and proteomic tests, which we now are using to look at the inherent genetic capability of an individual to repair their DNA, as well as the status of their DNA repair. This is included in the Life Raft Index testing that we perform. We then look at markers of DNA damage.

One that is readily available is to measure 8-hydroxy-2-deoxyguanosine (8-OHdG) levels in white blood cells. Measuring 8-OHdG gives us insight into DNA damage levels related to excess oxidative stress. To optimize these levels, we look at reducing factors that increase oxidative stress, like heavy metals. Heavy metals interact with oxygen to increase oxidative stress.

We also utilize H2 to balance the redox system and decrease overall oxidative stress. In fact, we formed a new company between Gladden Longevity and Neo7 Bioscience called Genesis Longevity Bioscience to build out the transcriptomics and proteomics of aging and to be able to test for these in order to understand where a person struggles and to make precision interventions. The additional transcriptomic and proteomic markers we've developed for DNA damage and repair, along with other Hallmarks of Aging, have now given us the ability to be more precise with our supplement recommendations. In addition, we can formulate custom-built peptides to modulate gene expression to optimize oxidative stress and improve DNA repair. Gladden Longevity has also created a blend of mushrooms in a tincture to turn down inflammation, the inflammatory signaling of Nf-Kb, called the Anti-Inflammatory Shroom Formula.

We also utilize Curcumin and PEA in more precise ways based on an individual's test results. In working with Neo 7, we are working to reestablish a youthful balance of genetic expression. Some inflammation is necessary and good, some oxidative stress is necessary and good. We are using more precise diagnostic and therapeutic tools to more precisely balance the ecosystem—not attack any one process. We are now in an age where we have never before seen strategies when it comes to addressing and balancing Hallmarks of Aging, and the drivers of aging.

CHAPTER THIRTEEN

Mitochondria

Our mitochondria generate most of the energy needed for cells to function. To get a handle on mitochondrial function—and, therefore, your mitochondrial age—we look at it through several different lenses.

Fat is an efficient way to store energy; it's also an efficient way to provide energy to the body, particularly in a resting state. Our ability to store glucose is much more limited. Glucose stores are typically reserved for short bursts of intense effort. When healthy mitochondria are at rest, they burn predominantly fat for fuel. When we burn fat, we get a total of thirty-four energy-containing molecules known as *adenosine triphosphate* (ATP). When we exercise and have healthy mitochondria, we transition from primarily burning fat to burning glucose exclusively at peak exercise. This is true no matter what your diet is or how "keto" you are trying to be. The reason we transition from fat to glucose in high-intensity activities is that we can get thirty-six ATPs from glucose.

Think of fat as regular gas and glucose as premium. At rest, ideally, eighty percent of the energy comes from burning fat, and the rest is from carbohydrates. By pushing ourselves into a state of peak performance, like during intense exercise, all of us transition to burning 100 percent glucose. This happens regardless of your food intake, including keto and low-carb diets. The benefit of low-carb diets is that it trains the mitochondria to burn a higher percentage of fat relative to carbs at rest. That being said, when we do intense exercise, we deplete our stores of glucose, called glycogen, and they need to be restored so they will be available the next time you need them. The muscles are particularly receptive to rebuilding the glycogen stores in the thirty minutes immediately following exercise; if you are ever going to eat some simple carbs that quickly turn to sugar, this thirty-minute time slot is the time to do it.

Another way to look at mitochondria is the rate at which they transition from burning fat at rest to burning 100 percent glucose. When we're at rest, fat—our "regular gas"—keeps us going, but as we push ourselves toward maximal effort, we transition by gradually adding more "premium gas" to the mix. The rate at which your body makes this transition from burning regular to premium is a very precise indicator of your mitochondrial health, i.e., your mitochondrial age.

It's important to note that the oxidative damage theory of mitochondrial aging is no longer felt to be true. The theory posited that because mitochondria are making ATP by utilizing oxygen and, in the process, generating reactive oxygen species as a byproduct, these free radicals were the source of mitochondrial aging.

While it's true that too much oxidative stress can be damaging to the mitochondria, the mitochondria also age if they are not exposed to oxidative stress. The ecosystem loves to be stressed. It keeps it in balance and healthy. These stresses are called "hormetic" stresses. Exercise, saunas, fasting, and cold plunges are all examples of moderate stresses, hormetic stresses, that fall in the "Goldilocks zone" of making us stronger and more antifragile. They don't damage us beyond what we can repair.

Keep in mind the body was built to be used like a car was built to be driven. We have a lot of built-in enzymatic systems to manage those oxygen free radicals and neutralize those particles, just like the catalytic converter on a car manages the exhaust. Three enzymes are primarily involved: superoxide dismutase, glutathione, peroxidase, and catalase. They basically take the mitochondrial exhaust of energy production, known as reactive oxygen species, and neutralize them, turning them first into hydrogen peroxide and then back into water. Reactive oxygen species (ROS) are also necessary, signaling molecules that instruct the body to upregulate repair mechanisms, make more mitochondria, and build muscle, tendons, ligaments, bones, blood vessels, and heart muscle. Blocking these with antioxidants like Vitamin C pre-workout robs you of the benefits of exercise. Using H2 to balance them allows you to minimize damage but get the full effect of the signaling you want to get stronger.

When mitochondria *do* become damaged and dysfunctional, they produce less energy and contribute to inflammation. Failing mitochondria contribute to a general decline in energy and health, and, in the nervous system, neurodegenerative diseases like ALS and Alzheimer's, chronic fatigue syndrome, neuropathy, MS, and many others.

Note that when telomeres shorten, they signal the mito-chondria to make less ATP. Poor mitochondrial function is one of the reasons older people feel tired and cold all the time. One antidote to this is to activate our AMPK pathway through protracted cardiovascular exercise, fasting, saunas, cold plunges, metformin, and berberine. Activating AMPK—think restorative functions—and down-regulating mTOR—think anabolic growth functions—triggers both autophagy and mitophagy. Autophagy recycles or disposes faulty or worn-out components in the cell, and mitoph-agy induces the production of new, better-performing mitochondria.

Measurement and Optimization

A Cardiopulmonary Exercise Test (CPET) shows us the percentage of fat-burning at rest and maps the transition that occurs with exercise from predominantly fat burning to 100 percent glucose-burning at peak exercise. This rate of transition from fat-burning to glucose-burning with exercise is critical to knowing your mitochondrial health. It is referred to as the RER curve, or respiratory exchange ratio curve.

RER is the ratio of carbon dioxide produced in making ATP relative to the oxygen consumed in making the ATP. This is rarely ever measured at "longevity clinics" but is an essential metric in understanding the health of your mitochondria.

At Gladden Longevity, we measure it on everyone we see. It turns out that the slower you transition from fat-burning to carb-burning, on your way from being at rest to maximal exercise, the healthier and younger your mitochondria are. It can be that simple!

In addition, CPET measures VO2 -max, which tells you how much blood your heart can pump in a minute. The more blood you can pump, the younger your heart is, the longer you live, and the healthier you are while you're alive.

When the mitochondria are healthy, that transition from burning fat to burning carbs is slow and linear. When the mitochondria are weak, and one is in a state of poor cardiovascular fitness, the transition is abrupt and occurs at a lower level of exercise. Our testing has shown that in addition to several supplements, regular, thirty to sixty-minute sessions of cardiovascular training, four or five days a week—with both steady state and interval training—is critical for improving the RER curve and restoring mitochondrial health.

Another window into mitochondrial health comes from the Krebs Cycle—also known as the Citric Acid or Tricarboxylic Acid (TCA) cycle—which looks into a biochemical pathway inside the mitochondria.

Named for German-British physician and scientist Hans Krebs, we are able to look at the intermediates, cofactors, and obstructing factors. There are appropriate levels of intermediates and cofactors that are required for that cycle to work properly. We can identify whether there are deficiencies or obstructions to the cycle functioning normally and make recommendations on how to restore its function.

It's not enough to just take a bunch of antioxidants and think that will solve the problem; it doesn't. It has been shown that exercise, which increases reactive oxygen species, and even the use of ozone, which increases reactive oxygen species, actually *stimulates* the cell to adapt to oxidative stress, enabling us to handle more of it. We will never get away from the need for exercise because it is a "hormetic" stress that allows us to get stronger.

We talk a lot about chronic stress and how bad it is for us, but intermittent, hormetic stress enables us to get stronger and is a *required* stress. I find most people don't exercise hard enough; if you can carry on a conversation during all your cardio training, you are not pushing hard enough.

Hormetic stressors are important because they stimulate the body to become more youthful. Yes, exercise increases the number of reactive oxygen species, but we're also signaling the body to upregulate its ability to handle them. And ultimately, that makes us stronger. When the mitochondria are healthy, you feel great; when they are not, you feel tired and cold all the time.

Finding ways of incorporating hormetic stressors into your daily life, like exercise, fasting, sauna, and cold plunge, keeps our mitochondria and us much healthier. Make this a priority!

Another company has developed a test, Mito Swab, that gives us insight into another part of the mitochondria—the respiratory transport chain. This is the assembly line that utilizes oxygen as an electron-receptor to set up a cascade of electrons moving down an energy gradient, resulting in the production of ATP from ADP. Gaining insight into the steps along this cascade gives us insight into what supplements, precursors, and interventions to use to optimize energy production. NAD and H2 play a role here, along with CoQ10 and other cofactors.

PEMF mats can also revitalize mitochondrial function. We have found that it takes testing with a variety of assessments to get a handle on a person's mitochondrial status and to be able to make the appropriate recommendations. Looking at the mitochondria through multiple lenses enables us to create better more comprehensive solutions for our clients.

A few key supplements, peptides, and devices that promote enhanced mitochondrial function are listed below, many of which can be stacked together as needed.

- The NAD/NADH ratio optimization:
  - o NAD Precursors are used, such as Niacin, Nicotinamide D Riboside, NMN, and Nuchido Time™.
  - o Nuchido Time™ combines supplements to optimize NAD production, recycling, and minimize its loss. Internal data shows that with regular twice-daily use, there was a clinically significant increase in intracellular NAD levels.
  - o 5Amino-1MQ is a peptide that can keep nicotinamide from being siphoned out of the NAD salvage pathway to boost NAD.
  - o MOTS-c is a peptide that translocates to the nucleus in relationship with AMPK and also improves The NAD/NADH ratio.
- Activated B vitamins: B vitamins are consumed with energy production. If you are athletic, they will be consumed faster, and your requirements may be higher. The Genova NutrEval® test can give you insight into your ongoing need for these vitamins.
- L-Carnitine or Acetyl-L- Carnitine: promotes the utilization of fat for fuel.
- Urolithin-A (MitoPure): Promotes mitophagy to replace damaged mitochondria with new ones.
- CoQ10: An antioxidant and cofactor in the respiratory transport chain that enhances mitochondrial energy production.

- Alpha Lipoic Acid: A cofactor for the enzymes that participate in intermediary cell metabolism resulting in ATP production.
- H2: Modulates the redox status of the cell to bring it into balance and optimize its function.
- PEMF (Pulsed Electro-Magentic Frequency) Devices: These devices push magnetic energy into the body in an attempt to optimize the body's internal energy fields. The results are increased ATP production through the electron transport chain and modulation of genes associated with inflammation and anti-inflammation. Pain reduction or resolution also occurs.
- Red Light Therapy: Red light therapy has been shown to enhance electron transport chain function in the mitochondria. This results in more energy production for the cell.
- Methylene Blue: Can also increase ATP production directly but should not be used by those taking SSRI anti-depressants, as it may cause too much serotonin activity in the brain. This results in mild shivering and/or diarrhea to severe muscle rigidity, elevated body temperature, and seizures. Note: Severe serotonin syndrome, if not immediately addressed, has been associated with death.

CHAPTER FOURTEEN

Altered Proteostasis and Autophagy

A s of 2022, proteostasis and autophagy are both considered Hallmarks of Aging. *Proteostasis* refers to the life cycle of a protein, and *autophagy* refers to the cell recycling its proteins and other components to keep the cell in a youthful condition. Autophagy occurs when AMPK is activated, as in times of fasting or protracted exercise, and is shut when mTOR is activated. Things like when growth hormone and testosterone are increased, and in times of plentiful nutrients, like protein and amino acids. Because proteostasis and autophagy are related, and we will touch on both of them here.

For a protein to be made properly, the DNA that codes for the protein needs to be intact, and the messenger RNA transcribed from the DNA needs to be error-free. The protein needs to be assembled properly from the mRNA at the ribosome. Then, the protein needs to fold properly into a three-dimensional structure in order to perform its function. Finally, when the protein is at the end of its life, it needs to be disposed of properly so it doesn't clutter the cell and become misfolded into a clump that is toxic to the cell.

Proteins are made of amino acids. Amino acids have a basic (as in acid-base) amino group, NH2, on one end and an organic carboxylic acid group, COOH, on the other. This gives each amino acid an electrical charge which means when they are linked together into a protein, the charged amino acids will configure themselves into a stable low-energy state where positive charges attract negative charges, and like charges repel. Based on this, the protein will fold into a very specific, three-dimensional structure. The protein can then function as a receptor, a signaling agent (think lock-and-key), a structural component, or micromachines that perform work in the cell.

If the amino-acid chain contains over one hundred amino acids, it is called a *protein*. Between two and fifty amino acids, it's called an *oligopeptide* or simply a *peptide*. A chain between fifty and one hundred amino acids is referred to as a *polypeptide*.

The folding of proteins is not always perfect. Proteins, along with previously misfolded proteins, can be chaperoned to fold or refold properly with the help of heat-shock proteins. Heat-shock proteins are up-regulated with intermittent sauna use. Hence, one of the reasons saunas are such a great longevity hack. The amino acid serine also aids in chaperoning protein folding. You might want to consider taking some serine; it dissolves in water and tastes good while you're in the sauna!

Proteins are marvelous to watch in action. If you haven't seen them in action, go to YouTube and search for "The Inner Life of the Cell Animation," a video posted by XVIVO Scientific Animation.

There are many examples of misfolded proteins, resulting in suboptimal cell function and associated with disease. Alzheimer's Disease is associated with Beta-Amyloid and Tau proteins. Parkinson's Disease is associated with Alpha Synuclian. ALS (Lou Gehrig's Disease) is associated with several dysfunctional proteins, SOD1, TDP-43 Ubiquilin-2, p62, etc. Even common cataracts are the result of misfolded proteins.

The final component of proteostasis involves getting rid of proteins at the end of their life via autophagy. Through autophagy, old proteins and other cell components are recycled, and amino acids are reused. Misfolded proteins that can't be salvaged with chaperone-mediated refolding are also targets for autophagy. There are various strategies to augment autophagy that we should all utilize: fasting, sustained cardiovascular exercise, saunas, and taking spermidine all enhance this process.

Measurement and Optimization

To identify the proteomic status of an individual, we are currently developing at Gladden Longevity more extensive transcriptomics and proteomics technologies to look beyond DNA structure and examine how the DNA is expressed and gauge the fidelity of that expression into mRNA and the final protein product. In addition, we can look at the relative levels of protein production.

In terms of longevity optimization, saunas are a mainstay. A study done in Finland followed 2,300 men between the ages of forty and sixty for twenty years. The men were grouped by their use of a dry Scandinavian sauna once a week, two or three times a week, or four or more times a week. The study showed that to get a benefit, one needs to be in the sauna at greater than 170 degrees for longer than nineteen minutes. The men who used the sauna four or more days a week experienced a 65 percent reduction in Alzheimer's, a 65 percent reduction in dementia, a 50 percent reduction in heart attack and stroke, and a 40 percent reduction in all-cause mortality in comparison to those who used it just one day a week. These are spectacular numbers!

What about eating protein? Turns out middle-aged people die sooner on high-protein diets, and older people die sooner on low-protein diets. If the reason for eating protein is to build protein-like muscle, then using a product like BodyHealth's Perfect Amino, combined with hormone replacement therapy, works well as a base. Note that when we eat protein, the majority of that protein does not go into building protein in our bodies. For example, when we eat egg whites, the gold standard biological dietary protein replete with all the essential amino acids, only 50 percent of that protein is utilized to build protein. With collagen protein, it is closer to 18 percent. With Perfect Amino, it is 99 percent. If you want to build protein, Perfect Amino works great without overstressing your system with too much protein.

When it comes to optimizing your health and longevity, it is critical to cycle between building protein, that is, being anabolic and, alternately, being catabolic. We want to stimulate the mTOR and anabolic pathways to build bone and muscle. But if we do it all the time, the pathways get down-regulated, and longevity data shows we don't live as long and have a higher incidence of cancer. Note that mTOR activation turns off autophagy. On the other hand, AMPK activation turns on autophagy as well as mitophagy and other important pathways that keep us young. For example, when AMPK is activated, DNA repair and telomere maintenance are up-regulated.

So how do we balance these two helpful but seemingly mutually antagonistic pathways? We alternate between the two. The idea is that if you are going to be anabolic, be anabolic. Augment testosterone, growth hormone release, IGF-1 levels, protein intake, resistance training, etc., but then seven to ten days later, take rapamycin to block mTOR and use supplements like hydroxy-berberine, Gynostemma pentaphyllum, Hesperidin, Resveratrol as Vinia or Pterostilbene, NMN, and NAD to activate AMPK. AMPK is also activated with exercise and fasting. These are very powerful; every study that looked at calorie restriction done correctly or exercise done correctly shows improved health and longevity. While activating AMPK, stay away from testosterone, growth hormone, and high-protein diets.

Regardless of whether you are anabolic or catabolic, things you should always do are meditation, some cardiovascular and some resistance exercise, balance training, prioritizing sleep, and so on. Getting this right for you is something you need to work through with your practitioner because there are many variables to take into account to get this right. The idea of cycling between mTOR and AMPK activation, however, is a solid recommendation and is a major rhythm in playing the Symphony of Longevity.

CHAPTER FIFTEEN

Glycan Age

When we talk about our Glycan Age, we are referring to the age of the immune system and its inflammatory tendencies. When proteins are made, they can then be modified to further differentiate their function. It's analogous to buying a car and adding options or accessories to make it perform better in specific circumstances. Proteins are similar; they can be modified to enhance certain functions or adapt to new situations. It's far more efficient for the body to code for and build a single protein and then modify it than to code for and build many different proteins.

Proteins are modified with endogenous sugar molecules. Some examples of sugars used to modify proteins:

- Fructose
- Galactose

- GalNac (N-Acetylgalactosamine, is an amino sugar derivative of Galactose.)
- Glucose
- Inositol
- Manitol
- Xylitol

These and other sugar derivatives are attached to proteins in a way that changes the function of the protein. Glycan Age refers to the modifications of our IgG antibodies by these sugars.

The Glycan Age test measures glycated patterns of our IgG antibodies and correlates it to a biological age. The idea is that the more anti-inflammatory the IgG antibody glycation patterns are, the younger you are. Conversely, the more inflammatory the patterns are, the older you are.

Measurement and Optimization

Lifestyle optimization seems to be the best way to affect the Glycan Age, but we are currently exploring other possibilities as well. Gladden Longevity has developed an alcohol mushroom extract designed to down-regulate NFkB. NFkB is a prime mover in upregulating inflammation. In addition to using the Life Raft Index, we are working with Neo7 Bioscience to develop custom peptides to modulate inflammatory genetic expression back into a more youthful state.

CHAPTER SIXTEEN

Glycation and Cross-linking

I ndependent of the Glycan Age, a high-sugar diet leads to cross-linking of the proteins with the sugars in our diet. These cross-linked proteins cause protein stiffness, which we experience as stiff joints, lack of flexibility in our muscles, tendons, and ligaments, inflammation, and pain. A low-carb diet with plenty of healthy fats can relieve this "age-related" stiffness and soreness.

Measurement and Optimization

We currently do not have a blood test beyond HbA1C to measure protein-to-sugar cross-linking or other Advanced Glycation End (AGE) products. HbA1C is used primarily to give us a three-month running average of blood sugar levels but it should be noted that it can also provide some insight into AGE levels.

Why are AGEs important? When we consume sugar before bed, the next morning, we will likely wake up with stiff joints and tendons, making it difficult to move around. This is because a diet rich in fast-release carbs or sugar leads to cross-linking of proteins. L-Carnosine helps to protect us from this cross-linking. In addition, L-Carnosine decreases senescent cells and protects muscle strength and volume.

Consuming healthy fats, leafy greens, and little or no sugar, we'll awaken with joints that don't hurt and tendons that are not stiff. This is an easy, clinical way to gauge the glycation, or cross-linking, of your proteins. We have recently come across a remarkable product called Sugar to Fiber that, if taken one to two hours before a meal, will enzymatically transform the sugar you ate into fiber and fructose by using plant enzymes. Studies at Harvard report that 50 to 80% of the consumed sugar will be turned into fiber. As you know, fiber is excellent for gut health. We have used Sugar to Fiber in conjunction with a continuous glucose monitor and have seen no rise in blood sugar when eating foods that previously spiked blood sugars.

CHAPTER SEVENTEEN

Inflammation

nflammation is now a stand-alone Hallmark of Aging. It is also related to other hallmarks, like Altered Intracellular Communication and Senescence Associated Secretory Phenotype (SASP). Inflammation is a problem because, ultimately, it increases the level of oxidative stress at the cellular level. The downward spiral of aging results in ever-increasing amounts of inflammation, tissue damage, and dysfunction. It is a key driver in the exponential acceleration of aging.

Dysregulation of the immune response is a leading cause of this chronic systemic inflammation. These drivers of inflammation lead to dysregulated proinflammatory mediators, cytokines, and chemokines that are major culprits in mediating the development of chronic inflammation and the immunosenescence process collectively known as *inflammaging.* In order to understand inflammaging better, we need to break it down into its component parts.

The first part is that the immune system response is modified, resulting in a lack of inflammation resolution. Chronic inflammatory diseases, including autoimmune disorders like rheumatoid arthritis, lupus, and eczema, are examples, along with chronic inflammatory response syndrome (CIRS) found in protracted Lyme Syndrome, mold, and Actinomyces exposure. It is the result of the innate immune system not being turned off after the initial insulting agent has been removed.

The second part is excessive wear and tear. Exercise and repeated trauma set up chronic inflammation in joints, tendons, and ligaments. These insults become compounded and lead to ever-accelerating cycles of damage, inflammation dysfunction, and more damage.

The third part is the Senescence Associated Secretory Phenotype (SASP). SASP is a major contributor to the accelerating current of aging. It results from senescent cells, which transform from quiescent inert zombie cells into active secretory cells. SASP is directly involved in many diseases of aging, such as heart disease, high blood pressure, cancer, and dementia. Normal cells trying to function in this toxic, inflammatory environment find it harder and harder to do so. Sadly, stem cells and repair mechanisms don't work as well in this toxic, inflamed environment making endogenous rejuvenation or even exogenous rejuvenation with various stem cell or PRP procedures impossible. Consequently, decline continues. As inflammaging continues, we can get to a point of no return.

Measurement and Optimization

Testing panels have been and are being developed to look at inflammation from the various vantage points outlined above. For example, panels to look at inflammatory markers directly impacting cardiac events have been developed. Panels to look at the cause and effects of Chronic Inflammatory Response Syndrome (CIRS) triggered by Lyme, mold, and actinomyces are available. Autoimmunity panels are available, and SASP panels are also available. Transcriptomics and proteomics are proving to be very helpful in aiding our understanding of the cause of inflammation and the best ways to target it. Once the knot is unraveled, the sources can be addressed individually, and the fire put out. This approach works and goes well beyond the simplistic strategy of relying solely on measuring hsCRP and prescribing curcumin and a healthy diet.

Removing old plasma by donating plasma or by plasmapheresis can play an important role here as well. The removal of inflammatory cytokines lowers the inflammatory environment in the body and is a critical area to focus on.

If young people want to stay young, one of the best things they can do is to donate plasma on a regular basis. For older individuals, plasmapheresis—where old plasma is removed and replaced with albumin, the primary protein in the blood—has been shown to be helpful. Ongoing studies are looking at combining plasmapheresis with plasma from young adults ages eighteen to twenty-five. This appears to give an even bigger boost in reversing inflammaging.

At Gladden Longevity, we are actively involved in this research. Interestingly, it appears that based on plasma protein analysis across the decades of life, we begin the aging process at twenty-six, with spikes at thirty-five, sixty, and a massive spike between sixty-three and seventy-eight. Plan accordingly. You'll be rewarded!

There are many approaches to lowering inflammation.

1. Eat a low-inflammatory diet is a great way to begin

   - Red meat
   - Processed meats, like you would buy at a deli or in a package
   - Refined grains, including white bread, white rice, refined grain pasta, and breakfast cereals
   - High-glycemic foods, like chips, cookies, crackers, and pastries
   - Sodas and other sweetened drinks
   - Fried foods
   - Sugar in all forms
   - Vegetable and seed oils

2. Eat more anti-inflammatory foods

   - Leafy green vegetables, spinach, kale, arugula, and collard greens
   - Nuts, like almonds, pistachios, and walnuts
   - Healthy animal fats like fatty fish: salmon, trout, herring, mackerel, anchovies, and sardines
   - Healthy plant fats like avocados and olives
   - Use olive oil daily, but avoid heating it to higher temperatures or cooking with it as it can be damaged and form aldehydes, which can be cancer-producing. Note: Olive oil and avocados contain oleic acid, which activates sirtuins and enhances DNA repair and longevity.

- Low-glycemic fruit, like organic strawberries, blue-berries, cherries, and oranges

3. Get heavy metals safely out of your system with metal-free, activated charcoal, PEMF mats, and see a biological dentist to get metal fillings safely out of your teeth.
4. Red Light Rx lowers inflammation
5. Curcumin
6. GL Inflammation Shroom formula modulated NFkBeta
7. H2 modulates cellular redox (remember, inflammation cause excess oxidative stress)
8. All antioxidants at lower doses are anti-inflammatory: Vitamins A, C, E. Vitamin D is a master modulator of immune system function, strengthening healthy responses to infections and eradicating malignant cells to strengthen regulatory processes to decrease excessive inflammation. Optimal levels are critical, yet they are not enough to fully manage age-related "inflammaging."
9. SPMs derivatives of fish oil with anti-inflammatory properties
10. Sulforaphane from broccoli to up-regulate anti-inflammation and detox genes
11. Melatonin reduces inflammation and preserves hypothalamic stem cells critical to youthfulness
12. BPC 157 SQ or Oral will modulate cellular redox and lower inflammation while promoting healing
13. KPV peptide immune system modulation; helpful in autoimmunity
14. Focusing on the gut by removing foods the immune system is sensitive to; diagnosing and treating malabsorption; diagnosing and treating bacterial and yeast overgrowth; diagnosis and treating parasites; and critically healing leaky gut with peptides Oral BPC 157, Lorazatide, and KPV.

CHAPTER EIGHTEEN

Oncogenic Potential

ancer arises from many causes, which unfortunately accumulate as we age.

- External DNA damage, like radiation exposure
- Internal DNA damage, like replication errors and oxidative damage to DNA
- Metabolic abnormalities that lower energy production and enable other forms of energy production to arise that favor cancer formation
- Loss of immune system function and surveillance to identify and kill malignant cells
- Genetic predispositions BRAC1 BRAC2

The problem with cancer is that it is always diagnosed too late. How many times have you heard, "He or she was doing well but then was diagnosed with stage 3 or stage 4 cancer"? It's because routine cancer screenings are inadequate to identify malignant cells early enough to take preemptive action.

The traditional cancer markers routinely screened in the blood are:

- CA 125 is associated with ovarian cancer.
- CA 15-3 is associated with breast cancer.
- CA 19-9 is associated with monitoring for recurrence in pancreatic, hepatobiliary, or gastrointestinal malignancies.
- CEA, a high level of CEA can be a sign of certain types of cancers, including colon, rectum, prostate, ovary, lung, thyroid, or liver.
- Prostate Specific Antigen, or PSA, and %Free PSA are associated with prostate disorders, one of which is cancer. PSA is a poor marker for the detection of prostate cancer, as a normal PSA does not preclude disease, and a high PSA does not make the diagnosis of cancer. In fact, PSA can be elevated after sex, riding a bicycle, or with prostatitis. If someone has been diagnosed with prostate cancer, PSA can be used to follow regression and progression. %Free PSA is a way to add color to the PSA as a lower %Free indicates a higher probability of underlying malignant cells. Ideally, PSA is low <1, and %Free PSA is high >30.

According to the National Cancer Institute, the PSA test was used routinely in the past to screen men for prostate cancer. However, as more was learned about the limitations of the test (including relatively low specificity), medical groups began to recommend against using it for routine population screening.

Several liquid biopsy-based assays that test for multiple tumor markers to detect cancer early in people without symptoms are in development.

- PapSEEK identifies ovarian and endometrial cancer-related alterations in DNA obtained from fluids collected during a routine Pap test. In a study that included women already diagnosed with cancer, the test was able to detect some endometrial and ovarian cancers at early, more treatable stages.
- CancerSEEK is a blood test that detects DNA mutations and protein biomarkers linked to multiple types of cancer. In a large trial of women with no history of cancer that combined the blood test with whole-body PET imaging, 65 percent of the cancers that were detected were at an early stage.
- UroSEEK is a urine-based test that detects the most common alterations in 11 genes linked to bladder and upper tract urothelial cancers. In a study that included patients not yet diagnosed with bladder cancer but at high risk of the disease because of symptoms, UroSEEK identified 83 percent of those who developed bladder cancer.

The National Cancer Institute states that "although these tests are able to detect early cancers, it is not yet known whether treating those cancers would reduce deaths from these cancers." Our feeling is that early detection is critical. It is infinitely easier to deal with a problem if it's detected early.

Other Liquid Bx tests have been developed, like Grail, and despite the media hype, sensitivity and specificity are still not where we would like to see them. New tests, however, are in the pipeline and should be available very soon. Being able to diagnose the presence of malignant cells is critical, and detecting them at stage 00 gives us the opportunity to treat early and potentially avoid clinical cancer development.

Imaging with an MRI is of some use, but with a resolution of 1–2 mm, MRI is inadequate to identify early preclinical malignancy, and some people can be falsely reassured that they are "fine," when in fact, they have early cancer that could not be detected because the resolution of the images. Think about trying to see fine details on the moon when the image is slightly out of focus. You can see why with MRI, things are missed, and conversely, things are suggested that are not there.

Full-body MRIs are not diagnostic for prostate cancer. A prostate-specific MRI is required to see the prostate adequately. The results are reported on a PI-RADS scale of one to five, indicating the probability of cancer.

Pooled results from a number of prostate-specific MRI studies indicate the chances of having prostate cancer are as follows:

- 2 percent for PI-RADS 1
- 4 percent for PI-RADS 2
- 20 percent for PI-RADS 3
- 52 percent for PI-RADS 4
- 89 percent for PI-RADS 5

There are also exosome tests for prostate cancer detection. An exosome is information sent from one cell to another. Think of it as a letter; it has information in the form of RNA, DNA, protein, or lipids wrapped in an envelope of a cellular membrane with a characteristic signature.

The information is sent to inform and instruct other cells. Cancer cells release exosomes, and these can be detected and result in a probability score for the presence of clinically identifiable cancer.

In addition, newer tests are being developed to identify transcriptomics, i.e., mRNA, proteomics, i.e., proteins, and exosomes in the blood to identify and characterize malignant cells sooner.

Circulating tumor stem cells can also be identified through several companies and, in many cases, give the tissue of origin for the tumor. This is not a perfect technology, but we have found it to be very, very good in most situations. That being the case, using several tests to detect malignant cells early is the strategy we have adopted. We have used this approach to identify malignancies at stage zero, i.e., at a preclinical stage, many times.

Identifying malignancy early creates a world of treatment options outside the dreaded "Bermuda Triangle" of surgery, chemo, and radiation. It is beyond the scope of this book to discuss all the things we have at our disposal, but there is a world of diagnostic treatments available that we are happy to discuss and apply in individual cases. In addition, there are exciting new tests that hold the promise of higher near-perfect sensitivity and specificity being developed to bring real hope in the battle of early detection of cancer.

It is important to note that balancing mTOR and AMPK is critical to reducing the risk of cancer. To this end, Gladden Longevity is involved in a trial utilizing rapamycin and other interventions to see if, by using this strategy, we can decrease cancer risk.

Measurement and Optimization

Our approach begins with a family and personal history, along with full genome sequencing to see if there is a genetic predisposition for cancer, and, if so, what type or types. We look at traditional cancer markers and screen for circulating tumor stem cells. Based on the findings, we prescribe imaging and go down specialized custom pathways for each client and, if needed, preemptively treat as precisely as possible in collaboration with other oncology practitioners.

The key is to be preemptive in the prevention and diagnosis and bring therapy within an ecosystem of support and intervention that leaves no stone unturned. Numerous advances, such as immunotherapy and cancer vaccines, are beginning to appear. Gladden Longevity is currently working with a company Neo7 Bioscience, which has developed advanced transcriptomic and proteomic testing to characterize cancer in patients already known to have it. In addition, they can identify circulating tumor cells or use cells from a biopsy and understand the pathways the tumor is using to proliferate. They then create custom peptides to modulate or shut down cancer gene expression. Using this technology, they are reporting 75 percent remission rates in patients who have failed everything else.

Keep in mind cancer is the ultimate survivor and finds ways to mutate around most interventions. It is important to understand that if you have a type of cancer, you have a thousand cancers—in the sense that all cancers are a mosaic of cell types, and a single strategy will almost never be enough.

A strategy to decrease cancer risk should be:

- Know your genetics
- Daily exercise

- Eat an anti-inflammatory, plant-based diet, but not necessarily vegan or vegetarian
- Cut alcohol consumption
- Use a sauna four or more days a week for twenty minutes at 170 degrees Fahrenheit or hotter
- Maintain an ideal body weight
- Boost your immune system with peptides like thymulin and thymosin alpha 1
- Consider starting an intermittent Rapamycin protocol in conjunction with appropriate supporting supplements and peptides to modulate AMPK activation and inhibit mTOR.

CHAPTER NINETEEN

Epigenetic Ages: Urine, Intrinsic, Extrinsic, Rate of Aging, and More

We tend to think of DNA as a blueprint, but it's not—it's a set of adaptable instructions that can respond to its environment. So the environment, defined as the epigenetic environment, that the DNA resides in goes a long way towards determining what DNA expression will be.

This is why lifestyle is so important. Good or bad, healthy or unhealthy, our lifestyle creates an epigenetic environment in which our DNA is reacting and is subsequently expressed. In some cases, living a healthy lifestyle creates an environment where cancer cells are shut down, vascular health is improved, and DNA replication and repair are improved—all without us even feeling these things are taking place. Likewise, when the effects of an unhealthy lifestyle and bad habits wreak havoc on our DNA expression, we don't feel it until we are diagnosed with something.

Lifestyle will always be a part of the longevity equation, period.

A few terms that will enrich our discussion on epigenetic ages:

- *Double-stranded DNA* is Chromatin made up of double-stranded DNA intertwined with functional histone proteins and structural components called *lamina*.
- *Methyl Groups:* The molecule CH3, attached or unattached to the DNA at the location of specific genes to upregulate or downregulate that gene's expression.
- *Acetyl Groups:* COCH3 are attached to Histone proteins that are interlaced with the DNA. The addition of an acetyl group typically upregulates a specific gene's expression.

Our DNA age, one of our biological ages, is measured by analyzing the DNA's methylation patterns. These methylation patterns are dictated by both internal and external factors. Interestingly, methylation patterns are also inherited, like genes.

These patterns can carry stress responses dating back several generations. Yes, you carry not only your great-grandparents' genes but their traumas and successes, too. Things in our life—like childhood trauma, worry, stress, smoking, excessive alcohol consumption, depression, to name a few—all create the internal environment that impacts our DNA methylation patterns and, ultimately, how genes are expressed.

Likewise, exercise, meditation, loving, nurturing relationships, great sleep, sunshine, and healthy, nutrient-dense food all lead to youthful DNA methylation patterns. It should be noted that histone acetylation levels are negatively correlated with age, meaning the more acetyl groups added to the histone proteins, the older our DNA is.

As we age, the methylation pattern of more or fewer methyl groups takes on a characteristic pattern correlating with an older pattern of DNA expression, making an impact on many bodily functions. The methylation pattern starts to create a clock that was initially focused on predicting chronological age. These clocks have been shown to correlate with chronological age across all mammalian species—dogs, cats, horses, primates, and humans.

Dr. Steve Horvath, currently at UCLA, is credited with this work. Following his work on predicting chronological age, he began to work on using the clocks to determine when someone might die. This clock was named after the Grim Reaper and was named the Grim Age. Dr. Horvath's work is complex but boils down to the direct correlation between DNA methylation patterns, our chronological age, and our biological age.

Epigenetic DNA methylation patterns can also be correlated to other parameters of aging, such as the heart's VO2 max (maximin blood pumping ability) or the level of the brain's neuroinflammation. Using "omics"—transcriptomics, proteomics, and metabolomics—as the gold standard for understanding aging, the "omics" have been identified that correlate with "omics" methylation patterns. This theoretically allows one to look at the DNA methylation patterns and infer what the "omics" would be without directly having to directly measure the "omics."

As of this writing, these test reports are on the verge of being available, and we will be more than curious to see how they stack up. We know in other areas that there has been no substitute for direct measurement, but we shall see. Epigenetic age is a very useful tool when looking at biological age, but I hope you are seeing that it's not the only biological age that matters—we are all a *mosaic* of ages.

While the epigenetic clock is good—a better clock than the telomere at predicting chronological age—the telomere clock is still important, as is the mitochondrial clock, the age of your heart and blood vessels, and so on. In short, it is important not to hang your hat just on one measure of your age. Looking at it through a risk lens, we are only as young as our oldest age.

We have also seen that when a client has cancer that the epigenetic age goes up rather dramatically. Epigenetic clocks are now also reporting on cell division activity to give us another clue as to whether malignant cells are present or not.

Epigenetic age is a hallmark of aging. In some respects, it reveals the cumulative effects of the aging process. It's possible to have a DNA methylation age that is much younger than your chronological age. If you take a DNA methylation test and the results are "younger" than your biological age, you likely look younger. That's because your rate of aging is slower than others who share your biological age. It turns out that the rate of aging (DunedinPACE) is very important in understanding when you are likely to die. In fact, it's as predictive as the Grim Age, possibly even more precise.

A paper published in July 2023 by David Sinclair's Group at Harvard, demonstrated a technique to reprogram cells to a younger age with a cocktail of drugs and supplements. Utilizing NCC as a means to identify senescent cells and a transcriptomic clock to measure cellular age they demonstrated that in a matter of days old skin fibroblasts could be reprogrammed to a youthful transcriptomic age without loss of cell identity, integrity and without causing tumor formation.

This study is a milestone stone built on the epigenetic theory of aging. The epigenetic theory of aging postulates that there is a backup of epigenetic information in the cell that when accessed can reboot a cell and make it young again. Sinclair's group had previously shown that using gene reprogramming Yamanaka factors OCT4, SOX2, and KLF4 (OSK), it was possible to reprogram the genome to express itself in a youthful manner, decreasing the cell's DNA methylation age, restoring youthful DNA methylation patterns, transcript profiles, and tissue function, all while maintaining cellular identity.

What is exciting about this particular study is that this deep level of reprogramming was accomplished without direct genetic reprogramming but with a relatively simple cocktail of chemical factors. The implications are that by using a simpler less expensive technology, we may be able to reprogram cells and avoid the risk of tumor formation which can occur with exposure to Yamanaka factors. Translating the use of this cocktail to animals will be the next step.

When it comes to DNA Methylation another important paper published in 2022 gave us more insight into what epigenetic age can tell us and what it can't tell us. The paper demonstrated that epigenetic age is distinct from cellular senescence, telomere attrition, and genomic instability, meaning that when these hallmarks are addressed the DNA methylation age will not be impacted. This suggests to me that DNA methylation age is not the be-all and end-all in defining where someone is in the aging process.

Interventions that impact nutrient sensing, mitochondrial activity, and stem cell composition however are represented in the DNA methylation age and therefore can be a more reliable measure of progress being made relative to those hallmarks.

CHAPTER TWENTY

DNA Methylation and Grim Age

M ethyl groups are one-carbon and three-hydrogen atoms clustered together that can be added or subtracted to a section of DNA to upregulate or downregulate that section's expression. The DNA Methylation clocks developed by Steve Horvath, Ph.D., found that DNA methylation patterns could predict the chronological age of the individual. Subsequently, a new question arose: Can we describe an individual's biological age using these DNA methylation patterns? The answer is yes. Grim Age was the original attempt by Dr. Steve Horvath to understand and predict when an individual might die based on these DNA methylation patterns.

In addition, Dr. Horvath took into account eleven other blood-based markers, along with smoking, and added them to the algorithm. In a retrospective analysis, it turned out to be a fairly accurate predictor of when someone is likely to die; hence, the reference to the age at which the Grim Reaper might appear. Age or Grim Age stuck as a name. Subsequently, the eleven markers were reduced to seven:

- **Adrenomedullin:** A fifty-two AA peptide with several functions, including vasodilation, regulation of hormone secretion, promotion of angiogenesis, and antimicrobial activity.
- **Beta-2 microglobulin (Beta2M):** A biomarker of chronic kidney disease and end-stage renal disease as well as Cancer, Lymphoma, Myeloma, and Leukemia.
- **Cystatin C:** A muscle mass-independent marker of kidney function. A decrease in kidney function is associated with a shorter life expectancy.
- **Growth Differentiation Factor 15 (GDF-15):** GDF15 is a stress-response cytokine induced by injury and inflammation. It has a strong association with many diseases, including inflammation, cancer, cardiovascular diseases, and obesity, and potentially serves as a reliable predictor of disease progression and risk of mortality. A functional role for GDF15 has been suggested in cancer, cardiovascular disease, kidney disease, and metabolic disease.
- **Leptin:** A fat and small intestine enterocyte hormone, leptin is a hormone predominantly made by adipose fat cells as well as enterocytes in the small intestine. It helps regulates energy balance

by inhibiting hunger, which in turn diminishes fat storage in adipocytes.

- **Plasminogen Activation Inhibitor 1 (PAI-1):** Stops fibrinolysis or blood clot dissolving. Elevated plasma PAI-1 levels have been indicated as a strong risk factor for stroke in old age. PAI-1 functions as the principal inhibitor of tissue plasminogen activator (tPA) and urokinase (uPA), the activators of fibrinolysis or clot dissolution.

- **Tissue Inhibitor Metalloproteinase 1 (TIMP-1):** 1) Plays a vital role in carcinogenesis, and 2) Patients with median TIMP-1 levels >37.6 ng/ml have an increased incidence of major adverse cardiac events. Matrix metalloproteinases (MMPs) are a family of zinc-dependent enzymes that includes 25 current members. MMPs degrade the structural components of the extracellular matrix and are bioactive molecules, including cytokines, chemokines, and growth factors. MMP activity is tightly controlled by the endogenous tissue inhibitors of metalloproteinases (TIMPs) comprising four homologous members (TIMP-1, TIMP-2, TIMP-3, and TIMP-4). The dynamic balance between MMPs and TIMPs controls extracellular matrix turnover and maintains tissue homeostasis. Alterations in the balance between MMPs and TIMPs are implicated in the pathogenesis of cardiovascular disease.

- **Smoking Pack-Years (PACKYRS):** This is a major risk for mortality. Higher numbers of pack years at baseline were associated with an increased risk of all-cause, CVD, COPD, any cancer, lung, colorectal, and prostate cancer mortality.

Measurement and Optimization

A DNA Methylation test is now being used in place of Grim Age called DunedinPACE, named after a New Zealand town where the data was longitudinally collected. It was developed using a cohort of persons born in 1972 and 1973 to identify their rate of aging.

Using this information, we can see the rate at which someone is aging. It turns out the rate of aging is as predictive as the Grim Age's predictions regarding how long we are likely to live.

Lifestyle choices play a huge role in our rate of aging, but there are also genetic factors at play. The bottom line is that you want to know this age—not because it is the final word on aging, as we are a mosaic of ages—because it is modifiable and provides excellent feedback on how well your interventions are working. As of this writing, TruAge is a company that utilizes DunedinPACE testing. What is even reported to be many times more precise, however, at predicting life span than DunedinPace is the "omics" clocks being developed by TruAge. We will be curious to see these as they will be available shortly.

If my epigenetic age was tested and the results determined that I was five years younger than my chronological age, and from that, I believed that I was "good for my age" and "aging well," that would be a naive conclusion. We are only as young as our oldest age. Unless you know the full mosaic of your ages, you don't really know where you stand with regard to aging. The idea that one test result is all you need does everyone a disservice, yet it's quite prevalent in the anti-aging and longevity communities. Failure to fully characterize what's going on is why we have so many physically healthy people drop dead from a "mysterious" or "surprising" disorder while others who have been diagnosed with chronic illness live well into their eighties or nineties.

Some feel that DNA methylation may be a go-to test that can help estimate many different biological ages, not just DNA methylation age. We work closely with TruAge. They also have an algorithm for estimating telomere lengths, though we have found that there is no substitute for direct measurement of telomere lengths to characterize them accurately.

We are also currently involved in research looking at whether epigenetics can predict someone's VO2 max is (cardiovascular health and the heart's blood-pumping capacity), body composition, blood sugar, and so forth.

You can also measure DNA methylation as it relates to different bodily fluids, namely, blood and urine. Gladden Longevity measures DNA methylation age in the urine. If we see that the DNA methylation pattern in the cells coming through the bladder and the urethra has an elevated age, we have seen it correlate with bladder cancer.

In many cases, lifestyle changes have a significant impact on making us young again, but despite having the best lifestyle, we still age, and so more is needed to keep us thirty as we chronologically approach age 100.

The lifestyle intervention with the greatest effect on the DNA methylation DunedinPace test is calorie restriction—chronic calorie restriction of 11 percent. We will be curious to see if intermittent fasting will have a great or a greater effect on the soon-to-be-released "omics" clocks. In addition to calorie restriction to gain a bit of control over our mTOR activation and its acceleration of aging, we use rapamycin intermittently to suppress it. This is a drug more commonly used to prevent organ transplant rejection, and there is a lot of animal data that shows that it can improve lifespan and health without causing immunosuppression when used on an intermittent basis.

Note that a new supplement Mimio containing PEA OEA Spermidine and Niacin has been developed from research done to identify the key molecules that confer the benefits of fasting and caloric restriction. While there is no long-term data use of the supplement seems to provide the benefits of fasting without having to fast. The OEA interfaces with the endocannabinoid system and decreases appetite. Escalating doses also increase reverse cholesterol transport after a meal which may have major implications for preventing cardiovascular disease as we now understand that it is the ability to transport cholesterol out of plaque and cell membranes that is most protective against cardiovascular events. This will be discussed in more detail in the Health section looking at optimizing the cardiovascular system. Spermidine is up-regulating autophagy, which is turning out to be a major player in enhancing longevity.

Gladden Longevity is beginning a new IRB-approved trial that includes DNA methylation as a marker of aging. Genesis Longevity Bioscience (GLB), the partnership between Gladden Longevity and NEO7 Bioscience, is dedicated to unraveling the knot of transcriptomics and proteomics as they relate to the drivers of aging. Beginning with eight drivers of aging, what we are seeing so far is fascinating. We see that people are not only aging at different rates but by different primary mechanisms. This is groundbreaking work!

The areas we are focusing on first are

1. Longevity,
2. Telomere maintenance,
3. Oncogenic Potential,

4. Inflammation and oxidative stress,
5. Mitochondrial function and Mitophagy,
6. Senescence and SASP,
7. Autophagy, and
8. DNA Repair

For the first time, we are seeing behind the curtain that is behind the curtain. Armed with this information, we are developing strategies utilizing client-specific custom-designed peptides to massage and modulate the ecosystem of genetic expression into a more balanced and youthful state. Remember, biology is an economy of balance. It does not respond well to being pushed into extreme states of no inflammation or hyper-elongation of telomeres. This is truly playing the symphony of longevity at the next level. Stay Tuned!

CHAPTER TWENTY-ONE

Deregulated Nutrient Sensing

Deregulated Nutrient Sensing is one of the Hallmarks of Aging that directly affects epigenetic age and is easily approachable. The nutrient-sensing system is vital for both growth and longevity. When nutrients are plentiful, the body goes into growth mode. Being in growth mode all the time, when nutrients are available all the time, is associated with a shorter life and more cancer. When nutrients are not plentiful, however, the body moves away from growth mode into recycle, restore, and conserve mode. Being in this conservation mode all the time leads to longer life and less cancer, but more frailty.

Part of the symphony of longevity is cycling into and out of these phases in a rhythmic way. Doing so in an optimal fashion significantly contributes to allowing us to stay strong and live long.

When playing this symphony of longevity, cycling through growth mode (mTOR activation), and restore mode (AMPK activation), can help do the following:

- boost the immune system by regulating the balance of nutrients and energy in the body. This helps reduce inflammation and fights off infections and diseases;
- improves cognitive performance by increasing blood flow to the brain and providing energy for neurons to function;
- enhances metabolic processes and helps the body break down and process food more efficiently, optimizing digestion and nutrient absorption;
- lower blood sugar levels and reduce the risk of developing diabetes;
- reduce the risk of cardiovascular disease by improving cholesterol and triglyceride levels;
- boost weight loss and maintenance by regulating the body's energy balance and improving its ability to burn fat and build muscle; and
- increase lifespan by optimizing cellular health, reducing oxidative stress, and improving mitochondrial function.

The nutrient-sensing system is composed of things you are likely familiar with, but you may not be aware of their roles in mTOR and AMPK activation.

mTOR activation is initiated by:

- Growth Hormone, and its primary effector, IGF1, is responsive to amino acids.
- Insulin release in response to sugar consumption and glucose levels.

- Testosterone and its metabolites, like Dihydrotes-tosterone, and their anabolic effects.
- DHEA with its anabolic effects.

AMPK Activation and its downstream effects on longevity are initiated by:

- The AMP/ATP ratio with low-energy levels, i.e., more AMP less ATP activates AMPK.
- The NAD/NADH ratio, more NAD activates AMPK.
- Metformin and Berberine decrease ATP production, leading to more AMP and hence AMPK activation.

When mTOR is activated, it tends to down-regulate things like autophagy and FOXO gene expression, both very important in the activation of our longevity genetics. So when you're activating mTOR, you are growing and building but also decreasing the activation of longevity genetics, and if it is out of balance, it is a big deal. That's why I put such emphasis on the symphonic and rhythmic timing of mTOR and AMPK activation. When it comes to cracking the code on aging, we need both mTOR and AMPK activation, but at different times and for different reasons. We need mTOR for bone density, muscle mass, and healthy connective tissue, but without AMPK, our immune systems weaken, telomeres shorten, autophagy is not turned on, and DNA repair is not performed. We will ultimately be less healthy and die sooner without AMPK. We need intermittent AMPK activation to "build" longevity.

Think of it this way—why build all those beautiful bones and muscles just to keel over? Likewise, what good is a long life without the benefit of those beautiful bones and muscles?

Some people make the mistake of finding something that they think is good—in this case, longevity—and then wanting to do more of it. I don't think there is any better example than ketosis. While it's true that being ketotic can be very helpful, people without a specific medical indication, like cancer, seizures, or neurodegeneration, are mistakenly trying to be ketotic *all the time* or the vast majority of the time. Biology does not like to be pushed into a corner.

Here's another way of looking at it. Money is an economy of scarcity; there is never enough, and when there is, we fear losing it. Love is the true abundance economy; the more love you give away, the more you have. Biology, however, is an economy of balance. When you try to push your biology into one state or another and hold it there, the body will find a way to work its way back to equilibrium, or if it can't, it will simply break down and not function optimally.

Our bodies love cycling between states and experiencing moderate amounts of stress—good stress, hormetic stress.

- Being fed followed by fasting, exercising followed by recovery.
- Being hot followed by being comfortable.
- Being cold followed by being comfortable.
- Stimulating growth hormone release and testosterone release and letting them fall or blocking their mTOR activation with Rapamycin.

The magic is in the symphonic cycling, not in any given sustained state.

One of the reasons that we encourage our clients to avoid lots of sugar in their diet is because it does boost insulin levels. Insulin is a driver of cellular senescence. A more plant-based diet encourages a slow release of insulin.

Several eating plans out there encourage high-protein consumption, it's important to understand that middle-aged people on high-protein diets die sooner. Older individuals need protein, but the most efficient way to build protein is not eating tons of protein but consuming amino acids in the right ratios. In Chapter Fourteen, I mentioned BodyHealth's Perfect Amino. This product is designed to build new proteins and collagen. Everyone out there trying to consume large amounts of protein to build muscle is *not* doing themselves any favors. This can be particularly true for carnivore diets.

I want to take a relevant detour to explain how mTOR and AMPK factor into epigenetics. We will explore these in greater detail in the next section, but both play a role in ultimately how our messenger RNA molecules are expressed.

The sum total of the expressed messenger RNA molecules transcribed from our DNA at any given time is known as the transcriptome. mTOR and AMPK are protein complexes that mediate their effects under certain circumstances. An abundance of amino acids activates mTOR—typically through a high-protein diet. When mTOR is activated, it results in cell growth and cell division—anabolic activity, building muscle and bone. Testosterone, growth hormone, and insulin are anabolic hormones that activate mTOR when we are in a fed state, i.e., we have plenty of amino acids around. Weight training and HIIT (High-Intensity Interval Training) increase growth hormone release and activate mTOR. We need mTOR to be activated for proper muscle mass, bone density, brain function, heart function, and so on. Many even consider muscle mass a currency of aging and to some degree it is, but using muscle as the metric of how well you are aging is short-sighted.

One might conclude that mTOR should always be activated—wouldn't that be optimal? Bodybuilders think so. Humans (or other mammals), however, will die sooner and have a higher incidence of cancer if mTOR is activated all the time. So we know that mTOR is important, but we know that we want just the right amount of it. Cycling mTOR on and off in conjunction with alternatively cycling AMPK on and off is one of the key rhythm lines in the symphony of longevity.

AMPK is activated when cells are depleted of ATP. This occurs during protracted endurance exercise, fasting, and calorie restrictions. You may recall that AMPK is also activated by saunas, as are heat-shock proteins. (*Yea, saunas!*) AMPK activation unlocks all of our longevity genetics, and heat-shock proteins help proteins fold or re-fold properly. When an organism is stressed by lack of water, food, or exercise, as long as it is getting adequate sleep and enough nutrients not to starve to death, these hormetic stressors activate AMPK and make the organism much stronger, i.e., robust and resilient, and they turn back our epigenetic age. AMPK activation will also re-lengthen telomeres. The body will recycle old proteins and cellular components via autophagy that otherwise may be hanging around and disrupting optimal cell function.

Like mTOR, however, we don't want our AMPK to stay activated all the time. The goal is a balance between the two. Think of mTOR and AMPK as a teeter-totter, as they have an inverse relationship—when one goes up, the other comes down, and vice-versa. When we modulate mTOR and AMPK, we can make our epigenetic age younger. A paper by K. Raj was published demonstrating that the use of Rapamycin to modulate mTOR and AMPK had a significant impact on epigenetic age. This is very exciting.

Measurement and Optimization

Our hormone levels can easily be measured in blood and saliva. Hormone metabolite levels are easily measured in urine. IGF-1 is easily measured in the blood. It is important to test to get the proper baselines. It's also important to cycle strategies and measure. My regimen is more elaborate than this, but I'll give you a simplified example to give you a feel for how I cycle things. I focus on using testosterone twice a week and GH-releasing peptides the night after I inject testosterone and the following evening.

So let's say I inject testosterone on Monday; I will inject CJC/Ipamorelin Monday night to boost growth hormone releases and activate mTOR. Tuesday, I'll take BioPro+™ to boost IGF-1 and consume its trophic growth factors. I'll do strength training with blood-flow restriction, utilizing Vasper™ or B Strong® Bands, followed by using Perfect Amino. Tuesday night, I'll inject CJC/Ipamorelin to boost growth hormone release again. On Wednesday, I'll take BioPro+™ and do a cardio workout to build endurance, followed by Perfect Amino. Wednesday and Thursday nights, I don't use CJC/Ipamorelin and will take Spermidine. I avoid BioPro+™ Thursday and Friday. I'll do more cardio, like surfing, mountain biking, or an Elliptigo ride followed by a sauna and cold plunge on Thursday and Friday. Finally, I'll inject testosterone again on Friday evening, then restart the cycle.

After two weeks of this, I take 10mg of rapamycin on Sunday. On Monday and Friday of the following week, I'll use testosterone but not CJC/Ipamorelin or take BioPro+™. That week, I will focus more on fasting, saunas, Spermidine, AMPK-activating supplements like resveratrol, and peptides to activate AMPK. After a week to ten days of this, I go back to cycling between being more anabolic and alternating with being more catabolic. I'll describe this in more detail at the end of the book, but to give you an idea, there is a daily, weekly, and monthly rhythm being played.

Sometimes, I take rapamycin every other week and modify the cycle accordingly. I use transcriptomics and proteomics, DNA methylation testing, as well as other lab and performance tests like mitochondrial function assessments, VO2 max testing, and glucose monitoring along with wearable data for sleep, HRV, and recovery, to coach me on how I'm doing and where to adjust. This regimen works well for me, enables me to cycle between states, and gives my body a series of hormetic stressors.

The above is for illustration purposes as, again, my regimen is more involved, and I've left many pieces out but will put them in tabular form at the end of the book. I hope this gives you the basic rhythms of the symphony as it relates to this one Hallmark of Nutrient Sensing and mTOR and AMPK modulation.

CHAPTER TWENTY-TWO

NAD/NADH

N icotinamide adenine dinucleotide (NAD) is important for energy production in the mitochondria, immune-cell function, neurotransmitter health, and sirtuin activation. Sirtuins enable DNA repair, control of inflammation, metabolic control, cell survival, circadian rhythm, and healthy cell death. NAD also impacts epigenetic modifications, although it and the use of its precursors have not been shown to impact epigenetic age directly.

As we age, senescent cells, immune cells, and other sources secrete a protein called CD38, which has the ability to avidly utilize nicotinamide adenine dinucleotide (NAD), lowering the available NAD for other critical anti-aging activities, like DNA repair. Increasing levels of CD38 is part of an interwoven feedback loop of drivers working together to accelerate the aging process. It is part of the reason that older people don't seem to have any energy. It contributes to the exponential process of aging.

The ratio of NAD to nicotinamide adenine dinucleotide with hydrogen (NADH) is critical for energy production, DNA repair, sirtuin activation, immune-cell function, and neurotransmitter health. Being able to boost NAD through precursors, like nicotinamide mononucleotide (NMN), nicotinamide riboside, and niacin is beneficial, but being able to make an impact on the entire biochemical pathway by which NAD is made and recycled is even better. In addition, decreasing the activity of CD38 with apigenin, which comes from parsley or with Cyanidin-3-O-glucoside (C3G), is also important. Nuchido Time+ is a food supplement that provides NAD precursors, NAD salvage pathway enzyme enhancers, and apigenin.

Measurement and Optimization

Directly measuring NAD is very difficult to do. Until recently, you had to have a mass spectrometer in the room next door from where you're drawing the blood in order to capture it. Dr. Jin-Xiong She, formerly at the University of Georgia, has developed a technology he believes can measure the composite of NAD and NADH. He also developed a product to raise NAD levels. As of this writing, we are in the process of testing it. This is exciting because if we can decrease the degradation of NAD by blocking CD38 *and* augment its production using a product like Nuchido Time. We know that when combined with other interventions, like exercise, fasting, calorie restriction, and mitigating mTOR, it gives us a better chance to activate sirtuins, which will then help to keep us young. NADMED in Finland has also developed a NAD test, which may be even better. We are currently testing it. Remember, we are only married to the questions, not our current answers.

Dr. David Sinclair has done a tremendous amount of work in the NAD space in conjunction with sirtuins. Sirtuin activation requires NAD as a cofactor. Sirtuins are signaling proteins that help regulate metabolism, DNA repair, and telomere maintenance. Sinclair and his research group have been able to reverse aging in mice using NAD to boost sirtuin levels. His regimen includes a combination of metformin and Beta NMN as a primary anti-aging strategy. NMN may soon no longer be available as a supplement, based on a patent and an FDA submission by Sinclair.

In the meantime, the company Nuchido Time™ may emerge as the best, if not better, alternative.

Our current strategy is to use C3G in conjunction with Nuchido Time.

SALVAGE PATHWAY

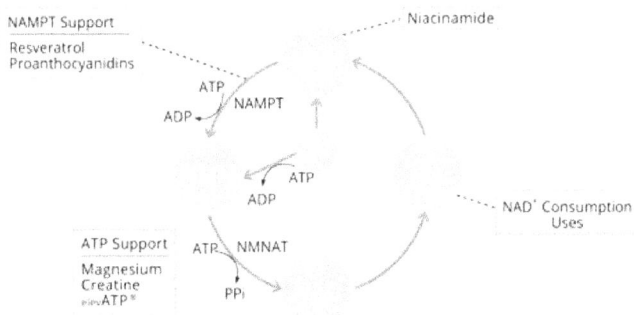

NAMPT Support
Resveratrol
Proanthocyanidins

Niacinamide

ATP
NAMPT
ADP

ATP
ADP

NAD⁺ Consumption
Uses

ATP Support
Magnesium
Creatine
pqqATP®

ATR NMNAT

PPi

NEUROHACKER
COLLECTIVE

Nuchido Time ingredients

- Nicatinamide + Apigenin + quercetin, rutin, and troxerutin for NAMP Salvage Pathway activation
- ALA to Activate AMPK & Increase the conversion of NADH to NAD
- EGCG for inhibition of NNMT. NNMT blockade enables more efficient NAD Recycling
- Vit C, Zinc for immunity, + Piperine for absorption and thermogenesis and fat cell destruction

NAD+ cannot be obtained from our diet. It must be made within our cells.

Nicotinamide (a form of niacin) is one of the raw materials that the body uses to make NAD+. It is sometimes referred to as an "NAD+ precursor".

CHAPTER TWENTY-THREE

Stem Cell Exhaustion

Stem cells and progenitor cells are cells that are held in reserve to repair the worn-out cells in the body. Having a supply of these is critical and there is a limit to how many we have. When the supply is exhausted, we are no longer able to repair damage and our demise is close at hand.

It is important to note that there are stem cells, and then there are stem cells. What I mean is that stem cells with true pluripotency, the ability to become any other cell type, are limited to embryonic stem cells, induced stem pluripotent stem cells, or very small embryonic-like stem cells. All other stem cells, such as mesenchymal or hematopoietic stem cells—found in fat or bone marrow, respectively—can only become a few types of differentiated cells. Progenitor cells are stem cells specific to one tissue.

Stem cells have telomerase turned on, which keeps their telomeres long and keeps them young. According to a joint article written by researchers at Harvard University, Joslin Diabetes Center, Massachusetts General Hospital, and Howard Hughes Medical Institute: "Depletion of the stem cell pool with age may occur because these cells lose self-renewal activity and terminally differentiate, thereby exiting the stem cell pool, or because they undergo apoptosis, meaning cell death or senescence induced by exposure to cellular stress, although it is not exactly clear what mechanisms inform the choice."

When stem cells are exhausted, we can no longer repair and rejuvenate ourselves. Although stem cells have their own telomerase to stay young, over time, they still become depleted due to oxidative stress and external factors like toxins and radiation. We are currently exploring whether telomerase keeps stem cells young. If it does, it could play a key role in allowing our stem cell population to last potentially years and decades beyond what they are currently able to do.

For many years, stem cells from cord blood could be harvested at birth and stored in the event that their host needed them later in life. Dr. Anthony Atala has identified placental stem cells that are also pluripotent and have no tumorigenicity like embryonic and induced pluripotent stem cells do. Dr. Movlia from Argentina is also doing fascinating work harvesting white blood cells and exposing them to a particular tissue like the neurons in the spinal cord. The white cells are then used to program mesenchymal stems harvested from fat to instruct the stem cells on what tissue to repair. Using this approach, significant strides are being made in the ability of mesenchymal stem cells to heal injuries like spinal cord injuries which previously were not able to be healed.

Dr. Todd Ovokaitys has found a way to liberate very small embryonic-like stem cells, known as VSELs, living in our blood in hibernation. VSELs are attached to a protein ligand that keeps them inactive. Since they are hibernating, they're not dividing and not aging.

Dr. Ovokaitys has also developed a highly patented, low-energy red light laser that can liberate those very small, embryonic-like stem cells from the protein holding them in hibernation. The VSELs reside in the platelet-rich plasma fraction of the blood known as PRP. The laser focuses on the stem cells located in the PRP to liberate them.

According to Dr. Todd Ovokaitys, these very small, embryonic-like stem cells contain some unique properties that enable them to heal any cell in the body, making them unique, especially when combined with signaling peptides like BPC157.

This is where the stem cells harvested at birth—through cord blood, placenta, and so on—differ from the stem cells Dr. Ovokaitys discovered. The former has never been able to become another tissue. Instead, they orchestrate healing. In the case of VSELs, they can become any tissue in the body. So is capturing the cord blood at birth still necessary? I would not discourage anyone from this practice as a means to protect their children, but we cannot ignore the magnitude of Dr. Ovokaitys's work.

In addition, the same laser can be focused on the body part needing rejuvenation and activate adhesion molecules, which attract the VSELs to go directly to where they are needed. The VSELS then go to the specific body part and differentiate into those local cells, such as brain cells, heart cells, etc.

This is exciting work! At Gladden Longevity, we couple VSELs with supplements and ozone to boost NAD levels and use select peptides to enhance the effectiveness of the repair.

Measurement and Optimization

While it's important, it is also difficult to measure stem-cell levels. CD34 are bone-marrow-derived stem cells, and therefore, they can be measured in the blood. We are also collaborating with Neo7 Bioscience to measure stem-cell function with the transcriptomics and proteomics indicative of stem-cell activation.

Optimizing stem-cell use is critical. Stem cells don't work in a vacuum, and we get the best results by creating a cocktail of agents and procedures to prep the body, optimize the VSELs or mesenchymal stem cells, and then create a therapeutic environment to enhance the stem cells' function. This "stacking" of technologies makes the difference between good and great outcomes. BPC157, GHK-Cu, CJC1295/Ipamorelin, NAD Boosting technologies, and peptides specific to the target, in addition to client-specific agents and adjunct procedures, can all add a great deal.

The intentions and expectations of the recipient also play a large role in how effective the treatment is. Placing positive energy and good intentions into the process by the staff and the recipient enhances the outcomes. The power of this cooperative, positive, energetic environment cannot be overstated.

In addition, plasmapheresis is used to clear out inflammatory cytokines and other proteins that sabotage stem-cell function. Adding young plasma while doing plasmapheresis to infuse rejuvenating factors sets the stage for the injection of the stem cells and optimal stem cell rejuvenation results.

Our use of the VSELs complies with the patented processes and is done inside an IRB-approved trial.

What about PRP? PRP, or Platelet-Rich Plasma, does have factors that enhance healing. As a standalone procedure, it can be helpful. When combined with a comprehensive approach, however, it works much better.

CHAPTER TWENTY-FOUR

Senescent Cell Burden and Senescence Associated Secretory Phenotype (SASP)

W hen cells are damaged in any manner, they can become senescent. Senescent cells no longer divide and no longer contribute to the optimal function of their tissue of origin; they take up space and resist apoptosis or cell death. "Zombie Cells" is a colloquialism used to describe them.

Senescence, however, serves a number of purposes. They are part of the healing and regeneration process, and function as a self-protective mechanism by removing damaged cells with the potential for malignant transformation from circulation. Think of it this way: the body identifies that this cell will become malignant, so it intelligently shuts down its ability to divide. This places the cell in a state of senescence so it doesn't propagate, transform, and become clinical cancer.

So far, so good, but when these senescent cells accumulate and begin to secrete inflammatory cytokines, SASP, it creates a problem for the tissue where they reside, along with the rest of the body. What's not good is that these SASP cells not only pollute the environment that normal cells are trying to function in but potentiate the development of cancer. Self-protection has now turned into potential self-destruction. As we age, the burden of senescent cells increases and begins to cause dysfunction in the surrounding normal cells, leading to muscle weakness, bone loss, reduced brain function, slower healing, and so on.

Senescent cells exist not only as a Hallmark of Aging but also as a key driver of aging. In fact, they are a major player in the exponential acceleration of aging. Interestingly, while senescence and SASP are major drivers of aging, they do not directly impact epigenetic age. This indicates that DNA methylation or epigenetic age is not the be-all and end-all of describing the aging process.

Here is an analogy I like to use to explain the impact of senescent cells. Let's say you have a company with one hundred employees and twenty of them are *senescent*. What does that mean? It means they come to work and collect a paycheck but don't do any actual work—they just put their head on their desk, occupying space. Your company's productivity goes down.

But then it gets worse. When senescent cells become SASP cells and secrete inflammatory cytokines into the environment, its analogous to senescent employees becoming toxic, turning off the wifi, locking the doors, closing people's laptops, and beginning to recruit other employees to become senescent, making a severe impact on your company's productivity. When 20 percent of your senescent employees become 30, 35, or 40 percent, there is an exponential decline in the ability of the company to perform. This example is analogous to the ever-increasing impact SASP cells have on the body's health, resilience, robustness, and performance. It plays a key part in the exponential decline that occurs with aging.

Biology being an economy of balance implies that senescent cells are not uniformly bad, but they do need to be modulated for the ecosystem to remain healthy.

Imagine that when you're young, your internal biological ecosystem is pristine and in balance—analogous to having an Olympic-sized swimming pool that you swim in, train in, and set new personal records in, so well-constructed and maintained that an Olympic swimmer could use it to set a world record. Over time, the swimming pool fills up with trash—a combination of leaves, dead animals, sticks, and so on. As the garbage accumulates, it's no longer a desirable environment to swim in, and certainly not conducive to setting world records. Even an Olympic swimmer, like a stem cell, would have a hard time functioning here.

As these senescent cells secrete inflammatory *cytokines* into our system, it is like polluting the swimming pool that all the other cells are trying to work in. One of the key strategies in making 100 the new 30 is to recognize that senescent cells are accumulating and understanding their secretory burden on the environment is critical. In other words, understanding what sort of cytokines are being released, and in what amounts.

Having an effective strategy to remove the senescent cells and their cytokines—to clean up the swimming pool—is essential. Removing toxic cytokines with plasmapheresis, modulating their production with senomophics like rapamycin, resveratrol, and metformin, and killing off a portion (but not all) of the senescent cells with senolytics like fisetin or dasatinib and quercetin appears to be key. Without an effective strategy to deal with senescent cells and their secretory products, we will never make 100 the new 30.

Measurement and Optimization

Previously, when measuring senescent-cell burden, we only had access to measuring beta-galactosidase. The challenge with beta-galactosidase is that it is not entirely specific to senescent cells, and the levels can be misleading. In conjunction with Neo7 BioScience, we have developed new transcriptomic and proteomic tests to determine the senescent cell burden and their secretory status. The transcriptomics and proteomics focused on eight Drivers of Aging are available in the LIFE RAFT Protocol.

Once we know the senescent-cell burden, we want to attack the problem from multiple angles. Understanding what leads to senescent cell formation in the first place—DNA damage, short telomeres, reduced mitochondrial function, deregulated nutrient sensing, lack of proteostasis, and so on—enables us to target these processes to maintain youthfulness instead of only treating senescent cells themselves. We've discussed the way to optimize each of these factors in other portions of this section.

There are other factors that also induce senescence, such as pathogen-associated molecular structures (PAMPs), expressed by pathogens such as bacteria and their products, and damage-associated molecular products (DAMPs), consisting of proteins or nucleic acids released by necrotic cells at the site of necrosis (tissue destruction). Mechanical stress, hypoxia, too little oxygen, and hyperoxia, too much oxygen, can also induce senescence.

Beyond preventing excessive senescent cell formation, there are also strategies that use senolytics to induce apoptosis, or cell suicide, in senescent cells. For example, dasatinib—a chemotherapy drug for treating Philadelphia chromosome-positive (Ph+) acute lymphoblastic leukemia and chronic myeloid leukemia (CML)—and quercetin, a plant flavonol, have been used in combination to decrease the senescent cell burden and shown clinical benefit in treating idiopathic pulmonary fibrosis, a lung condition characterized by an increase in senescent cells in the lung tissue. There are other senolytics available, like fisetin from strawberries and the peptide FOXO4 DRI, that can also eliminate senescent cells.

Elimination of too many senescent cells, however, is not beneficial. The body will rebound and reform senescent cells at an even faster rate, so once again, a balanced-system approach is required. The forty-thousand-foot overview of the strategy that we have implemented at Gladden Longevity is:

- Screen for cancer.
- Measure the senescent cell burden with transcriptomics and proteomics and beta galactosidase.
- Mitigate the drivers of senescence and use agents to decrease senescent cell formation, like rapamycin, and re-lengthening telomeres, optimizing DNA repair by improving the NAD/ NADH ratio.
- Activate AMPK and Sirtuins.
- Control glucose and insulin levels, which drive senescence.

- Use senolytics in appropriate doses and monitor the results.
- Clean up the swimming pool's senescent cytokines and senescent cell debris with plasmapheresis.
- When appropriate, replace old plasma with young plasma.
- Consider rejuvenation strategies with stem cells, PRP, Peptides, etc.
- Repeat the testing and monitor.
- If there is an element we are not adequately addressing, create custom peptides to address these areas in conjunction with our Neo7 BioSciemce partner.

If you're going to make progress here, it's important to clean up the secretory cytokines that have been put into the system, and plasmapheresis is the best way to do it. Plasmapheresis has been used to treat autoimmune diseases and is now being used in the anti-aging community. Depending on vein size and hydration status, the process takes two to four hours. It pulls blood from one arm and separates the plasma from the blood cells by removing the old plasma that contains those senescent-cell cytokines. Then, infuse either albumin, saline, or young plasma into the other arm.

Research shows that if this is done on a fairly regular basis, you can change the internal environment. In changing the internal environment, you can reboot endogenous stem cells across all biological tissues.

The takeaway is that we can reboot our own stem cells, increase the effectiveness of other stem cell procedures, and improve organ function when plasmapheresis is used as part of a comprehensive systems approach.

Plasmapheresis has also been used in treating neurodegenerative diseases like Alzheimer's and other types of dementia and has been shown to improve liver, kidney, and heart function. More applications are currently being tried in different experimental models.

Much of this work—demonstrating that plasmapheresis could reboot endogenous stem cells in all three tissue types—was pioneered by Drs. Irina and Michael Conboy at UC Berkeley and Dr. Dobri Kiprof, an internationally renowned pioneer and expert in therapeutic apheresis. A leader in using plasmapheresis for the last thirty years, Dr. Kiprov has published papers that show the slowing of the Alzheimer's process. This is an exciting technology, and more research is underway to see if adding young plasma to plasmapheresis will improve the results even further.

Regularly donating plasma is a great hack for rebooting your system at any age. You can typically donate twice a week. Plus, you get paid to do it! For the first month, twice a week would be ideal, and after that, once a week. You'll need a healthy, nutrient-dense diet with high-quality protein to rebuild the proteins you have lost, and you will need to replace the electrolytes, trace minerals, and nutrients you lose in your donation. The reported health benefits are lower blood pressure, lower risk of heart attack, improved energy and mood, lower cholesterol, and accelerated detox.

Note that there is a risk of low immunoglobulin levels because it takes time for the levels to replenish them. Those who donate frequently and long-term may also be at risk for anemia from incidental loss of red cells during donation.

Donating blood also boosts your health as long as you have enough iron. According to the Red Cross, you can donate blood every 56 days.

Despite all these innovations and exciting developments, I still cannot stress enough that plasmapheresis, with or without young plasma, is not enough to optimize our biology and keep us young. If you haven't stopped the formation of senescent cells and you aren't killing off senescent cells responsible for the secretory cytokines in the first place, you're not reaching your full potential. You will arrive right back at your starting point in a very short time. It takes a very comprehensive systems approach to make durable progress.

As you can see, a critical piece of the puzzle is preventing senescent cells from forming in the first place. To do that, we are studying the use of rapamycin to decrease mTOR activity in conjunction with low-carb diets—because elevated levels of insulin, glucose, IGF 1, and mTOR are all drivers for senescent-cell formation. Regarding shortened telomeres driving senescent cells, our strategy is to re-lengthen telomeres, which we will examine more closely in Part Three.

At Gladden Longevity, we are currently testing a product that appears to be more effective than any other product we've ever seen in terms of re-lengthening telomeres. If we succeed, we think we can decrease the rate at which senescent cells form cellular replication. This may be important in unraveling the knot and balancing the senescent cell population with their cytokine burden. This is incredibly exciting work in the whole area of senescence and SASP!

CHAPTER TWENTY-FIVE

Immune System Senescence

One of the reasons that many people die of cancer, pneumonia, or urinary tract infections later in life is because their immune system has become dysfunctional. In order to reboot the immune system, lowering the senescent cell burden is critical because the immune system itself will develop senescence. Cancers are so much more prevalent later in life because the immune system is failing to remove malignant cells from the body.

We're very excited about coupling the technologies of plasmapheresis and rapamycin together, where we can minimize senescence throughout the body, clean up the swimming pool from the senescent cell cytokines, and reboot the immune system simultaneously. Playing all these different instruments in the orchestra is essential to the symphony.

Your immune system contains two major compartments: the innate immune system, which carries genetically programmed immunity like natural killer cells, and the adaptive immune system, which can adapt to new threats. The adaptive immune system has many different cell types that are produced in different tissues. Examples are Thymus, or T cells from the thymus gland, and B cells, which produce antibodies from the bone marrow. T cells are divided into several populations with various roles such as T Reg cells to regulate the immune system, and T Helper cells present foreign structures to Cytotoxic T Cells, which kill foreign invaders. In addition, T Helper cells present foreign material to B cells so they can make protective antibodies. There are many control mechanisms and feedback loops to keep the immune system working well and to keep it from attacking us. Autoimmunity is when those mechanisms fail and we are attacked by the immune system. Earlier, we mentioned that telomere lengths are measured in white blood cells, and shorter telomeres are associated with immunosuppression and disease.

Interestingly enough, pushing hard on exercise acutely reduces your immune system function. So if you feel like you are coming down with something, that's not a good time to go to the gym or run and "power through." It's a good time to rest and take the things that will boost your immune system.

Running and aerobic exercise transiently suppress the immune system because they put stress on the body, and cortisol is released in response. Your immune system comes back stronger and healthier, however, as a result.

We have also observed that the immune system itself can become senescent. Several things can destroy the immune system.

- High levels of chronic stress, anxiety, depression, or any kind of mental disorder will weaken the immune system. Unlike aerobic exercise, where the immune system makes a comeback, the excess cortisol released from chronic stress dampens immune system function, therefore making us more susceptible to viral diseases (like COVID-19), bacterial infections, or cancer.
- Steroids are given to people when they have an inflamed joint or autoimmune disease with excess inflammation. Steroids also weaken the immune system response. And the same is true for us—when we run high levels of cortisol, it decreases our immune response.
- Alcohol has long been rumored to be good for the heart, and the French are often credited with longevity because of their red wine consumption. Actually, alcohol is *not* beneficial beyond perhaps one drink a day or less, and even that is suspect for many of us. Alcohol also suppresses the immune system. I remember my grandfather used honey, sugar, and brandy to treat a cold or sore throat, but we now understand that concoction probably doesn't help.
- Lack of sleep is another immune-system killer. Our immune systems need adequate, deep, restorative sleep.
- Lack of social contact also depresses the immune system, as social contact is key to lowering stress and raising oxytocin levels, the love or bonding hormone.

So when we think about measuring and optimizing our immune systems, it's important to understand how the above can lead to immuno-senescence.

Greg Fahy, Ph.D., has done important work to rejuvenate the immune system utilizing growth hormone, DHEA, and Metformin. Using serial MRI scans, this combination was demonstrated to rejuvenate the Thymus gland while slightly lowering epigenetic age.

Measurement and Optimization

At Gladden Longevity, we currently look through a variety of lenses to assess immunity. One lens is sending samples to UCLA to determine the youthfulness of the immune system. A youthful immune system has more young, "naïve" cells and a greater number of Helper T cells, cells that gather and present new information to the immune system. In comparison, there are fewer Cytotoxic T cells, resulting in a favorable T Helper to T Cytotoxic ratio. An older immune system has a higher number of differentiated cells and fewer helper cells and is, therefore, less able to adapt to new threats. Having cells that are not committed to a particular course of action—"naïve" cells—is critical because when a new virus shows up like COVID-19, for example, the cells provide the adaptability to respond swiftly. Testing tells us a lot about whether you have young cells in your immune system or how much damage has already been done.

Just because you are young does not mean your immune system is. Remember, aging is a symphony, not a few individual notes. There are teenagers with suboptimal immune levels. Unless you live in a warm climate and stay outside all the time where your body absorbs plenty of sunshine and makes Vitamin D, I strongly recommend getting your immune system tested—regardless of your chronological age.

In addition, we can also test the robustness of the immune system's response to a known mitogen. A mitogen is something that causes cells to divide. Think of it this way. You know a dog will go after a specific kind of bone. The question is how aggressively will it go after that specific bone. The mitogen is the bone; it induces a response from the immune system that can cause immune cells to divide. The dog is the immune system. By measuring the aggressiveness of the mitotic response, we can get an idea of how robust the immune system is.

We currently test 63+ ages that an individual has—ages that we all have—and that's not including chronological age. The mosaic of ages can give us a tremendous amount of information about the status of someone's brain, bones, muscles, heart, liver, kidneys, and so on.

Yet, there are still parts of the puzzle that we don't see as clearly.

We formed a joint venture—Genesis Longevity Bioscience—with Neo7 BioScience to develop testing that has traditionally been used in the cancer space. It is used to understand how the DNA of a cancer cell is being transcribed and which proteins are being manufactured. When you understand this, it's possible to develop very specific therapies that can migrate into the nucleus of the cancer cell and modulate its genetic expression to decrease malignant expression. Essentially, it hits the off switch for the cancer cell.

It is vital to understand that part of the problem with treating cancer is that cancer is not composed of one cell type—it's a mosaic of different cell types, each of which has a unique set of genes that are activated. You can think of it this way: If you are diagnosed with cancer, you have a thousand different variations of the cancer cell types comprising your particular cancer. Finding the common denominator that will kill most of these cells takes a very focused and concerted effort. It takes a broad base of interventional targets within the DNA of the cancer cells to effectively attack multiple cell types simultaneously and have a hope to wipe out the cancer.

Our new company, Genesis Longevity Bioscience, is utilizing the same processes of transcriptomics and proteomics and custom-designed targeted therapies to unravel the knot of aging and then apply targeted therapies to alter DNA expression in areas where other more conventional interventions are found to be falling short. In essence, we are creating a client-specific, custom-fit approach to address aging and youthfulness pathways that previously could not be addressed.

Old cells express DNA differently than when they are young. We are using this technology to be able to map how an individual's genome is expressed as they age. From this, we will be able to better understand where you are in the aging process, what youth looks like for you, and whether you are truly making progress when it comes to making yourself younger. This is in addition to measuring telomere lengths, epigenetic ages, mitochondrial function, levels of inflammation, etc. It helps us map the pathway between youth and age, enabling us to know what to target and accurately measure age reversal through another lens. This approach becomes an important component in playing the symphony of longevity.

What else can we do to boost our immunity?

Looping back to the Life Energy Mosaic, we see another reason to minimize and manage stress, as stress makes a massive impact on your immune system. Secondly, we see the impact social contact has on our immunity. Good relationships lower stress and raise oxytocin levels.

Oxytocin is a hormone released when a woman is breast-feeding a child. Known as the "milk let-down hormone" and "love hormone," it is triggered as the baby starts to suckle. Oxytocin is released in both the mother and baby, which enables the milk to release and feed the infant, increasing their social bond. Oxytocin also has some amazing benefits that modulate the immune system—it lengthens telomeres and decreases extraneous inflammation. In fact, children with autism are deficient in oxytocin, and a lot of their symptoms can be improved by giving them exogenous oxytocin. This enables them to have greater social bonding.

There are supplements available that can also help the immune system. Recently, I hopped on a flight to attend a conference in California and felt fine as I boarded. By the time I landed, however, I had shaking chills, fatigue, and dizziness. I wasn't sure that I would be able to attend at all. I stopped at Whole Foods en route to my hotel and bought a series of supplements: primarily echinacea, astragalus, zinc, and Vitamin C.

I took big handfuls of them and went straight to bed around six o'clock that night. When I woke up at midnight, I took another handful, then woke up again at five o'clock in the morning and took a third handful. The next morning, I was no longer feeling sick. I attended the conference feeling stronger as the day went on and was able to go for a nice run the next morning, feeling completely well.

This is the beauty of having a strong immune system. Feel a challenge, give your immunity some help, and get well quickly. Other helpful interventions are SQ injections of Thymulin or thymosin alpha 1 and oral drops of NES Health "Immune."

Reviewing the list of things that can destroy the immune system in the preceding section, it's a given that when you feel yourself coming down with something, staying away from alcohol and getting adequate sleep are a huge help. We'll talk more about sleep specifics in Part Three, but for now, understand that restorative sleep is vital for immune health, and many people do not get enough of it.

When you have senescent cells in the immune system, your immune system is dysfunctional. As we age, the population of natural-killer cells increases, but their efficacy goes down, making it easier for cancer to evade them. The UCLA testing also gives us insight into the senescent status of the immune system and the number of natural killer cells present.

By looking at immunosenescence through this lens and understanding where you are on this aging spectrum, we have found that re-lengthening telomeres can help slow and reverse immunosenescence. There are several products that can do this: TA 65, Isagenix, and TAM 818. At Gladden Longevity, we have had a great deal of success in simultaneously re-lengthening telomeres and making the immune system younger for our clients. As I mentioned in the previous section, we are developing a new product that, if early testing is any indication, will be significantly stronger and more beneficial than any product currently on the market when it comes to re-lengthening telomeres.

All that said, there is no escaping a nutrient-rich diet when trying to strengthen your immune system: especially Vitamins B, C, and D vitamins. Taking a Vitamin D supplement will significantly contribute to keeping the immune system healthy.

Final Thoughts on Longevity

For the first time, we have effective strategies to address most of the currently known Hallmarks of Aging and a number of the sub-issues related to them. We are rapidly progressing in our ability to measure and understand the biological aberrations that occur within the aging process, enabling us to therapeutically intervene with far greater precision.

In this respect, we are the luckiest generation of all time. Think about it: We can take action at key points that can significantly slow, arrest, or potentially even reverse the aging process for us, but the strategy takes a very comprehensive systems approach, one that allows us to play this symphony in a fuller, more complex and melodic way.

We will never succeed with just one technology; it takes playing the *entire* symphony. Plasmapheresis will never get you there. Just lengthening telomeres will never get you there. Optimizing your NAD levels alone will never get you there. Doing cellular reprogramming with Yamanaka factors or a cocktail of agents won't get you there either. It takes an all-encompassing defensive strategy to avoid getting sick and dying, and it takes an all-encompassing offensive strategy to go straight at the drivers of aging.

At Gladden Longevity, we continue to refine and develop great defensive and offensive strategies specifically for you and then help you to execute them with the right timing, frequency, intensity, and duration, coupled with your optimization mindset, we believe it is possible for you to Live Young for a Lifetime!

Longevity Notes

Svetlana Ukraintseva et al., "Decline in Biological Resilience as Key Manifestation of Aging: Potential Mechanisms and Role in Health and Longevity," *Mechanisms of Ageing and Development* 194 (December 16, 2021): 111418, https://doi.org/10.1016/j.mad.2020.111418.

Hanae Armitage, "'Ageotypes' Provide Window into How Individuals Age, Stanford Study Reports," Stanford Medicine News Center, January 13, 2020, https://med.stanford.edu/news/all-news/2020/01/_ageotypes_-provide-window-into-how-individuals-age--stanford-st.html.

Apratim Bajpai, Rui Li, and Weiqiang Chen, "The Cellular Mechanobiology of Aging: From Biology to Mechanics," Annals of the New York Academy of Sciences 1491, no. 1 (November 24, 2020): 3–24, https://doi.org/10.1111/nyas.14529.

Carlos López-Otín et al., "The Hallmarks of Aging," *Cell* 153, no. 6 (June 6, 2013): 1194–1217, https://doi.org/10.1016/j.cell.2013.05.039.

Tomas Schmauck-Medina et al., "New Hallmarks of Ageing: A 2022 Copenhagen Ageing Meeting Summary," *Aging* 14, no. 16 (August 29, 2022): 6829–39, https://doi.org/10.18632/aging.204248.

Daniel M. Davies et al., "Cellular Enlargement - a New Hallmark of Aging?," *Frontiers in Cell and Developmental Biology* 10 (November 10, 2022), https://doi.org/10.3389/fcell.2022.1036602.

Jae-Hyun Yang et al., "Chemically Induced Reprogramming to Reverse Cellular Aging," *Aging* 15, no. 13 (2023): 5966–89, https://doi.org/10.18632/aging.204896.

Laura Salvador et al., "A Natural Product Telomerase Activator Lengthens Telomeres in Humans: A Randomized, Double Blind, and Placebo Controlled Study," *Rejuvenation Research* 19, no. 6 (December 1, 2016): 478–84, https://doi.org/10.1089/rej.2015.1793.

Darren J. Baker et al., "Increased Expression of BUBR1 Protects against Aneuploidy and Cancer and Extends Healthy Lifespan," Nature Cell Biology 15, no. 1 (December 16, 2012): 96–102, https://doi.org/10.1038/ncb2643.

María Carolina Barbosa, Rubén Adrián Grosso, and Claudio Marcelo Fader, "Hallmarks of Aging: An Autophagic Perspective," Frontiers in Endocrinology 9 (January 9, 2019), https://doi.org/10.3389/fendo.2018.00790.

"The Inner Life of the Cell Animation," YouTube, July 11, 2011, https://www.youtube.com/watch?v=wJyUtbn0O5Y.

"What Happens to the Brain in Alzheimer's Disease?," National Institute on Aging, May 16, 2017, https://www.nia.nih.gov/health/what-happens-brain-alzheimers-disease.

Leonidas Stefanis, "α-Synuclein in Parkinson's Disease," *Cold Spring Harbor Perspectives in Medicine* 2, no. 2 (February 2012), https://doi.org/10.1101/cshperspect.a009399.

Azin Amin et al., "Amyotrophic Lateral Sclerosis and Autophagy: Dysfunction and Therapeutic Targeting," *Cells* 9, no. 11 (November 4, 2020): 2413, https://doi.org/10.3390/cells9112413.

Tanjaniina Laukkanen et al., "Association between Sauna Bathing and Fatal Cardiovascular and All-Cause Mortality Events," *JAMA Internal Medicine* 175, no. 4 (April 2015): 542, https://doi.org/10.1001/jamainternmed.2014.8187.

BodyHealth.com LLC, "Does Perfectamino Work?," BodyHealth. com LLC, accessed April 12, 2023, https://bodyhealth.com/pages/ perfectamino-customer-reviews?gc_id=9504877412&h_ga_id= 102253920412&h_ad_id=421220557906&h_keyword_id=kwd-314497497298&h_keyword=perfect+amino&h_placement=&gclid= Cj0KCQjwnrmlBhDHARIsADJ5b_nSYqE644Z4k74Axf60gE c9fvvRWTvvJIkeAH0aPG6XvnCtI5Vt83UaAr8nEALw_wcB.

Hae Young Chung et al., "Redefining Chronic Inflammation in Aging and Age-Related Diseases: Proposal of the Senoinflammation Concept," Aging and Disease 10, no. 2 (April 1, 2019): 367, https://doi. org/10.14336/ad.2018.0324.

"Prostate-Specific Antigen (PSA) Test," National Cancer Institute, March 11, 2022, https://www.cancer.gov/types/prostate/psa-fact-sheet.

"Study Examines Whether Blood Test Can Identify Early Cancers,"National Cancer Institute, June 2, 2020, https://www.cancer.gov/news-events/ cancer-currents-blog/2020/cancerseek-blood-test-detect-early-cancer.

Regan Wong and Charles J. Rosser, "UroSEEK Gene Panel for Bladder Cancer Surveillance," Translational Andrology and Urology 8, no. S5 (December 2019), https://doi.org/10.21037/tau.2019.12.41.

"Tumor Markers," National Cancer Institute, May 11, 2021, https://www.cancer.gov/about-cancer/diagnosis-staging/diagnosis/ tumor-markers-fact-sheet.

Benedict Oerther et al., "Cancer Detection Rates of the PI-RADSv2.1 Assessment Categories: Systematic Review and Meta-Analysis on Lesion Level and Patient Level," Prostate Cancer and Prostatic Diseases 25, no. 2 (July 6, 2021): 256–63, https://doi.org/10.1038/s41391-021-00417-1.

"What Cancer Screening Tests Check for Cancer?," National Cancer Institute, November 10, 2022, https://www.cancer.gov/about-cancer/ screening/screening-tests.

NCI Staff, "Study Examines Whether Blood Test Can Identify Early Cancers," National Cancer Institute, June 2, 2020, https://www.cancer.gov/news-events/cancer-currents-blog/2020/cancerseek-blood-test-detect-early-cancer.

Maxime Blijlevens, Jing Li, and Victor W. van Beusechem, "Biology of the Mrna Splicing Machinery and Its Dysregulation in Cancer Providing Therapeutic Opportunities," International Journal of Molecular Sciences 22, no. 10 (May 12, 2021): 5110, https://doi.org/10.3390/ijms22105110.

"Measuring Age: Steve Horvath, Ph.D., and Epigenetic Clocks," The Institute for Functional Medicine, August 10, 2021, https://www.ifm.org/news-insights/measuring-age-steve-horvath-phd-and-epigenetic-clocks/.

Sylwia Kabacik et al., "The Relationship between Epigenetic Age and the Hallmarks of Aging in Human Cells," Nature Aging 2, no. 6 (May 16, 2022): 484–93, https://doi.org/10.1038/s43587-022-00220-0.

R. Waziry et al., "Effect of Long-Term Caloric Restriction on DNA Methylation Measures of Biological Aging in Healthy Adults from the Calerie Trial," Nature Aging 3, no. 3 (February 9, 2023): 248–57, https://doi.org/10.1038/s43587-022-00357-y.

Jae-Hyun Yang et al., "Chemically Induced Reprogramming to Reverse Cellular Aging," Aging 15, no. 13 (2023): 5966–89, https://doi.org/10.18632/aging.204896.

Ake T. Lu et al., "DNA Methylation GrimAge Strongly Predicts Lifespan and Healthspan," Aging 11, no. 2 (January 21, 2019): 303–27, https://doi.org/10.18632/aging.101684.

Merry L. Lindsey, Andriy Yabluchanskiy, and Yonggang Ma, "Tissue Inhibitor of Metalloproteinase-1: Actions beyond Matrix Metalloproteinase Inhibition," Cardiology 132, no. 3 (October 2015): 147–50, https://doi.org/10.1159/000433419.

Griselda A Cabral-Pacheco et al., "The Roles of Matrix Metalloproteinases and Their Inhibitors in Human Diseases," International Journal of Molecular Sciences 21, no. 24 (December 20, 2020): 9739, https://doi.org/10.3390/ijms21249739.

"The Birth of the Dunedin Study: The Dunedin Study - Dunedin Multidisciplinary Health & Development Research Unit," The Dunedin Study - DMHDRU, accessed July 12, 2023, https://dunedinstudy.otago. ac.nz/studies/assessment-phases/the-birth-of-the-dunedin-study.

"Nuchido Time+ Nad Supplement," Nuchido, accessed July 13, 2023, https://nuchido.com/.

NAD Research, "Boosting Intracellular NAD Levels: An Interview with Dr. Jin-Xiong She," Nad Research, Inc., January 5, 2023, https://nadresearch. org/dr-she-describes-his-research-into-testing-and-supplementing-intracellular-nad-levels/

Nadmed Ltd, June 26, 2023, https://www.nadmed.com/.

Yuancheng Lu et al., "Reprogramming to Recover Youthful Epigenetic Information and Restore Vision," Nature 588, no. 7836 (December 2, 2020): 124–29, https://doi.org/10.1038/s41586-020-2975-4.

"Answers to Your Questions about Stem Cell Research," Mayo Clinic, March 19, 2022, https://www.mayoclinic.org/tests-procedures/bone-marrow-transplant/in-depth/stem-cells/art-20048117.

Juhyun Oh, Yang David Lee, and Amy J Wagers, "Stem Cell Aging: Mechanisms, Regulators and Therapeutic Opportunities," Nature Medicine 20, no. 8 (August 6, 2014): 870–80, https://doi.org/10.1038/nm.3651.

P Hollands and T Ovokaitys, "Human Very Small Embryonic like (Hvsel) Stem Cells: Little Miracles," CellR4, accessed July 13, 2023, https://www.cellr4.org/article/3304.

Jette Lengefeld et al., "Cell Size Is a Determinant of Stem Cell Potential during Aging," Science Advances 7, no. 46 (November 12, 2021), https://doi.org/10.1126/sciadv.abk0271.

Huayong Zhang et al., "Sustained Benefit from Combined Plasmapheresis and Allogeneic Mesenchymal Stem Cells Transplantation Therapy in Systemic Sclerosis," *Arthritis Research & Therapy* 19, no. 1 (July 19, 2017), https://doi.org/10.1186/s13075-017-1373-2.

Benoit Lehallier et al., "Undulating Changes in Human Plasma Proteome Profiles across the Lifespan," Nature Medicine 25, no. 12 (December 5, 2019): 1843–50, https://doi.org/10.1038/s41591-019-0673-2.

Daehwan Kim et al., "Old Plasma Dilution Reduces Human Biological Age: A Clinical Study," GeroScience 44, no. 6 (August 24, 2022): 2701–20, https://doi.org/10.1007/s11357-022-00645-w.

Mercè Boada et al., "Feasibility, Safety, and Tolerability of Two Modalities of Plasma Exchange with Albumin Replacement to Treat Elderly Patients with Alzheimer's Disease in the AMBAR Study," *Journal of Clinical Apheresis* 38, no. 1 (October 28, 2022): 45–54, https://doi.org/10.1002/jca.22026.

Chris Thrive, "Benefits of Donating Plasma," ABO Plasma, March 11, 2023, https://aboplasma.com/benefits-of-donating-plasma/.

Karthik Kumar, "Is Donating Plasma Good for Your Body? Benefits & Drawbacks," MedicineNet, September 20, 2022, https://www.medicinenet.com/is_donating_plasma_good_for_your_body/article.htm.

"Donating Plasma for Money: Is It Healthy?: Shine365 from Marshfield Clinic," Shine365, June 28, 2023, https://shine365.marshfieldclinic.org/wellness/plasma-donation/.

"Frequently Asked Questions," Questions About Donating Blood | Red Cross Blood Services, accessed April 13, 2023, https://www.redcrossblood.org/faq.html.

Cristina Fantini et al., "Vitamin D as a Shield against Aging," International Journal of Molecular Sciences 24, no. 5 (February 25, 2023): 4546, https://doi.org/10.3390/ijms24054546.

Gregory M. Fahy et al., "Reversal of Epigenetic Aging and Immunosenescent Trends in Humans," Aging Cell 18, no. 6 (September 8, 2019), https://doi.org/10.1111/acel.13028.

Melod Mehdipour et al., "Rejuvenation of Three Germ Layers Tissues by Exchanging Old Blood Plasma with Saline-Albumin," Aging 12, no. 10 (May 30, 2020): 8790–8819, https://doi.org/10.18632/aging.103418.

Yalin Zhang et al., "Hypothalamic Stem Cells Control Ageing Speed Partly through Exosomal Mirnas," Nature 548, no. 7665 (July 26, 2017): 52–57, https://doi.org/10.1038/nature23282.

Alan A. Cohen et al., "A Complex Systems Approach to Aging Biology," Nature Aging 2, no. 7 (July 20, 2022): 580–91, https://doi.org/10.1038/s43587-022-00252-6.

Lucas Paulo de Lima Camillo and Robert B. Quinlan, "A Ride through the Epigenetic Landscape: Aging Reversal by Reprogramming," GeroScience 43, no. 2 (April 2021): 463–85, https://doi.org/10.1007/s11357-021-00358-6.

Mohammed S Razzaque, "Therapeutic Potential of Klotho–FGF23 Fusion Polypeptides: WO2009095372," Expert Opinion on Therapeutic Patents 20, no. 7 (May 12, 2010): 981–85, https://doi.org/10.1517/13543771003774100.

Paola Sanese et al., "FOXO3 on the Road to Longevity: Lessons from Snps and Chromatin Hubs," Computational and Structural Biotechnology Journal 17 (June 13, 2019): 737–45, https://doi.org/10.1016/j.csbj.2019.06.011.

Jan M. van Deursen, "The Role of Senescent Cells in Ageing," Nature 509, no. 7501 (May 21, 2014): 439–46, https://doi.org/10.1038/nature13193.

M. Shawkat Razzaque, "The FGF23–Klotho Axis: Endocrine Regulation of Phosphate Homeostasis," Nature Reviews Endocrinology 5, no. 11 (November 2009): 611–19, https://doi.org/10.1038/nrendo.2009.196.

Zhou Jiang, Qianpei He, and Warren Ladiges, *A Cocktail of Rapamycin, Acarbose and Phenylbutyrate Prevents Age-Related Cognitive Decline in Mice by Altering Aging Pathways*, September 9, 2022, https://doi.org/10.1101/2022.09.07.506968.

Norbert Guettler, Kim Rajappan, and Edward Nicol, "The Impact of Age on Long QT Syndrome," *Aging* 11, no. 24 (December 28, 2019): 11795–96, https://doi.org/10.18632/aging.102623.

Brian J. Morris et al., "*Foxo3:* A Major Gene for Human Longevity - a Mini-Review," *Gerontology* 61, no. 6 (March 28, 2015): 515–25, https://doi.org/10.1159/000375235.

Premranjan Kumar, Ob W. Osahon, and Rajagopal V. Sekhar, "Glynac (Glycine and N-Acetylcysteine) Supplementation in Mice Increases Length of Life by Correcting Glutathione Deficiency, Oxidative Stress, Mitochondrial Dysfunction, Abnormalities in Mitophagy and Nutrient Sensing, and Genomic Damage," *Nutrients* 14, no. 5 (March 7, 2022): 1114, https://doi.org/10.3390/nu14051114.

Timothy V. Pyrkov et al., "Longitudinal Analysis of Blood Markers Reveals Progressive Loss of Resilience and Predicts Human Lifespan Limit," *Nature Communications* 12, no. 1 (May 25, 2021), https://doi.org/10.1038/s41467-021-23014-1.

Robert Podstawski et al., "Effect of Repeated Alternative Thermal Stress on the Physiological and Body Composition Characteristics of Young Women Sporadically Using Sauna," *Physical Activity Review* 11, no. 1 (2023): 49–59, https://doi.org/10.16926/par.2023.11.07.

Christopher D. Wiley and Judith Campisi, "The Metabolic Roots of Senescence: Mechanisms and Opportunities for Intervention," *Nature Metabolism* 3, no. 10 (October 18, 2021): 1290–1301, https://doi.org/10.1038/s42255-021-00483-8.

Hyun Jung Hwang et al., "Factors and Pathways Modulating Endothelial Cell Senescence in Vascular Aging," *International Journal of Molecular Sciences* 23, no. 17 (September 4, 2022): 10135, https://doi.org/10.3390/ijms231710135.

Salvatore Fusco, Giuseppe Maulucci, and Giovambattista Pani, "Sirt1: Def-Eating Senescence?," *Cell Cycle* 11, no. 22 (November 15, 2012): 4135–46, https://doi.org/10.4161/cc.22074.

Nimisha Lingappa and Harvey N Mayrovitz, "Role of Sirtuins in Diabetes and Age-Related Processes," *Cureus*, September 4, 2022, https://doi.org/10.7759/cureus.28774.

Marcia C. Haigis and Leonard P. Guarente, "Mammalian Sirtuins—Emerging Roles in Physiology, Aging, and Calorie Restriction," *Genes & Development* 20, no. 21 (November 1, 2006): 2913–21, https://doi.org/10.1101/gad.1467506.

E. Dambroise et al., "Two Phases of Aging Separated by the Smurf Transition as a Public Path to Death," *Scientific Reports* 6, no. 1 (March 22, 2016), https://doi.org/10.1038/srep23523.

Diane H. Russell, Vicente J. Medina, and Solomon H. Snyder, "The Dynamics of Synthesis and Degradation of Polyamines in Normal and Regenerating Rat Liver and Brain," *Journal of Biological Chemistry* 245, no. 24 (December 1970): 6732–38, https://doi.org/10.1016/s0021-9258(18)62595-5.

Junying Wang et al., "Spermidine Alleviates Cardiac Aging by Improving Mitochondrial Biogenesis and Function," *Aging* 12, no. 1 (January 6, 2020): 650–71, https://doi.org/10.18632/aging.102647.

Tobias Eisenberg et al., "Cardioprotection and Lifespan Extension by the Natural Polyamine Spermidine," *Nature Medicine* 22, no. 12 (November 14, 2016): 1428–38, https://doi.org/10.1038/nm.4222.

Paula Martínez and Maria A. Blasco, "Role of Shelterin in Cancer and Aging," *Aging Cell* 9, no. 5 (September 16, 2010): 653–66, https://doi.org/10.1111/j.1474-9726.2010.00596.x.

Raul Sanchez-Vazquez et al., "Shorter Telomere Lengths in Patients with Severe Covid-19 Disease," *Aging* 13, no. 1 (January 11, 2021): 1–15, https://doi.org/10.18632/aging.202463.

Bruno Bernardes de Jesus et al., "Telomerase Gene Therapy in Adult and Old Mice Delays Aging and Increases Longevity without Increasing Cancer," *EMBO Molecular Medicine* 4, no. 8 (May 15, 2012): 691–704, https://doi.org/10.1002/emmm.201200245.

Mariela Jaskelioff et al., "Telomerase Reactivation Reverses Tissue Degeneration in Aged Telomerase-Deficient Mice," *Nature* 469, no. 7328 (November 28, 2010): 102–6, https://doi.org/10.1038/nature09603.

Richard C. Allsopp, Samuel Cheshier, and Irving L. Weissman, "Telomerase Activation and Rejuvenation of Telomere Length in Stimulated T Cells Derived from Serially Transplanted Hematopoietic Stem Cells," *The Journal of Experimental Medicine* 196, no. 11 (December 2, 2002): 1427–33, https://doi.org/10.1084/jem.20021003.

Mayya Razgonova et al., "Telomerase and Telomeres in Aging Theory and Chronographic Aging Theory (Review)," *Molecular Medicine Reports* 22, no. 3 (June 25, 2020): 1679–94, https://doi.org/10.3892/mmr.2020.11274.

JinWoo Hong and Chae-Ok Yun, "Telomere Gene Therapy: Polarizing Therapeutic Goals for Treatment of Various Diseases," *Cells* 8, no. 5 (April 28, 2019): 392, https://doi.org/10.3390/cells8050392.

Calvin B Harley, "Telomerase Is Not an Oncogene," *Oncogene* 21, no. 4 (January 21, 2002): 494–502, https://doi.org/10.1038/sj.onc.1205076.

A. Mojiri et al., "Human Telomerase M-RNA Treatment Restores Functions in Progeria IPSC- Derived Endothelial Cells," *Canadian Journal of Cardiology* 35, no. 10 (October 25, 2019), https://doi.org/10.1016/j.cjca.2019.07.191.

Julio Aguado et al., "Inhibition of DNA Damage Response at Telomeres Improves the Detrimental Phenotypes of Hutchinson–Gilford Progeria Syndrome," *Nature Communications* 10, no. 1 (November 18, 2019), https://doi.org/10.1038/s41467-019-13018-3.

Jingwen Zhang et al., "Ageing and the Telomere Connection: An Intimate Relationship with Inflammation," *Ageing Research Reviews* 25 (January 2016): 55–69, https://doi.org/10.1016/j.arr.2015.11.006.

Benoit Lehallier et al., *Undulating Changes in Human Plasma Proteome across Lifespan Are Linked to Disease*, September 1, 2019, https://doi.org/10.1101/751115.

Rong Hu et al., "In Vivo Pharmacokinetics and Regulation of Gene Expression Profiles by Isothiocyanate Sulforaphane in the Rat," *Journal of Pharmacology and Experimental Therapeutics* 310, no. 1 (February 26, 2004): 263–71, https://doi.org/10.1124/jpet.103.064261.

Kara Turner, Vimal Vasu, and Darren Griffin, "Telomere Biology and Human Phenotype," *Cells* 8, no. 1 (January 19, 2019): 73, https://doi.org/10.3390/cells8010073.

Ake T. Lu et al., "DNA Methylation-Based Estimator of Telomere Length," *Aging* 11, no. 16 (August 18, 2019): 5895–5923, https://doi.org/10.18632/aging.102173.

Alexandra Barbouti et al., "Implications of Oxidative Stress and Cellular Senescence in Age-Related Thymus Involution," *Oxidative Medicine and Cellular Longevity* 2020 (February 5, 2020): 1–14, https://doi.org/10.1155/2020/7986071.

Peng An et al., "Expanding Tor Complex 2 Signaling: Emerging Regulators and New Connections," *Frontiers in Cell and Developmental Biology* 9 (July 30, 2021), https://doi.org/10.3389/fcell.2021.713806.

Giuseppina Rose et al., "Further Support to the Uncoupling-to-Survive Theory: The Genetic Variation of Human UCP Genes Is Associated with Longevity," *PLoS ONE* 6, no. 12 (December 27, 2011), https://doi.org/10.1371/journal.pone.0029650.

Leigh Goedeke and Gerald I. Shulman, "Therapeutic Potential of Mitochondrial Uncouplers for the Treatment of Metabolic Associated Fatty Liver Disease and Nash," *Molecular Metabolism* 46 (April 2021): 101178, https://doi.org/10.1016/j.molmet.2021.101178.

Anurag Singh et al., "Direct Supplementation with Urolithin a Overcomes Limitations of Dietary Exposure and Gut Microbiome Variability in Healthy Adults to Achieve Consistent Levels across the Population," *European Journal of Clinical Nutrition* 76, no. 2 (June 11, 2021): 297–308, https://doi.org/10.1038/s41430-021-00950-1.

Davide D'Amico et al., "Impact of the Natural Compound Urolithin A on Health, Disease, and Aging," *Trends in Molecular Medicine* 27, no. 7 (July 2021): 687–99, https://doi.org/10.1016/j.molmed.2021.04.009.

Tetsuo Shioi et al., "Rapamycin Attenuates Load-Induced Cardiac Hypertrophy in Mice," *Circulation* 107, no. 12 (April 2003): 1664–70, https://doi.org/10.1161/01.cir.0000057979.36322.88.

Danusha Vellasamy et al., "Targeting Immune Senescence in Atherosclerosis," *International Journal of Molecular Sciences* 23, no. 21 (October 27, 2022): 13059, https://doi.org/10.3390/ijms232113059.

A M Wang et al., "Use of Carnosine as a Natural Anti-Senescence Drug for Human Beings," *Biochemistry* 65, no. 7 (July 2000): 869–71.

Ivana Jukić et al., "Carnosine, Small but Mighty—Prospect of Use as Functional Ingredient for Functional Food Formulation," *Antioxidants* 10, no. 7 (June 28, 2021): 1037, https://doi.org/10.3390/antiox10071037.

Benoit Lehallier et al., "Data Mining of Human Plasma Proteins Generates a Multitude of Highly Predictive Aging Clocks That Reflect Different Aspects of Aging," *Aging Cell* 19, no. 11 (October 8, 2020), https://doi.org/10.1111/acel.13256.

Jonathan A. Lindquist and Peter R. Mertens, "Cold Shock Proteins: From Cellular Mechanisms to Pathophysiology and Disease," *Cell Communication and Signaling* 16, no. 1 (September 26, 2018), https://doi.org/10.1186/s12964-018-0274-6.

Daniel W Belsky et al., "Quantification of the Pace of Biological Aging in Humans through a Blood Test, the Dunedinpoam DNA Methylation Algorithm," *eLife* 9 (May 5, 2020), https://doi.org/10.7554/elife.54870.

"BEN'S DUNEDINPOAM REPORT The Study Explained & Where You Land," *TruDiagnostic*, July 24, 2020.

Amalio Telenti, Brad A. Perkins, and J. Craig Venter, "Dynamics of an Aging Genome," *Cell Metabolism* 23, no. 6 (June 2016): 949–50, https://doi.org/10.1016/j.cmet.2016.06.002.

Yasaaswini Apparoo et al., "Ergothioneine and Its Prospects as an Anti-Ageing Compound," *Experimental Gerontology* 170 (December 2022): 111982, https://doi.org/10.1016/j.exger.2022.111982.

"Cognitive Vitality Reports®," Alzheimer's Drug Discovery Foundation, September 4, 2018, https://www.alzdiscovery.org/.

"Focus on Aging," *Cell Metabolism* 23 (June 14, 2016): 951–56.

Huarui Cai et al., "Recent Advances of the Mammalian Target of Rapamycin Signaling in Mesenchymal Stem Cells," *Frontiers in Genetics* 13 (August 30, 2022), https://doi.org/10.3389/fgene.2022.970699.

For more references, please visit GladdenLongevity.com/Book100.

Part Three

Health

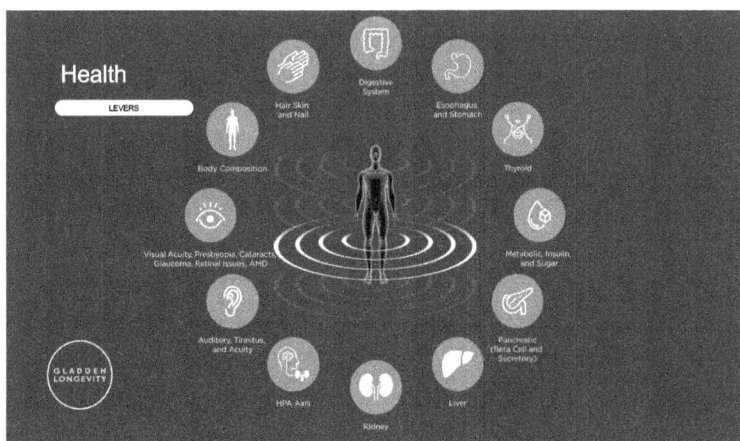

How Do We Make 100 The New 30?

What is the definition of *health*? In the traditional, medical, sick-care system, it is the absence of identifiable disease. The "Hallmarks of Health," published in *Cell* in 2020, reiterates this definition: "Health is the absence of pathology." Health becomes equated to wellness, which can also be defined as the absence of identifiable disease, and wellness becomes traditional medicine's highest goal.

At Gladden Longevity, we not only define health as the absence of identifiable disease or pathology but also as the optimal function of the individual with regard to Life Energy, Longevity, Health, and Performance. Although we do not have a religious affiliation, we are all about optimizing mental, spiritual, and relational health as a critical feature in realizing your optimal health, longevity, and performance levels. In doing so, we are optimizing a youthful mindset and functional capabilities, which create the opportunity to pursue, do, and achieve anything you want.

In essence, optimal health enables you to make your biggest impact. This is such a critical distinction in the definition of health. The mindset of the medical professional you seek out will land you in a wellness camp, a functional medicine camp, a pseudo-longevity camp, or a life-energy, longevity, health, and performance optimization camp. Be careful who you work with, as they will define the ceiling of how far you can go. Which camp appeals to you?

As noted in "Hallmarks of Health," there are three keys required for health:

1. **The ability to have and maintain structural integrity.** Think not only in terms of bones, muscle, and proteins but cell membranes that enable communication with other cells and maintain the structural integrity of that particular cell. This structural integrity is as critical for the small structures in the cell as it is for the macroscopic structural components of the body.

2. **The ability to stay in, return to, and maintain homeostasis, a state of equilibrium or balance found in a smoothly operating organism.** Homeostasis is transiently interrupted in the face of challenges that cause perturbations to the system, such as COVID, an accident, or a toxin. Homeostasis can be lost in the aging process and other non-terminal or terminal conditions. As we described earlier, one's ability to return to homeostasis is directly related to their robustness and resilience.

3. **An appropriate and adequate response to stress.** With the right amount of stress—not too little and not too much, known as *hormetic stress*—we achieve the ability to recover, repair, regenerate, and get stronger. Hormetic stress enables us to get stronger, experience robust health, and maintain resilience and robustness.

Woven together, these keys become the underlying principles of health. In order to stay healthy, we must experience challenges and stresses, such as infections, microbes, toxins, exercise, heat, cold, and so on. Without these stimuli to recover, repair, regenerate, and get stronger, we get weaker. Being strong and able to withstand stressors builds resilience and robustness; living in a bubble does not.

Stressors are key to us becoming antifragile. But despite doing everything right and exposing ourselves to the right amount of health-promoting stress, we lose resilience and robustness due to the unaddressed drivers of aging and their cumulative toll on our physiology. Avoiding good stress compounds the problem, like being seduced by a life of ease and luxury, where things are done for us—elevators replace stairs, vehicles replace walking, bellmen carry our bags . . . . By taking every opportunity to enjoy small physical stresses, you protect your capabilities and youthfulness.

One final thought is to change the way you think about healthcare today and understand what healthcare in the future will look like. I have created a new construct to understand this. In this construct, there are three strata of medical care.

- The surface level is our standard healthcare/sick-care system and its symptom and "sign"-driven approach, like your blood pressure is up, so you take a pill to lower it, or you feel poorly, so you see the doctor. Likewise, if we "feel" fine, we are less likely to visit the doctor because we wait for a sign or symptom—like a mole getting bigger or shortness of breath—to prompt us to go.
- One stratum deeper is functional medicine, driven by its root-cause approach—a desire to understand what is causing the problem and not just treat the symptoms. An example might be if your eczema is related to your dietary allergies and leaky gut. Let's fix your gut, clean up your diet, and watch your eczema improve.
- The foundational strata, however, is longevity med-icine, focused on understanding and addressing the

drivers of aging, known and unknown. This is the stratum where aging is accelerated due to things like changes in DNA methylation patterns, shortening telomeres, increasing inflammation and oxidative stress, mitochondrial dysfunction, increasing numbers of senescent cells, and so on. It is at this strata that the battle needs to be waged because these drivers of aging, if not addressed, create an exponentially increasing current that exponentially increases our rate of aging.

These drivers of aging at this lowest stratum are the true root cause of disease and decline. Standard or functional medicine doesn't adequately address this deepest stratum. As such, the results from treatments recommended by traditional and functional medicine, even regenerative treatments like stem cells and exosomes, will be short-lived. Resilience and robustness will not be durably enhanced or even fully restored.

The medicine of the future will address all three levels beginning with the drivers of aging, the root causes of the ailment, and the symptoms simultaneously. This creates the most comprehensive and durable healing. It optimizes resilience and robustness.

Gladden Longevity takes this approach. When we look around, we realize we are pioneers in this approach. Having set the stage, let's look at some of the key components of health.

CHAPTER TWENTY-SIX

Sleep

Sleep is one of the absolute cornerstones of health, and there is no place that is more evident than in looking at the health consequences and mortality rates of shift workers. Shift workers, particularly those working different shifts, have a disrupted circadian rhythm, are not going to bed with the sun and waking up with the sun. Instead, they are forced to switch between working days and nights. Their scheduled shifts rotate: overnight shift on Tuesdays and Wednesdays, day shift on Fridays and Saturdays, and then they're back on the night shift. Shift work plays havoc with our underlying circadian rhythm. Even working only graveyard shifts has an impact on longevity.

We are designed to go to sleep with the sun and wake up with the sun. For those whose work schedules are disrupted and do not follow this pattern, their mortality is significantly higher, not to mention their chances of getting cancer, heart disease, and diabetes. When our sleep is disrupted, especially on a continual basis, it derails our entire physiology.

When I was going through my medical training, disrupted sleep was a given. We kept crazy hours, often getting up in the middle of the night. During my internal medicine residency, in preparation for cardiology, we were on-call every third night while working on the regular hospital floors. In hospital intensive care units, we were on-call every other night, which meant we would go to work at seven o'clock in the morning and work until the nurses from the day shift went home. Then the afternoon nurses would come on shift, and we would work through their entire shift until eleven o'clock. Then the overnight nurses would come on shift, and we'd work through the night with them. Then the day nurses would come on shift, and you would hand off your patients to the incoming residents and physicians, who came on at seven in the morning. You'd make those rounds to ensure each patient was transferred appropriately and safely—that might take another three hours, so it would be ten o'clock in the morning before you finally got to go home. During that time, you might have picked up a couple of hours of sleep or, if it was a "quiet night," maybe even four hours.

That schedule was extremely difficult, and I shudder to think about the damage I was doing to my health. Surgical residents were taking calls every other night for their entire five-year residency. The irony of having young doctors work a schedule that destroys their health is not lost on anyone except those running the training programs. Keep in mind those who trained ten or twenty years prior to me had it even worse, but it shows you how a healing profession normalized going without sleep as just part of the job. It was a badge of honor; it showed your commitment and dedication. Fortunately, things have changed for current interns and residents. We did not give appropriate value to sleep back then, and unfortunately, some professions and industries still don't.

If you want to play the symphony of longevity and make 100 the new 30, getting enough quality sleep has to become one of your top priorities. It's as important as eating well, exercising, feeling loved, and having good relationships.

There are four stages of sleep: Light Sleep, Rapid Eye Movement Sleep (REM), Deep Sleep (also called "slow-wave" sleep), and awake. During REM sleep, we dream our most vivid dreams, process information, solve problems, and pull up fragments from the past or previous days.

It's critical that we get slow-wave sleep in order for the brain to reset itself. As we age, particularly over fifty, many people do not experience deep, slow-wave sleep, which is the stage in which our neurons regenerate. The brain needs to go into this deep state to rejuvenate itself for the next day. When sleep is disrupted, and you never really get to go through all the stages of sleep in a sequence, it disrupts your brain function.

There is a system in the brain called the Glymphatic System (GLS) that cleans out the physiological debris, trash, and toxins from the brain that accumulate from activity during the day. The system only works at night during slow-wave sleep, and it works best if you are sleeping with your right cheek on the pillow. (Try this, and see if you don't wake up more clear-headed.)

Sleep is important for recovery, and while we'll discuss heart-rate variability (HRV) in Part Four, we need to highlight its relationship to sleep here. Heart-rate variability is a measure of how much stress the body is under; both psychological and physical stress make an impact on it.

HRV is not the change in heart rate that occurs when you go from sitting in your chair to climbing a flight of stairs, and your heart rate goes up from sixty-five to ninety. HRV is the beat-to-beat variation in heart rate coupled to our respiration. Breathe in, and your heartbeats are slightly closer together, i.e., faster. Breathe out, and your heartbeats are somewhat further apart, i.e., slower. The less stressed and the more recovered your body is, the greater the variation in your heart rate between inspiration and expiration. A higher HRV means you are better recovered, and with more parasympathetic nervous system tone you have. You are more Zen.

HRV measures the balance between the sympathetic nervous system ("freeze, fight, or flight" responses) and the parasympathetic nervous system (involving rest, recovery, and repair). When stressed, the sympathetic nervous system dominates, and HRV is low. When we are relaxed, recovered, and have the capacity to take on stress, the parasympathetic nervous system is more dominant, and HRV is high. Stress management is massively important for good sleep, and good sleep is massively important for stress management. Those who struggle with stress, like PTSD or anxiety, have a lower HRV and often don't sleep as well.

The impact of stress on an individual varies based on their genetics, specifically the FKBP5, COMT, CHRNA5, CRHR1, and MAOA genes. These genes control how quickly we break down stress-related neurotransmitters and our susceptibility to past trauma and subsequent risk of addiction. The faster we break down the stress-related neurotransmitters, the less our psyches are affected by stress.

As previously noted, data shows that children who grew up in physically abusive families and had COMT and MAO configurations that quickly broke down stress neurotransmitters had a less negative long-term impact from the abuse. Conversely, children with COMT and MAO genes that broke down stress neurotransmitters more slowly suffered long-term consequences from their childhood trauma. Children with FKBP5, COMT, CHRNA5, and CRHR1 genes had a higher risk of PTSD (post-traumatic stress disorder).

If you suffer from stress or struggle with sleep after trying various techniques, it may be worth looking into genetics to get additional insight. Your nervous system may have greater sensitivity to stress.

As we have seen, heart-rate variability is very important in determining the overall recovery score. HRV can be measured at any point in the day. The World Health Organization has refined the measurement of HRV to occur during slow-wave sleep and only for a few minutes at night. There is a logic to this because, in slow-wave sleep, we are completely relaxed, paralyzed, not dreaming, and not thinking. It is when our brain is essentially shut down. By testing during slow-wave sleep, we get a "true read" on the stress levels we are under, and hence, a true indication of our recovery and, therefore, our state of readiness to take on new stress. Having a higher HRV indicates a healthier, better-balanced autonomic nervous system.

We can improve HRV in numerous ways, but great sleep is paramount to that list. We also know that going to bed earlier leads to a higher HRV, as well as protracted cardio—longer cardio sessions over time. We have learned that the following items commonly lower HRV:

- Ongoing infection
- injury
- alcohol

- relational or work-related emotional stress
- poor sleep
- working out very hard

Ideally, you want two or three sleep cycles per night, in sequence: light, REM, deep, and repeat. When sleep is disrupted, most of us feel fatigued the next day; very few people, genetically, can function on just four hours of sleep. Most of us need six to eight hours of sleep to feel good.

Two questions that often come up when it comes to sleep:

- **Quantity or quality?** The short answer is quality of sleep is more important than the number of hours. This dovetails into the second question.
- **Is there such a thing as too much?** Yes, there is such a thing as too much sleep. Those who sleep nine to eleven hours a day do not function as well, and the amount of sleep may be linked to other issues, like depression or some other illness.

Striving to hit that range of six to eight hours—seven being the magic number—is statistically associated with the best health benefits. Your magic number will likely be between six and nine hours, depending on your physical and mental activity levels.

Measurement and Optimization

Since sleep is so important, tracking it is essential. There are any number of sleep trackers to tell you how you're doing. There are even sleep-tracking mattresses that can track sleep. Sleep-tracking technology continues to improve, so if you're serious about your health, you need to find a way to track your sleep. Wearing a sleep tracker will show you how much time you spend in each sleep stage and how many interruptions you've had. You'll likely discover that you had interruptions that you were never aware of, and hopefully, you were able to get back to sleep.

Tracking gives you a baseline, a starting point for optimization. Since we are designed to wake up with the sun and go to bed with the sun, blue-light exposure—which comes from electronic devices like cell phones and televisions—stimulates the brain to go into a wakeful state, not a sleeping state. Yet most of us use these devices to unwind before bed.

Wearing glasses with blue-light blockers is helpful, and I recommend this, but I have also discovered the benefits of TrueDark® glasses, with their dark amber-reddish colored lenses that make everything look red. I put them on in the evening, about an hour before bed, and they help to quiet my mind. Within ten to fifteen minutes, I start to feel tired. Further, I can feel a shift in my physiology—it feels like they are preparing my brain to sleep. They also make a lighter yellow lens to wear in the afternoon through the transition of sunset. If I'm going to be on my phone in the evening, I wear amber glasses to minimize the blue-light effect.

Sleeping in a cooler environment isn't just an old wives' tale; it improves sleep quality. Personally, I will turn my thermostat down to about sixty-four degrees at night to mimic sleeping in the mountains with the windows open. Cooling mattresses and cooling pillows are also helpful. Mattresses absorb heat, and as we go through the night, we get warmer and warmer. This doesn't take into consideration someone who might have a fever or a woman who is going through menopause and has hot flashes. More and more mattress manufacturers are adding cooling technology. It's not just a marketing gimmick; it really helps.

We have participated in podcasts with a company called Chilisleep®, which has developed a mattress pad that runs cool water to keep the bed cool. In my own experience, my body heat will still warm the mattress to some extent, but the idea is that it will help locate and regulate your ideal sleeping temperature.

I also recommend blackout curtains. Generally speaking, anything that will reduce light and lower the temperature of your sleeping environment will help you achieve better sleep quality. Keep in mind that illness or injury can disrupt your progress, so if you have the flu or experience a concussion, your recovery score will take a dive even if your environment is perfectly set up.

I am also a fan of grounding mats to improve sleep, as they keep me electrically grounded. They have also been shown to improve sleep quality.

Inevitably, people ask me about prescription and over-the-counter sleep aids. The problem with medications is that while they can get you to sleep, they also interrupt the stages of sleep. You never sleep well when relying on benzodiazepines like Xanax or Ambien, so we're not fans of sleeping medications. We are fans of optimizing melatonin levels. Melatonin is a hormone secreted by the pineal gland in response to sunlight and darkness, and it sets our circadian rhythm. This is another reason to spend some time in the sunshine each day and then in complete darkness at night—this practice helps synchronize your circadian rhythm.

If you take melatonin, understand that it will not make you sleepy; it helps with your circadian rhythm, which is the underlying substrate upon which you sleep. The other beautiful thing about melatonin is that it also feeds and keeps healthy a group of stem cells in the basal lateral hypothalamus, which is incredibly important for longevity.

Melatonin is an anti-inflammatory; it increases the expression of growth-hormone receptors, which can help maintain muscle mass and bone density; and it is a foundational supplement because it helps prepare you for sleep. The downside, however, is that too much will make you drowsy the next morning, and melatonin can also impair memory. On the flip side, melatonin can increase HRV. Start with one-half to one milligram in the evening to find what works for you. We know of people taking up to 200mg, but I certainly wouldn't recommend starting there. Importantly, you should know that taking melatonin does not decrease your body's ability to make it.

If you think about it, anything that you consume—food, sunshine, exercise, and so on—is actually information. This "information intake" interacts with the body, instructing it to do certain things, like turn on certain genes, turn off other genes, activate this pathway, deactivate that pathway . . . so really, you can boil all this down to information. Even melatonin is, in essence, a form of information. A company called NES Health™ has figured out how to imprint this information into salt water. They determined, at an energetic level, what the body needs and developed a series of products that help give that information back to the body.

With this in mind, one of the most interesting supplements I'm using currently is produced by NES Health™, called Sleep. When I first heard about it, I was incredibly skeptical, but the more I've used it, the more I have come to see that it works. I'm just taking a little bit of salt water, washing it down with some water, and I feel sleepy within five or ten minutes. I like the purity and simplicity of this approach.

Here are some other interventions that directly or indirectly assisted me with sleep.

- Be intentional about sleep.
- Avoid caffeine after lunch, even if you are a fast caffeine metabolizer.
- Avoid stimulant medications after you've taken a morning dose.
- Avoid alcohol in the evening; it makes you feel sleepy but disrupts your body's ability to go into deep, restorative sleep. All of our clients have noticed that their recovery scores and sleep scores are dramatically decreased when they drink alcohol in the evening.
- Plan your bedtime, your pre-sleep routine, and your sleep environment.

A note on sexual activity: An orgasm will release oxytocin for both men and women, which in and of itself has many longevity benefits and is to be encouraged. Oxytocin, however, has different effects in men and women. It makes men fall asleep and makes women more alert and awake, so plan accordingly when you are trying to optimize your sleep.

When improving sleep, you might also consider the following:

- **Alpha-Stim®:** An FDA-approved product rather than a supplement, Alpha-Stim can relieve stress, anxiety, and depression. It works by running a small electrical current through the brain that puts the brain into an alpha-wave state. We suggest a twenty- to thirty-minute session once a day, coupled with meditation. Even if your session is more than several hours ahead of bedtime, it still helps with sleep. In fact, Alpha-Stim® discourages bedtime sessions; however, a twenty-minute session effectively gets you back to sleep if you wake up in the middle of the night.

- **Taurine:** A supplement that is neuro-protective and blocks excess excitatory glutamate activity. This amino acid has been shown to alter GABA and glutamate brain levels in rodents. The glutamine-GABA balance in the brain is critical for sleep. You can take it in supplement form and get it naturally in meat and seafood. Taurine is frequently added to energy drinks but can improve sleep.

- **5-HTP:** Your body converts 5-HTP into serotonin, and serotonin can enhance GABA activity. 5-HTP is a synthetic form of tryptophan. Tryptophan is found in higher concentrations in turkey. (No wonder you're sleepy after a Thanksgiving dinner!) Food-based sources of tryptophan, however, are not thought to cross the Blood Brain Barrier the way 5-HTP does.

- **L-Theanine:** This precursor of glutamate appears to lower glutamate activity in the brain by blocking receptors while also boosting GABA levels. It's found naturally in tea and also is available as a supplement. About 200mg (usually two pills) of L-theanine at bedtime improves sleep and HRV.

- **Alpha Gaba:** Improves sleep and can be used again if you wake up in the middle of the night. It contains L-theanine and melatonin.

- **Chamomile Tea:** Drink at bedtime to help improve sleep quality, recovery, and blood sugar. Chamomile tea or valerian root tea calms the nervous system.

- **Glycine:** One scoop of the amino acid glycine in water at bedtime can be effective on heavy workout days or if you have restless leg syndrome. Glycine has also been shown to have a longevity benefit.
- **Magnesium Threonate:** Lowers neurotransmitter activity, so two magnesium threonate pills at bedtime can be helpful. Upgraded magnesium is another form of magnesium with good sleep data.
- **Ashwagandha:** An adaptogen for the adrenal gland and levels out stress. If chronic stress is the issue, we can end up with high cortisol levels and low melatonin levels at night—the opposite of what we want.
- **Relora®:** A trademarked combination of two Chinese tree barks, traditionally used to promote healthy stress reactions. Relora® combines a proprietary blend of *Magnolia officinalis* and *Phellodendron amurense*. Magnolia officinalis is known for supporting normal adrenal function, while Phellodendron amurense is known for supporting a calm state of mind. When used together, these Chinese tree barks are ideal for supporting well-being and stress management. The product Theanine Serene with Relora, by Serene Science®, works well.
- **NES Health™ Sleep:** From NES Health, I find it also improves sleep.
- **NES Health™ Chill:** From NES Health, had been shown to be relaxing. We have recently added Chill to H2. Our staff who use it love the feeling they have of being calm and relaxed.

Finally, there are some things to avoid when trying to improve your sleep quality. High-histamine foods—especially later in the day—might lead to poorer sleep for those with histamine intolerance. The following foods contain a high level of histamine:

- fermented dairy products, such as cheese (especially aged), yogurt, sour cream, buttermilk, and kefir
- fermented vegetables, such as sauerkraut and kimchi
- pickles or pickled veggies
- kombucha
- cured or fermented meats, such as sausages, salami, and fermented ham
- wine, beer, alcohol, and champagne are especially high
- fermented soy products such as tempeh, miso, soy sauce, and natto
- fermented grains, such as sourdough bread
- tomatoes
- eggplant
- spinach
- frozen, salted, or canned fish, such as sardines and tuna
- vinegar
- tomato ketchup

That doesn't mean you should avoid them altogether, but consider avoiding them as you get closer to bedtime or seek lower-glutamate alternatives (cheddar cheese, salmon, and blueberries, to name a few). Also, note that foods high in glutamate can worsen anxiety in sensitive people. An Intellxx DNA genetic test will tell you whether you're genetically sensitive. If you are, taking DAO, or diamine oxidase, will help to break down histamine in your diet.

CHAPTER TWENTY-SEVEN

Heart VO2 Max and Anaerobic Threshold

The number one killer in the Western world is still cardiovascular disease. We tend to think of heart disease as the development of plaque inside arteries. This plaque is associated with cholesterol deposited into the arteries. The arteries are susceptible to that deposit because the endothelium, the single-cell thickness of skin that lines the inside of the artery, is damaged by things we eat, drink, or inhale and becomes vulnerable.

Think about the anatomy of an artery like this: Visualize a garden hose composed of three layers. The outside layer is very tough, able to withstand being stretched, making contact with the pavement, etc. Inside the hose is something more supple, with enough strength so that water can pass.

Then, the very inner lining of the hose is a thin skin that allows the water to flow without any friction.

The artery has these three layers as well. With the artery, however, that middle layer, or media, is a muscle layer that expands and contracts to adjust blood flow. When exercising, your artery expands to allow more blood flow to your muscles, brain, and heart. The cool part is that the endothelium, or skin lining the inside of the artery, controls the media and arterial relaxation and contraction. The endothelium is just a smooth layer of cells one cell thick, but it has a sort of "fuzz" on the inner surface called a glycocalyx, which is made of proteoglycans and glycoproteins.

Think of the glycocalyx as moss at the bottom of a river; in the same way water in the river glides over moss, the blood cells will glide over the glycocalyx. The glycocalyx is electrically charged, so it repels molecules away from the endothelium, protecting it from damage and keeping the blood from clotting. When blood flow increases due to exercise or any stress that increases heart rate, it senses the increased flow and signals the endothelium to release nitric oxide (NO). NO then dilates the artery to accommodate more flow and optimize blood pressure and blood delivery to the areas that need it.

One of the secrets to great arterial health is maintaining a healthy glycocalyx. A healthy glycocalyx leads to a healthy endothelium, allowing the artery to dilate and constrict appropriately while making it resistant to the deposition of cholesterol and the development of atherosclerotic plaque and inappropriate blood clotting. Several different mechanisms can destroy the glycocalyx, but the biggest are sugar, toxins, and tobacco. The typical American diet is very high in sugar, and it destroys the glycocalyx.

When the glycocalyx is damaged—after we've eaten a meal high in sugar—nitric oxide production is limited. The arteries don't dilate appropriately. Sexual function is impaired, and over time, erectile dysfunction ensues. Exercise capacity and the heart's ability to pump blood are compromised. High sugar and high insulin build-up of senescent cells in the arterial wall makes them stiff and unresponsive. Blood pressure goes up, and sexual function gets even worse. Remember, excess insulin and growth hormones, such as IGF-1, increase cellular senescence throughout the body.

When you look at it through this lens, heart disease is a glycocalyx disorder that is largely controlled by what we eat.

Measurement and Optimization

There is a way to restore the glycocalyx. We use a supplement, Arterosil, to improve glycocalyx function we recommend taking it with every meal. Arterosil is made from a seaweed variety called Monostroma nitidum. The molecule rhamnan sulfate was isolated from Monostroma nitidum and has been shown to restore the glycocalyx and its function in humans.

There will always be something in a meal that's not perfect, so we take it with every meal. Arterosil can stabilize and reverse plaque in carotid arteries, which improves arterial function. When you have better arterial function, you have better exercise capacity, a healthier heart, better blood pressure, better sexual function, and better brain health and function.

We tend to think about heart disease formation as a long, slow, drawn-out process. But the glycocalyx and heart/cardiovascular disease is immediately caused when we eat, drink, or inhale something that damages the glycocalyx. We did a study in my practice where we tested twenty volunteers using a device called Max Pulse, which enables us to look at arterial blood flow and arterial status. After collecting a baseline test on each volunteer, we administered a dose of Arterosil, then tested them again after thirty minutes, sixty minutes, ninety minutes, two hours, and three hours. About 85 percent showed significant improvement in blood flow and arterial compliance, or elasticity, within thirty to sixty minutes of taking the Arterosil. Some of the gains were quite dramatic. When the glycocalyx is repaired, the artery will start to work better very quickly.

There is a flip side to this. Yes, you can think of heart disease progressing slowly and chronically, but when you break it down after seeing results like we observed, the arteries are being damaged when we eat sugar; so, when you think about eating that Big Mac®, fries, and a Coke®, you're causing heart disease with each bite and gulp. That's not a slow, chronic progression that will catch up to you years later; that's each moment, each second, an immediate response that destroys the glycocalyx causes cholesterol levels to go up, and triglycerides to go up. The endothelium is damaged and becomes dysfunctional. It can no longer dilate the way it is supposed to, which drives blood pressure up, and it becomes vulnerable to cholesterol being deposited inside of it; this is not an abstraction. The idea that "maybe just one won't hurt me" disappears when you realize how sensitive the system is.

Dr. Caldwell Esselstyn, a cardiothoracic surgeon at Cleveland Clinic, noticed some of his patients who had undergone bypass surgery were returning for second and third bypasses. They all had special heart scans that showed significant decreases in blood flow relative to normal. Physically, they were very limited in what they could do;

they had chest pain, could hardly walk, and had shortness of breath.

If you know how scarred someone's internals are after even one bypass surgery, a third or even fourth time is an almost-impossible task. Dr. Esselstyn got to a point where there was nothing left that he could offer these patients, so he put them on a vegetarian diet. Within about six to eight weeks, their scans had improved, and they could walk farther and do more. It just goes to show you the resilience of the human body when you remove the toxic standard American diet.

This is another key point, not only of cardiovascular health, but the whole process of making 100 the new 30 and staying 30 for the rest of your life: truly examining and answering the question, *What am I doing to myself that I should stop doing?* Then, think about what you can do to enhance your abilities. Instead, we tend to self-sabotage by thinking we'll address it "later" and shrug off choices, thinking one time won't hurt.

There are several different ways to test for cardiovascular health. Max Pulse gives us an idea of the heart's electrical power and also gives us an idea of arteries' elasticity and ability to constrict. These metrics are used to provide an index of arterial function.

In addition, we like EndoPAT®, a non-invasive, minimally uncomfortable endothelial dysfunction test that measures arterial stiffness and the artery's ability to dilate after a period of reduced blood flow. In this particular test, you wear a blood pressure cuff on your arm for about five minutes; when it's released, your arm is now hungry for blood. How vigorously and completely your arteries dilate in response to this gives great insight into the age of your arteries.

Other tests that may be administered include an ultrasound of an artery, an echocardiogram (an ultrasound of the heart), cardiac MRI, and coronary calcium scores. When looking at a coronary calcium score, it is critical to note that calcium is the tip of the iceberg when estimating plaque burden. It is possible to have a great deal of plaque with very little calcium. Also, keep in mind that calcium throws off the accuracy of a CT angiogram and a Cleerly CT angiogram.

A Cleerly CTA is a CT angiogram that is non-invasive and utilizes contrast to outline arteries like a coronary angiogram would do. In addition, the AI software can characterize any plaque found and create a three-D rendering of the artery the same way coronary ultrasound would do. This can be very useful in assessing high- and medium-risk individuals if you understand the limitations of the test. If someone has had a stent placed in a heart artery it will deflect the X-rays and the test is less reliable, especially in revealing what might be happening within the stented area. In addition, if someone has decreased kidney function the amount of contrast needed to do the test can be toxic to the kidneys. Limitations aside it can still be a very useful test to look at the anatomy of the heart arteries.

If you have a high calcium score, there is a higher probability that you'll have a cardiac event. Plaque starts as soft; over time, it becomes fibrotic and calcified. The body will calcify chronically inflamed areas. When I see the presence of calcium, I know that plaque is there. What's critical at that stage is whether soft plaque is present because soft plaque can be biologically active and rupture—that's how a blood clot forms, causing a heart attack.

The gold standard for assessing the anatomy and physiology of an artery is the use of intracoronary ultrasound coupled with fractional flow reserve measurements. The ultrasound lets us see through the arterial walls and determine plaque burden and the degree of narrowing. The fractional flow reserve enables us to measure the physiologic significance of a blockage in obstructing blood flow. The Cleerly CTA combines both assessments utilizing a contrast agent injected intravenously and a simultaneous CT scan of the arteries. There are pitfalls to this approach, and it is less precise when more calcium is in the arteries, but it can non-invasively give one a very good idea of the coronary anatomy and, to some extent, physiology. At Gladden Longevity, we are fans of looking at the heart through multiple lenses to get an accurate picture of endothelial function, coronary artery anatomy, blood flow, heart pumping function, heart rhythm, and response to exercise.

A quick detour on the calcification of the arteries: Taking calcium without Vitamin K2 may increase calcium deposition in your coronary arteries and raise your coronary calcium score. In addition, taking a statin drug virtually always increases the coronary calcium score while statistically decreasing heart-attack risk. You can see that if you simply want to define your risk by a coronary calcium score, you are missing the boat. It is a test with some utility but must be interpreted in a broader context of testing.

Too many people get full-body scans, thinking they eliminate risk or find problems early. While there is a modicum of truth to this, many people are being misled into thinking they are healthy when they are not or have a problem when they do not. Be skeptical if someone or an organization is promoting the scans they do as the major technology in helping you understand your health.

Plaque and cholesterol build-up in the arterial wall can be predominantly calcified, fibrous, or soft. Calcified plaque is rather inert. Fibrous plaque is more physiologically active, but soft plaque is the most physiologically active and most likely to cause an event like a heart attack or a stroke. If it turns out to be the soft plaque, it has a lot of Lp-PLA2, a platelet-activating enzyme that resides in soft plaque but can be detected in the blood; it increases the risk of a heart attack or stroke.

If the blood also contains elevated amounts of white-blood cell-derived myeloperoxidase, this can also increase the risk of heart attack and stroke. When elevated in combination, they are even more dangerous. A plaque has a fibrous cap that sits on top of the oxidized cholesterol, dead cells, and debris inside the plaque. The fibrous plaque can be either eroded from the inside-out by a LpPLA2, or outside-in, by myeloperoxidase. If this happens, the contents of the soft plaque spill into the blood. The passing blood thinks the artery has been "cut" when it contacts the eroded plaque and does what it is designed to do: form a clot.

Unfortunately, the clot cuts off blood flow to everything downstream from it, which causes tissue damage like a heart attack or a stroke. If the blood clot is big enough to close off the whole artery, the body will try to dissolve that blood clot.

To add another factor, if you have a particular form of cholesterol called LPa, you have less ability to dissolve the clot, which results in a bigger heart attack or stroke than if you had been able to dissolve the clot yourself. That's why you need to know not only your good and bad cholesterol but your LPa as well.

Angiography is another way to capture an image of the arteries, which involves placing a catheter into an artery and injecting dye to displace the blood. The result is a two-dimensional image of the inner contour of the artery. The technique is used to define the extent and location of blockages in the arteries. Additional evaluations can be done through a catheter.

Intracoronary ultrasound is a more accurate way to characterize arterial anatomy and blockages. I found it very helpful in understanding a patient's anatomy to achieve optimal results from a stent procedure. It can differentiate soft plaque, which is vulnerable to causing a heart attack, and more inert hard fibrotic or calcified plaque which is less apt to cause a heart attack.

It is critical to understand that properly evaluating heart function and blood flow requires assessments of both anatomy and physiology. Relying only on one or the other can be misleading. A Cleerly CTA, coupled with a Cardiopulmonary Exercise Test (CPET), is an ideal non-invasive way to make this assessment in higher-risk people. For screening purposes, a CPET is an excellent evaluation and, in my mind, trumps any other form of stress testing. As a cardiologist, I've learned that no one test is perfect or comprehensive enough to accurately characterize what is going on with the heart anatomically and physiologically. Don't be duped by anyone telling you all you need is a Cleerly CTA or a stress test and a cholesterol profile. The Cleerly CTA is a great test, but it is only part of the puzzle.

The carotid arteries in the neck may be used to evaluate the systemic arteries by using ultrasound to evaluate the carotid intima-media thickness. This test is called a CIMT. It measures the thickness of the artery, the plaque quality, and the burden. When older people have a "hardening of the arteries" and are prone to high blood pressure, this is due to senescent cells in the arterial wall making it thicker and stiffer. CIMT can give us an anatomic assessment of that thickening process and, subsequently, an anatomic age of the carotid arteries.

We rely heavily on The CPET test because it measures VO2 Max, anaerobic threshold, endothelial dysfunction, and lung function. In short, we can give your heart a functional age, assess your aerobic strength, understand if your glycocalyx and endothelium are working properly, and give you a lung age. VO2 Max is critical because it measures how much blood your heart can pump per minute. The more you can pump, the longer you live, the healthier you are while you're alive, and the less risk of dementia, cancer, Alzheimer's, and of course, heart disease you have. One critical message here is: *build your VO2.*

To build VO2, we have learned it takes both protracted cardio—thirty to sixty minutes of continuous cardio, three days a week, at 70 percent of your predicted maximum heart rate—and two days a week of interval training where you reach 90–100 percent of your predicted heart rate for 30–180 seconds repeatedly over twenty minutes.

Another key metric we like to check in the CPET is the "Peak O2 Pulse" or stroke volume. This indicates whether the left ventricle is able to increase its pumping ability in a linear fashion with the increasing level of exercise. As you exercise, your heart rate goes up, and the stroke volume, or amount of blood pumped with each beat, should also go up. When the increase deviates from this linear increase, it is indicative of an underlying pathology in the heart—any pathology can play a role—but typically, it will indicate microvascular, endothelial-mediated heart disease, where the arteries have enough endothelial and glycocalyx dysfunction that they can't dilate adequately to bring more blood to the heart muscle itself so that stroke volume can increase. Finding this deviation is one of the earliest signs of heart disease.

At Gladden Longevity, we love this test; I have been board-certified in cardiology, interventional cardiology, and nuclear cardiology, and I've done CT training. I've done stress tests, stress echos, PET scans, and the CPET test, by far, trumps all of those in terms of its ability to pick up early stages of heart disease and endothelial dysfunction. Likewise, the CPET can show progress in arterial function to let us know our interventions are working.

When we see that the left ventricle cannot increase its pumping capacity the way it should, we have observed that the heart rate will increase to compensate for it. This tell-tale increase in heart rate can be used to gauge severity and improvement in endothelial function and global heart function.

If I could only choose one biometric test to assess your heart, it would be the CPET test. There are other important tests, like genetics, blood work, and so on, but if you could only select one functional test, the CPET test is it.

When it comes to optimizing cardiac health, now is the time for you to start. Earlier, I mentioned that you can restore the glycocalyx, and the sooner you start, the better. Too often, I overhear someone reach for a high-sugar indulgence and say, "I know it's not good for me, but you know what? It's not a big deal."

No, it is a very big deal. The very second it reaches the arteries, the damage is being done. That indulgence matters. And I think when people start to understand that, they take a little bit different view of their diet.

Regarding cardiovascular health, it is hard to beat a plant-based diet—not a vegetarian or vegan diet, but a diet rich in a variety of plants. A common question is whether there is enough protein in a plant-based diet. If you mix beans and rice, you get plenty of protein. All of the essential amino acids are there. That's why rice and beans are a staple dish in so many different cultures.

Soy is also another source of complete protein, but it has a lot of other issues with regard to unwanted hormone modulation, along with GMO sources that make us want to consume it only in small quantities. You can get plenty of protein from plants, particularly if you're wise about it.

For most of us, heart disease is, in part, self-inflicted. If we are willing to adjust our diets and exercise patterns, we can do a lot to improve the function of many systems, not just the cardiovascular system. Remember, the mosaics are interrelated and make an impact on each other.

The element nitric oxide (NO) perfectly demonstrates the interrelationship of the mosaics and how its enhancement benefits a number of body systems. Nitric oxide is essential for men and women for arterial health and sexual function. When you have more nitric oxide, arteries dilate. Most of us have heard of Viagra®, a prescription that works by blocking nitric oxide degradation. Back in the 1960s, Viagra® was developed as a potential antihypertensive medication for lowering blood pressure. It wasn't a great antihypertensive, but a notable side effect was improved erections, which launched a new niche product.

In order to optimize nitric oxide, however, it's one thing not to degrade it, but it is even more important to generate more of it. You can't save what you don't have. So, how do you increase the amount of nitric oxide your body makes?

Start by eating foods high in dietary nitrate, like kale, arugula, spinach, beets, and chard. Eating foods rich in dietary nitrate is like putting gas in your car. You can also take supplements that activate nitric oxide release, like Citrulline or Neo40® Pro. Once you've put gas in your tank with your diet and added the spark plug with Neo40® Pro, you can start making nitric oxide immediately.

When someone has chest pain, there is an area of the heart that is blood-starved. When they take nitroglycerin, it initiates the production of NO, which increases the diameter of blood vessels around the obstructed artery to enable collateral blood flow, which carries blood to the affected area of the heart that is starved for blood, and relieves the pain.

Nitric oxide is critical. The glycocalyx is critical. The endothelium is the master conductor of the entire orchestra here. If you get those things right and decrease cellular senescence in the arterial wall, heart disease, and high blood pressure can be reversed.

We've had patients arrive at Gladden Longevity struggling with high blood pressure and taking two, three, or even four medications. When they take the telomerase product, which re-lengthens telomeres and subsequently moves cells out of a senescent status, their blood pressures fall dramatically. We have observed tremendous results, so we feel like heart disease is quite manageable, but it does take a lifestyle change regarding what goes in your mouth, how often you eat, and the supplements you might need to take.

Another factor that occurs with cardiovascular aging is the development of more arterial oxidative stress. A molecule called RNOX is released as we age, increasing oxidative stress on the arterial wall and generating senescent cells in the arterial wall.

RNOX starts to increase around age forty. We've seen some common supplements, like fish oil and Vitamin D, that can help slow this release, but the real secret weapon here are the Mediterranean herbs. For many years, we wondered about The French Paradox—so many of them smoke and eat fat-laden foods, yet they are generally heart-healthy people. Was it the red wine they were drinking?

No, it's the fresh herbs they eat that contribute to their heart health. In all the "blue zones" around the world—located in Italy, Japan, Costa Rica, and so on—people are eating very nutrient-dense herbs, whether in the form of algae or herbs they grow, with summer savory and basil being particularly heavy-hitters. Tarragon and rosemary also play a role, and together, they are even more potent. This explains why a ninety-five-year-old Mediterranean has the stamina to work in the garden. In many cases, they are also living in a vertically integrated family, where there are multiple generations at the dinner table, giving them a sense of connection and community.

When you consume those herbs, you inactivate RNOX for different periods of time and to different degrees. Gladden Longevity has combined the herbs into a tincture called The Blood Vessel Formula that can be added to tea or water, so you can get doses of summer savory, basil, tarragon, and EGCG throughout the day. Personally, I will add fresh basil to a variety of dishes or salads throughout the week. If I had to land on a "magic bullet" when it comes to arterial health, those fresh, nutrient-dense Mediterranean herbs would be it.

One thing you can do if you do decide to eat some sugar or quick-release carbohydrates is to take Sugar to Fiber 1-2 hours prior. This supplement mentioned earlier turns 50-90% of the sugar to fiber and fructose and will dramatically decrease the glucose and insulin spikes thereby protecting your arteries.

In order to Live Young, you must have a cardiovascular system that is in great shape and able to perform at levels decades younger than your chronological age. At Gladden Longevity, we have many clients, including myself, who are doing just that.

CHAPTER TWENTY-EIGHT

Lungs

D id you know that the astronauts who went to the moon in 1969 came back with a lot of respiratory issues? The dust on the moon was so fine that it got through their filtration systems and lodged in their lungs.

Since the heart and lungs work so closely together, after discussing heart health, lung health is a logical segue in the overall Health Mosaic of Living Young. To be frank, you do not want to lose lung capacity; having infections or smoking (including second-hand smoke) will decrease lung capacity but it also decreases with aging.

Air quality, particularly since most of us live in cities, is a very important factor to consider in the loss of lung function integrity and capacity. Populations aggregate into cities, and that creates a lot of pollution. Damage to our lungs is happening all the time, not only from vehicle and industrial exhaust but also from particulate matter in the air.

You can tell when you're exposing yourself to good-quality air, yet we don't readily seek it out. The cleanest air in the world right now can be found in Puerto Rico, New Caledonia in the Pacific Ocean, and the U.S. Virgin Islands. I happen to live part-time at the beach on the north shore of Puerto Rico, right next to the El Yunque rainforest. There is almost always a trade wind blowing east to west; the air quality here is exceptionally good—no smell of hydrocarbons. Frequent rainfall cleanses it, and I love breathing this air.

But I'm not always there to breathe this beautiful, clean air; you may live in a more polluted environment, too. So how can we clean up what we are breathing in?

Some companies will visit your home or office to analyze the air quality. Many will design filtration systems that fit the HVAC system to optimize your air. There are filtration systems that will filter particulate matter; the finer the filter's grid, the more force it takes to push air through it.

Some filtration systems use ozone to help purify the air. It makes the air smell a little bit like it does after a lightning storm, and there's not enough ozone to damage your lungs (ozone itself in the lungs is damaging). These systems will take out a lot of the particulates, bacteria, and viruses that are in the air. Other systems rely on filtration to remove particulates and other technologies to kill viruses, bacteria, inhibit mold growth, etc.

Having air purifiers in your home, investing in higher-grade HVAC filters, and not exposing yourself unnecessarily to fumes and smoke helps preserve lung function and control allergies. Decreasing particulate matter and reducing toxins is also helpful. The amount of air you can move—your lung capacity—typically goes down with age, so maintaining a large lung capacity is important.

Measurement and Optimization

We assess lung function via cardiopulmonary exercise tests. These tests measure lung capacity—the volume of air you can move in a single breath and how quickly you can exhale the air out of your lungs. Those metrics are key because different people have different chests and lung sizes. Some people are barrel-chested and have very large lung capacity. They can dive down below the water and hold their breath for five minutes without difficulty. Others have smaller chest cavities with smaller lungs and don't have the same capacity. Obviously, those with good lung capacity make better endurance athletes, but whatever your lung capacity is, having it measured will help you see where you fall relative to your chronological age and where you would fall relative to your youthful age. Your lung age is a function of how much air you can move and how quickly you can move it.

You can build lung capacity through aerobic exercise, but you can also build it by increasing the work that the lungs have to do. An Elevation Training Mask and a device called Aerofit are training devices that assist in this. When you breathe through either of these, there is resistance to airflow. You have to pull harder to get air through the device into your lungs and then exhale harder to get the air to go out so you can get the next breath.

Think of the lung anatomy as a tree. The main trunk is the trachea, which keeps branching and branching to the leaves. The leaves are the alveoli, where the action is—where the capillaries come in contact with the air. That's where the blood releases carbon dioxide, and oxygen is added to the hemoglobin in the red blood cells. The elevation training mask also adds dead space, which is the part of the airway not associated with gas exchange. The air has to travel through all that dead space before reaching the alveoli. That's just the cost of doing business, getting the air down there, and then getting it back out. So when you put a mask over your face, and now you've got a cavity in front of your face that you have to fill with air and then expel through, you've just added more dead space. It's more challenging to pull in the air because of the resistance that the mask is providing, but you also have to pull in *deeper* because you need more volume to fill the extra dead space. In doing so, you're expanding your lungs further and exercising your diaphragmatic and intercostal muscles (the muscles between your ribs).

Another metric of the cardiopulmonary exercise test is the maximum voluntary ventilation (MVV). This is a calculation of how much air you can move in a minute. You breathe hard, fast, and deep for about twelve seconds and then multiply by five to estimate how much air you could move in a minute at the maximal ventilatory effort. You don't perform this for a full minute, or you will hyperventilate and probably pass out. Your MVV indicates the strength of the diaphragm and the intercostal muscles and can be improved with training using the Elevation Training Mask or Aerofit.

CHAPTER TWENTY-NINE

Sex Hormones, Blood, Urine, and Saliva

I t's fairly common knowledge that when we go through puberty, our estrogen, progesterone, and testosterone levels go up, along with our libido, and sexual activity eventually follows. We also know that as we go through life, women go through menopause, and men go through andropause.

A decrease in hormone levels for a woman may lead to hot flashes, changes in skin tone, bone density, heart function, breast composition, and vaginal mucosal thickness and lubrication. Her libido and the ability to perform sexually without pain can become an issue.

In the past, a lot of anti-aging has been devoted primarily to hormone replacement therapy, which has led to a lot of controversy. About twenty years ago, a women's health initiative suggested that women who received post-menopausal hormones, synthetic estrogen, and progestin had an increased incidence of breast cancer. The study was flawed in many ways, and they used hormones that were not bioidentical. When the same study was conducted in Scandinavia using bioidentical hormones, the outcome was the exact opposite. (I need to state that we think synthetic progesterone is a bad choice because it increases breast cancer risk. It's worth mentioning that all birth control pills use synthetic progesterone.)

I think it's incredibly important for women to understand their genetic risk for cancer, heart disease, and dementia before they initiate hormone replacement. If you have a strong family history of breast cancer or other cancers, you definitely should request a conversation with your provider about whether or not hormones are right for you. I would recommend seeking a functional medicine doctor and having your hormones tested to see if they need to be replaced.

Generally speaking, women who undergo treatment with bioidentical hormone replacement, including estrogen, progesterone, testosterone, and DHEA, feel better. They have more vigor and energy, and their skin tone looks better. Their libido returns, and they are less ravaged by some of the emotional changes that occur with menopause, like anxiety and brain fog. They retain better bone density and muscle mass. However, balancing the hormones for an individual is an art and is not a one-size-fits-all solution.

It turns out that the sweet spot for starting BioIdentical Hormone Replacement Therapy (BHRT) is within ten years of menopause. It's not that they can't be started after that, but that seems to be the sweet spot for women to receive the best benefit. A younger age for the onset of menopause also correlates to a shorter life expectancy. The ovaries age at two and a half times the rate of the rest of the body. There are studies being done now to slow the ovarian rate of aging as a mechanism to slow aging in general for women.

The other important thing to know about hormones is that I think they are inappropriately tested most of the time, and traditional medical professionals in the female health space don't seem to understand how hormones are tested or replaced in the functional medicine space. Their concept of hormone replacement is to give somebody estrogen for hot flashes. We feel replacing estrogen without progesterone to counterbalance it is problematic. I have spoken with a number of these professionals through the years about this, and they are hung up on the fact that hormones are only indicated for symptom relief. They are missing the boat—many other health benefits are at play here.

The bottom line is that testosterone becomes estrogen for both men and women. Women make more estrogen from their testosterone than men do, but how that estrogen is subsequently metabolized has a lot to do with the risk factors for endometrial cancer, breast cancer, and prostate cancer. Those metabolic pathways can be managed with testing and supplements. Going into hormone replacement without having your hormone metabolites tested as part of the ongoing process potentially puts you at risk. Although hormone replacement isn't always indicated for men or women, it is critical, regardless, to have comprehensive hormone and hormone metabolite testing done. Given your underlying risk-benefit analysis, a conversation with your doctor will help you decide what is best.

Men go through andropause, which means lower androgen levels, like testosterone. Andropause also lowers DHEA and testosterone metabolites, like dihydrotestosterone (DHT), which on the downside, is associated with male-pattern baldness and prostate enlargement. DHT, however, is also associated with improved muscle mass and libido, so finding the right balance of DHT is critical.

Men in andropause can also become more estrogen-dominant. With reduced testosterone, they can also become more irritable and less able to handle stress. Too much testosterone, however, will increase aggression and irritability. For the sake of their intimate relationships, optimizing testosterone is generally helpful if it's done right. It's also beneficial regarding sexual function, libido, sense of well-being, and cardiovascular performance.

Just like women, it's very important for men to have their hormones and hormone metabolites tested—not just testosterone levels. You need to see the complete blood panel and your urine metabolites to understand where you are. Embryologically, breast and prostate tissue came from the same cells, making both tissues hormonally sensitive. This is why, when the wrong metabolites are building up—like 4OH Estrone, for example—it can increase the risk of breast cancer in women and prostate cancer in men.

One of the problems I see with most testosterone clinics is that they put men on testosterone without checking the hormone metabolites. They put them on anastrozole to keep them from converting testosterone into estrogen so they remain more "testosterone-dominant." In fact, men need estrogen just like women need testosterone; they just need it in different amounts. Estrogen helps men lose belly fat and is also great for brain function, cardiovascular health, and libido. Over-stimulation by androgens over time also decreases their effectiveness. Balance is key!

It's not about, *How much testosterone can I have?* It's about, *Do I have my hormone system optimally balanced?*

That's what you are going for. The health benefits of optimal balance are massive. The benefits of returning to sexual activity are compounded with oxytocin release, relational satisfaction, and improved resilience.

This book is not going into all the different types of testosterone replacement. I will say that topical testosterone is more heavily metabolized into dihydrotestosterone, which can cause prostate enlargement and potentially fan the flames of prostate cancer. It does increase libido and muscle mass but has the downside of having some of those prostate effects.

Also, be aware that injectable testosterone is not bioidentical. If injected once a month, you'll have a very high level and strongly activate the mTOR portions of your physiology, not the AMPK. Later in the month, as it wears off, you will be testosterone depleted. You'll go from feeling great to feeling poorly. The same can occur with pellets.

The release of testosterone from the pellets in men or women is a function of cardiac output. The more aerobically active you are, the faster you pull the testosterone out of the pellet and into your system. Your practitioner may tell you the pellet is good for three months, but that may or may not be true. You may run through it in six or eight weeks particularly if you're physically active.

Oral testosterone can be used, but it has some effects on the liver that aren't desirable. For some, however, that's the only form of testosterone they can tolerate.

At Gladden Longevity, we prefer dosing women with testosterone topically on an every day to every-other-day schedule. However, if they experience side effects, we will switch to intramuscular injections. We prefer to treat men with testosterone by injection twice a week to help them have smoother, more regulated testosterone levels.

When we are focused on longevity, healthy people may consider dosing with rapamycin on a once-every-three-weeks schedule to modulate mTOR expression. Rapamycin has a half-life, on average, of sixty hours. It takes four half-lives to eliminate the drug: 4 x 60 = 240 hours = 10 days. We use this information to currently suggest that rapamycin be dosed every other week or every third week.

Simultaneously, we focus on even more intense AMPK activation during the seven to ten days following the rapamycin. We use a client-appropriate choice of a five-day fast mimicking diet, intermittent fasting, saunas, Vinea (a more potent Resveratrol), Pterostilbene, Hydroxyberberbine, Metformin, Curcumin, Alpha Lipoic Acid, EGCG, Genistein, and Quercetin, all to activate AMPK. In addition, we recommend Mimio to enhance the benefits of fasting. It appears Mimio can provide the benefits of fasting even if you are eating normally.

When it comes to hormone replacement, there isn't an absolute right and wrong answer; you need to work with your practitioner to figure out what is best for you in order to end up in a balanced position.

Measurement and Optimization

Remember, biology is an economy of balance. This is not a question of "men's hormones" and "women's hormones." Hormones are interwoven and should be tested in a similar fashion—and then treated appropriately. I have already stressed the importance of speaking with your doctor and having your hormones properly tested. Here is a list of which hormones to test.

- Estrogen
- Testosterone
- DHEA
- Sex hormone-binding globulin
- Progesterone
- Testosterone Metabolites
- Dihydrotestosterone
- Growth Hormone/IGF-1
- Free testosterone

Those are all measured through blood tests, and most are also measured through saliva tests. This is a conversation for those who are not on any hormone replacement. You would also want a urine test that measures how you are metabolizing your hormones.

For post-menopausal women, I think having an annual vaginal ultrasound to look at the thickness of the endometrium is also very important, along with breast exams or breast MRIs. We're not big on mammograms because of the X-ray dose that is delivered.

Now for men, I strongly recommend they be proactive about optimizing prostate function. It is possible to get to a point where your testosterone levels are adequate for you to feel good, and your prostate is also working well through a combination of different interventions, either through supplements, like saw palmetto and boron, or medications like, low-dose finasteride, or procedures like steam therapy to reduce prostate size.

I think screening for cancer before and during hormone replacement is very important for both men and women—breast cancer and endometrial cancer for women and prostate cancer for men. For prostate cancer, a digital exam is almost useless as an early detection technique or preemptive diagnosis, and a prostate-specific antigen (PSA) test is not particularly sensitive or specific, either. PSA is most useful if someone already has prostate cancer, as it indicates whether it's getting worse or better, but as a preemptive diagnostic tool, it lacks sensitivity and specificity. A %Free PSA has been shown to be most helpful when PSAs are over ten, but we like to look at it to see how it is trending even with lower PSA numbers. Ideally, you want a low PSA (under one) and a high %Free PSA (over thirty). It's not a guarantee, however, that men with these numbers are safe, and we use additional follow-up testing described below.

There are exosome tests that can be done to look to see whether or not your prostate is secreting signatures of cancer cells into the urine. We've not been impressed with the sensitivity or specificity of heavily marketed blood tests for cancer, like Grail, and have used a lab in Greece to screen for circulating tumor stem cells. If they are present, there are no false positives; if they are not, false negatives are still possible. There are other tests on the horizon that we believe will be able to detect cancer accurately from a simple blood test.

Regardless, if you are going to use hormones, you want to be doing regular screenings at least once a year to make sure that you are not developing any cancer.

For men with suspicious findings, a dedicated 3T MRI can help define a PIRADS Score of 0–5.

PI-RADS classification	Definition
I	Most probably benign
II	Probably benign
III	Indeterminate
IV	Probably malignant
V	Most probably malignant

In the past, prostate biopsies were done blindly after an MRI showed a suspicious area, meaning the prostate was not imaged at the time of biopsy but randomly probed. Advancement led to ultrasound-guided biopsies after a 3T MRI. Co-registration to synchronize the ultrasound with the previously done MRI can be used to enable the urologist to target the suspicious area more precisely. Now things have progressed to where the biopsy can be done directly during the MRI. Using MRI guidance gives the best chance of precisely getting a sample of the suspicious tissue.

Some men are concerned that any biopsy may incidentally spread tumor cells and opt for alternative therapies without a biopsy. While there is risk in a biopsy, there is also a risk in not knowing what you are dealing with—and at this point, we are in favor of understanding the problem so we can devise the best treatment plan.

Therapy can now be done under direct MRI guidance using Trans-Urethral Ultrasound Ablation (TULSA). TULSA uses ultrasound energy to heat the prostate tissue and ablate the targeted cells effectively. Precision is key in ablating prostate tissue to minimize the collateral damage to the nerves and arteries essential for erectile function, and TULSA provides this level of accuracy. Using TULSA enables either a partial or complete prostate removal with real-time confirmation that the tissue was adequately heated and, therefore, ablated.

CHAPTER THIRTY

Sexual Function

One of the greatest gifts to our health, longevity, and psychology is sexual activity. The benefits of sexual activity are enormous, on par with exercise and good sleep. Those with more sexual activity and orgasms live longer, and men have less prostate cancer. Some would argue that this is true because healthier people have more sex. It works both ways; people who have more sex stay healthier, physically and psychologically; likewise, physically and psychologically healthier people have more sex.

If you think that health is a function of optimizing both the psychospiritual and physiological elements, then it stands to reason that sexual function does both—whether we are with a partner or, to a lesser extent, by ourselves. When we climax, oxytocin is released. Many people know oxytocin as "the love hormone," but, as mentioned previously, it is also known as the "milk let-down hormone" because it is released in both the mother and the baby during breastfeeding. Oxytocin increases the sense of social bonding, attachment, and connection. Oxytocin is low in autism, and replacing it can improve social bonding for people with autism.

When you think about older people that live in isolation—perhaps they've lost a spouse, lost their friends, or whatever the reason—isolation is one of the worst things that can happen to them. It's why prisoners are put in solitary confinement as the severest form of punishment. People in solitary confinement experience a dramatic decline in their health simply because of the lack of social contact. Remember, quality relationships, i.e., quality social contact, is one of the Life Energies we discussed in Part One, and oxytocin is one of the key elements that impact life energy, longevity, health circles, and their mosaic of ages.

When someone is isolated, there is lower oxytocin. Oxytocin has been shown to mitigate the shortening of telomeres. Oxytocin is also an anti-inflammatory molecule; if you're fighting aging and increasing inflammation, having oxytocin in your system is a great thing to have. Sexual activity is one of the best ways to release oxytocin, but it also happens with a twenty-second hug, an eight-second kiss, or seeing someone you love.

Erectile function is a great way to measure your cardiovascular-nervous system status. Erectile function is the first thing to go when the cardiovascular system starts to fail. In fact, think of erectile dysfunction as an early indicator of cardiovascular disease. When men start to notice that they need Viagra®, it's time to ask what's going on with the cardiovascular system.

When we work with couples, one of the first things we notice when one or both of them is going through the aging process, they have forgotten that to be successful in a relationship, you must continue to recreate it. To explore, create novelty, have fun, let go of the past, and find new joy in today. Instead, they fall into routines and familiar patterns, and suddenly, it becomes boring. Usually, someone is suffering from age-related sexual issues, like erectile dysfunction or vaginal dryness. In either case, the other partner doesn't want to impose or make the other person physically or psychologically feel bad, so they stop pursuing intimacy.

They start to pull away, and when the urge to have sexual activity arises, they repress it. This is one of the worst things we can do. For lack of a better analogy, it's a bit like constipation. The key to regular bowel movements is to give in to the urge; when you repress or suppress it, you are changing your nervous system in a way that will make it more difficult to have that bowel movement in the future. You can wind up with terrible constipation. Coming back to sex, repressing the urge for intimacy will diminish your ability to have and enjoy it. Use it, or lose it!

Measurement and Optimization

When it comes to measuring cardiovascular function, we love the cardiopulmonary exercise test because we get an early look at whether there is a problem with the endothelium. We do a CPET on anyone complaining of erectile dysfunction. Not all erectile or sexual dysfunction is due to cardiovascular issues; it can be linked to nerve damage due to diabetes or surgery and can also result from psychological issues like depression, anxiety, PTSD, and prior physical or psychological abuse. These things can obviously impair someone's ability to participate in sexual activity, but apart from them, sexual performance is an excellent indicator of vascular health.

In terms of optimization: If you have the urge to be close and intimate, it doesn't have to include sexual intercourse. As we said, you can boost oxytocin by hugging somebody for twenty seconds or kissing for eight seconds. Regardless, within the confines of your ethics and relationship parameters, if you have the urge to engage in any sort of sexual activity or intimacy, you should act on it—it enables the release of oxytocin, creates closeness, lowers your psychological stress, and also keeps your physiology working. You and your partner can find ways to make it fun and introduce creativity, romance, magic, and joy into it. It's okay to get a bit wild!

Sexual function is a metric of your physical and relational health. And just like exercise, the more you and your partner practice, the better it gets. All of a sudden, you're creating a really, really healthy, playful, fun, life-giving habit!

We have recently encountered a product that builds libido and sexual performance from BioProtein called BioPro+™. It contains numerous trophic or growth factors, as well as IGF-1. It works well, and it's not necessary to take it every day after an initial period of daily use for 7-10 days. Remember, too much of a good thing is bad, so if you use it, use it in moderation.

Earlier, we mentioned the benefit of a high-nitrate diet regarding heart health. Foods like kale, arugula, spinach, chard, and Mediterranean herbs found in the Gladden Longevity "Blood Vessel Formula" provide the fuel for us to release nitric oxide and keep our arteries healthy and our erectile function strong. These, plus Arterosil (which restores the glycocalyx) and Neo40® Pro, which causes instant nitric oxide production, and you're in business. Remember, everything that is good for your heart is good for your sex life, and almost everything good for your sex life is good for your heart.

CHAPTER THIRTY-ONE

Brain Function

Writer Joseph Campbell, author of *The Hero with a Thousand Faces,* deconstructed all the stories across all cultures, generations, and eras. He concluded that all stories can be boiled down to one story, which he called "the hero's journey."

Simply put, there are three components to the hero's journey:

1. Someone faces a challenge. In many cases, it is a coming-of-age, growth challenge, which is a challenge to reclaim a birthright.
2. In order to rise and meet the challenge, the hero leaves what is familiar and embarks on a journey that entails elements beyond their current capabilities, facing overwhelming odds to reclaim their

birthright. They learn something along the way and transcend the life they had before.

3. After completing the challenge—and having gone through an intense burst of personal growth to the point of transcendence—they return home, triumphant and transformed. They then share their story and the insights, wisdom, capabilities, and virtues they have learned and acquired. Doing so enables them and others to forge a new future where they can truly be their unencumbered, best version of themselves and elevate their community.

The number one thing the hero's journey requires is courage. It requires putting aside assumptions previously held to be true. It demands adaptation, growth, grit, and resilience to ultimately accomplish the challenge of reclaiming their birthright, being their unencumbered self, and living their best lives.

All of us are on our own hero's journey to reclaim our birthright of optimal health, longevity, performance, and life energy. I see myself as a participant and a mentor to you on this journey along with me. Each one of us faces challenges. We have all run a gauntlet of some sort, during which our brains were programmed to live in reaction to the "traumas" we have experienced. The environment in which we reside and the traumas we experience shape our sense of reality and possibility. Our hero's journey is to transcend those limitations. What we believe and think is possible *is* possible.

When we think about transforming our own life—our health, our longevity, our performance, and certainly our life energy—there is nothing more important than understanding that the brain's preprogrammed software is running the show. Therefore, our primary task in our hero's journey is to reprogram our brain's software. In doing so, we can optimize what we perceive reality to be. We can open the door to do what otherwise would have been impossible.

The programs running in our brains create a fictional reality. If the real key to unlocking life, energy, longevity, health, and performance is reprogramming the brain's software, what software is currently running in your brain? In other words, what is it that you believe to be true? I believe 100 can be the new 30, live well beyond 120, and live our best, most productive, generative, and impactful lives. The questions I'm asking drive the innovation to make it so. What questions are you asking? Are you married to your current answers? What are the unseen biases that are shaping your reality and your possibilities?

Confirmation bias is a term to describe how our software tends to prioritize information. It states that we are more apt to give credence to information that confirms what we already believe. These software programs were instilled during our upbringing and expanded on as we ran the gauntlet of obstacles in our path, leading us to a fabricated sense of security. Underneath it all, I find we all have a deep longing to know and be known, to love and be loved, and to be safe. The software currently running sabotages our opportunity to optimize our life energy, longevity, health, and performance. Some of the more common self-limiting software constructs are:

- *I'm not worthy.*
- *My parents died at this age, and so will I.*
- *It's in my genes; my fate is inevitable.*
- *I don't like to exercise, and I never will.*
- *Feeling stressed is the only way I can get things done.*

- *I need to have a few drinks tonight. It's the only way I can relax.*
- *I need a cigarette to think clearly.*
- *My loved one is sick, so I am not going to take care of myself because I need to take care of them.*

What that translates into, among other things, is:

- *I'm going to derail myself from winning the exponential game of staying young.*
- *I am depressed and anxious because I don't feel safe.*
- *I can't do this now because I don't feel like doing it.*

We have all this software running in the background, and many times, the biggest hurdle to achieving our goals is overcoming the self-sabotaging software that's running. When you think of it like that, almost *all health optimization requires software reprogramming.*

The second thing to look at concerning brain health is brain function—specifically, cognitive function. There are eight forms of intelligence:

- Logical-mathematical intelligence
- Linguistic intelligence
- Spatial Intelligence
- Musical Intelligence
- Bodily-kinesthetic Intelligence
- Intrapersonal Intelligence
- Interpersonal Intelligence
- Naturalistic intelligence

We tend to think of ourselves as smart based on the grades that we got in school. In fact, those who perform best in school are often not very successful in life; they simply adapted to a scholastic system of thought that rewarded them for getting the "right" answer. So school intelligence doesn't translate into success in life.

Cognitive function at Gladden Longevity is assessed through computerized tests that examine memory, executive function, reflexes, reaction times, and processing speed. We also look at the individual's gifts; this indicates where their intelligence shines and gives us a roadmap to optimize them.

The brain makes an impact on every other category of health; likewise, every category of health makes an impact on the brain. For example, if your thyroid is low, you won't have optimal brain function. There is a gene that codes for an enzyme called DIO2, which is responsible for converting up to 80 percent of the inactive thyroid (T4) into active thyroid (T3) in the brain.

Those with mutations of DIO2—whether they are heterozygous or homozygous—experience a decrease in the conversion of inactive to active thyroid in the brain. Fifteen percent are homozygous for this deficit which can lead to depression, anxiety, and cognitive impairment. Another 20 percent are heterozygous. This is extremely important because if you're trying to optimize brain function and don't know your thyroid status and the genetic status of DIO2, no matter what you try, it's still not going to work properly. Thyroid replacement with T3 or a combination of T3/T4 is required to restore optimal function.

Likewise, sex hormones are important for brain function, particularly growth hormone, estrogen, and testosterone. You'll recall from an earlier section that women who go through menopause and receive any form of hormone replacement for any period of time reduce the risk of dementia by 30 percent, so optimizing sex hormones is essential to brain function both pre- and post-menopause or pre- and post-andropause.

Cardiovascular disease affects the brain dramatically. When the endothelium of the arteries is dysfunctional, not only does it affect the heart, but it affects the brain. The micro-vasculature (small blood vessels) of both are affected. In the brain, this amounts to a lack of blood flow and oxygen. Remember, the brain is the highest utilizer of energy per gram of tissue in the entire body. When it comes to optimal brain function and risk of dementia, some of the most important genes are:

- APOE & APOC1 in combination
- TOMM40
- MTHFR 677 & IL6174 separately and in combination
- MTHFD1L
- TNF
- PEMT
- CYP19A1
- MME
- ABCA7
- ABCB1
- BCHE

Genetically, you get half of a gene or allele from Mom and half from Dad. When it comes to APOE, you can get a two, three, or four from either parent. That configuration, whatever it may be, is directly related to your risk for dementia, cardiovascular disease, and longevity.

For example, those with the 2-2 configuration, which is only 1 or 2 percent of the population, get an extra year and a half of life over those with a 3-3 configuration. Those who have the 4-4 typically see their lives reduced by the same amount compared to 3-3. The 3-3s account for about 65 percent of the population. APOE4 is only a problem if it is coinherited with APOC1. This happens 70 percent of the time. You can be misled if you don't test all the relevant genes.

When both APOE4 and APOC1 are present, however, you will have an issue with something called *reverse cholesterol transport*, which is the process of getting cholesterol out of your cell membranes and back to the liver.

In this instance, cholesterol accumulates in the neurons, which stiffens up the cell membranes. A chemical reaction in the cell membrane processes amyloid through either an alpha or beta pathway, the latter residing in the cholesterol-rich, stiff portions of the membrane. Reverse cholesterol transport occurs in the non-cholesterol-rich pliable portions of the membrane; if you have good cholesterol reverse transport like those with APOE2, you will process your amyloid through the amyloid alpha pathway and not be affected by it. On the other hand, if you don't have good reverse cholesterol transport, as is the case with APOE4, you will process your amyloid through the beta pathway, leading to amyloid-beta accumulation within the brain, a hallmark of Alzheimer's.

You can see how critical it is to unravel the knot of your genetics, reverse cholesterol transport, and brain function. There is much more to this story, but I want you to know that unless you are working with someone who can fully unravel your particular knot, you will never get the results you are looking for.

I would be remiss not to revisit Chapter Twenty-Six and omit the significance of sleep concerning brain health. Our brains require great sleep to function well. During slow-wave or deep sleep, the glymphatic system is responsible for cleaning out the debris and toxins the brain accumulated the previous day. In a way, it's like a "night crew" that carries out the garbage while we are in deep, non-REM sleep. The glymphatic transport is most efficient with your right cheek on the pillow (as previously mentioned), as more cerebral spinal fluid is cleared in this position compared to being supine and prone. Poor glymphatic drainage can increase the risk of dementia by 30 percent.

Alcohol inhibits brain function, and caffeine or hydrogen will improve it. There was a small study done on sleep deprivation where they took college students and tested their cognitive abilities at baseline. Then they deprived them of sleep overnight, allowing them to have just a few hours of sleep before retesting them. There was a noticeable cognitive decline. They gave them caffeine, which improved their cognitive abilities.

That doesn't mean we should start drinking coffee non-stop—that defeats the purpose of getting good sleep. Interestingly enough, when the study students consumed molecular hydrogen instead of caffeine, it also improved their intellectual and cognitive capabilities—to the same extent as caffeine, but through a different mechanism.

I have experienced seven concussions in all my athletic endeavors. Obviously, I take brain health very seriously and have done the work to rebuild my brain. I strongly encourage you to do the same. Given the tremendous scientific advancements we're about to dive into, I have such a sense of hope around brain health. Here are a couple of things I want to underscore:

- It is possible to reprogram the software. You're not stuck with how you're currently thinking or feeling unless you believe you are. Many kinds of therapy, especially those including ketamine and plant medicines (i.e., Psilocybin or 5 MEO-DMT), seem to be very helpful at rewiring the brain in a positive way. Be careful who you do it with, and be sure you are in a therapeutic setting. Johns Hopkins is pioneering this work with Roland Griffiths, Ph.D., leading the charge.

- Ketamine may also help treat resistant depression, but it is not for everyone. Contraindications include blood pressure exceeding 140/80, psychosis, panic attacks, autism, and cardiovascular disease.

- It's possible to rebuild your brain. Once you deconstruct the issues and systematically address them, remarkable results are possible.

- Brain Frequency™ is a new technique developed at Windmill Wellness Ranch by Founder Shannon Malish, MSW. It is used to rebuild the brain and typically requires between twenty and forty sessions. The patient reclines in a chair at the office, and a magnet is strategically placed at three to four locations on the head. Low-level electromagnetic therapy is painlessly applied through the skull to the brain. The energy awakens neurons and stimulates nerve growth and development. This application can be used effectively for anxiety, depression, PTSD, concussions, strokes, traumatic brain injury, and addiction. A baseline EEG is performed and will be repeated every ten sessions at which point the treatment protocol is adjusted. Patients can expect to spend twenty to thirty minutes per session. We have incorporated the technology into Gladden Longevity and have been pleased with the results.

- Spiritual and energetic experiences, like meditation and plant-based medicines, are another way to reprogram the brain. Some suggestions include Eckhart Tolle's *The Power of Now* and apps like Insight Timer and Headspace that can teach you how to meditate.

Measurement and Optimization

When discussing measuring and assessing someone's brain function, Gladden Longevity analyzes life energy through conversation. This helps us understand the software is running and determine the hurdles, limitations, and stresses you face. From there, we usually dive back into the Life Energy mosaic to help you resolve those problems, gain new perspectives, and understand that you are an eternal being with amazing capabilities. We help you reach a place where you can feel safe, known, and loved. You can now recognize that there is a path forward on your hero's journey to reclaim your brain, your birthright, no matter how challenging.

Many people come to us complaining of brain fog, anxiety, depression, and memory issues, so we also schedule EEGs, MRI scans, or CTs. EEGs look at brain function and see how the brain functions at rest and in response to performing certain tasks, while the MRI scan identifies structural defects, like thinning of the cortex, loss of neurons, and so on. This information is very helpful when determining what courses of action should be taken.

The advances taking place in neuroscience are moving quickly. Shelley Jordan, M.D., a colleague at UCLA, pioneered a new functional MRI exam, which maps neural connections throughout the brain and looks for early signs of dementia, Parkinson's, Alzheimer's, non-Alzheimer's dementia, PTSD, and traumatic brain injury. Once we analyze someone to determine the cognitive ability of their brain and any anatomic issues they are dealing with, we have a clearer pathway to optimization.

Plasmalogens are a healthy fat usually found in cell membranes and critical for optimal brain function. Prodrome neuro-testing elucidates specific fat metabolism pathways important for optimal brain function. In his book, *Breaking Alzheimer's: A 15-Year Crusade to Expose the Cause and Deliver the Cure,* Dr. Dayan Goodenowe has curated the data that shows when plasmalogens are optimized, it significantly decreases the risk of cancer, heart disease, and dementia. In fact, you can take somebody genetically predisposed to dementia with APOE4 and APOC1 and revert them to having the same risk as someone who is APOE3 simply by optimizing their plasmalogen levels. This is a very exciting discovery, and we have put it to good use.

Goodenowe's work shows that optimal plasmalogen levels change cellular function to compensate for APOE4 and APOC1. The plasmalogens increase reverse cholesterol transport, reverting the cells to membranes that function more like an APOE3 and dramatically reducing the risk for Alzheimer's.

If you have a family history of dementia, understanding your genetics is key. In my situation, I don't have APOE4 or APOC1, but my father died with dementia. So my issues reside in the methylation cycle, where I don't make certain neurotransmitters very efficiently, and my inflammatory genetics, where I'm prone to neuroinflammation. Upon testing this cycle regarding your health, the right combination of B vitamins and anti-inflammatory supplements, like H2, and mushrooms, like Lion's Mane, Cordyceps, and Reishi, can help that cycle work properly. Gladden Longevity has developed a blend of five mushrooms—Gladden Longevity Shroom Formula—to decrease neuroinflammation. PEA or palmitoylethanolamide also has data that it reduces neuroinflammation, especially when combined with Luetiolin. We use a product called Mirica, which has this combination.

Dr. Dale Bredesen, a neurologist and currently Chief Science Officer at Apollo Health, is best known for The Bredesen Protocol® and his best-selling book, *The End of Alzheimer's*. Dr. Bredesen takes a very comprehensive look at all the things in both the internal and external environments that can affect the brain—the specifics are beyond the scope of this book, but we routinely test for all of them at Gladden Longevity: toxins, mold, heavy metals, genetics, thyroid function, and so on.

Remember the study I mentioned earlier, where twenty college students were sleep-deprived and then given caffeine? When the brain is fatigued, it generates increased oxidative stress. Think about the fatigue your muscles experience after you exercise; drinking hydrogen balances out the oxidation-reduction system known as redox, which regulates a lot of metabolic functions in the cell. You need the same to reboot your brain. When you've been thinking and working all day, your brain gets tired; by drinking hydrogen, you are not only making a safer choice than caffeine, you are addressing the root cause of that brain fatigue.

Hydrogen is very accessible, and it's very portable. It comes in tablet form and has some magnesium in it. You drop it into a glass of water, and it starts to effervesce, releasing hydrogen gas into the water. Once the tablet has dissolved, usually within two to five minutes, you drink it immediately and feel the effects in a few minutes.

Another supplement regimen we like is oral theacrine combined with ProdromeNeuro™, a plant-based plasmalogen-enhancing product produced by Prodrome Sciences. It is now available in soft gels. We also add Neural Rx™, a proprietary product produced by Wizard Sciences, into the mix. Combining these with a NAD precursor, like Nuchido Time™ or Beta NMN, to boost NAD works very well. We are now also adding Mirica to the mix. In our experience, layering a twice-weekly ozone sauna with a NAD precursor is the best way to optimize NAD levels and the NAD/NADH ratio.

We like peptides because they increase the ability of the brain to regenerate and rejuvenate itself. Semax or Selank as a nasal spray and oral Dihexa can increase brain-derived neurotrophic factor, BDNF, which helps the brain grow new neurons and neural connections and improves neuroplasticity.

The peptide Selank has pronounced anxiolytic activity and acts as a stable neuropsychotropic, antidepressant, and anti-stress peptide that relieves aggression and fear reactions in humans and other animal species. Some clients do better with Selank due to its calming effects, and others with Semax, which increases brain regeneration to a slightly greater extent.

BPC 157 is a peptide that, when given by subcutaneous (under the skin) injection, can increase the healing of neurons and the brain while balancing the neurotransmitters.

The peptide Cerebrolysin® can easily penetrate the blood-brain barrier to reach neurons directly, allowing for neuronal stimulation, intracellular peptide synthesis, and neuronal protection. It can improve cognitive ability and help after brain trauma. (Note: As of this writing, the FDA forbids practitioners and compounding pharmacies to dispense Cererbrolysin.)

Gladden Longevity currently uses a couple of cutting-edge technologies to assist with brain health. The first is a proprietary form of neurofeedback developed and exclusively performed by Dr. Drew Pierson in Carlsbad, California. While wearing an electroencephalogram (EEG) cap, the patient looks at a screen while the brain is trained. The sessions retrain the brain and can overcome the effects of concussions. They can also increase intuition, sense of balance, and cognitive ability. It requires a qualified practitioner who understands the best way to conduct your sessions. Patients who undergo this technique should plan for about two sessions per week because it's like a workout for your brain. You should also expect to feel tired immediately following each session. We drink molecular H2 after either a Brain Frequency session or after Neuro Feedback.

Another technology that we like to enhance cognitive ability is Brain Frequency, which, as we mentioned earlier, can be used to treat addiction, depression, and anxiety. Again, you will likely need twenty to forty sessions to get the full benefit.

Brain Frequency stimulates neuron growth, and many have seen a dramatic improvement in patients with traumatic brain injury, like multiple concussions, who have been incapacitated. Their patients now lead normal lives, start businesses, have good relationships, and feel cognitively sound. In addition, it is used to treat addiction and alcoholism. In our hands, combining these treatments with H2 and Nuchido Time or Beta NMN works well.

Trials are underway to demonstrate its benefits; from personal experience, I can tell you that my intuition and cognitive ability have improved significantly. When I combine Brain Frequency with neurofeedback, Nootropics, and peptides, I am much quicker and think much faster than

I used to. My brain is getting better. I test this by playing games on Lumosity and a game called Dual N-Back, studied at Johns Hopkins, which has been shown to improve cognitive ability. Both are available in your app store.

When it comes to optimizing your brain health, you have to understand its anatomy, physiology, and genetics. When you get all of that in order, you can bring the right technologies and therapies to rejuvenate your brain. In fact, it can function better than it has ever functioned up to this point!

There is also a role for stem cells, and we have had great results with these in rebuilding the brain, especially as technologies are intelligently layered together.

Optimizing trace minerals is also important and can be looked at with hair mineral analysis and repleted with products from Upgraded Formulas.

One final thought on microdosing. Microdosing Psilocybin in conjunction with Lions main mushrooms, B vitamins, and NAD precursors, has been shown to significantly increase neuroplasticity and creativity. It can accelerate the reprogramming process.

Some are also using microdoses of LSD and getting similar effects.

CHAPTER THIRTY-TWO

Bone

My mother was ninety-three and lived in a retirement community. She fell frequently and reported that others in her community were frequently falling. Over a three-year span, she broke both hips and her ribs. Her last fall resulted in a broken femur requiring surgery, and at age ninety-three, she did not have the physiologic reserve or will to rehab and passed away three weeks later.

Bone loss is a major contributor to the morbidity of aging; surprisingly, however, bone is a very active, metabolic tissue. Osteoblasts are constantly forming bone, and osteoclasts are constantly reabsorbing and remodeling bone. It is the balance between these two activities that determine our bone density.

The gold standard for measuring bone density is a dual-energy X-ray absorptiometry scan, better known as a DEXA scan. It is a very low-energy X-ray that maps body composition as well as bone density. We do it roughly once a year for our clients who have bone loss.

Osteoblasts are stimulated to make bone by weight-bearing exercise. OsteoStrong® is an exercise weight-loading system that builds bones by loading a person's body with a strong but controllable load for sixty seconds using a variety of dedicated, machine-based exercises. There are other ways to mimic this bone loading: an ARX machine, a squat rack, and free weights can all be used. The bottom line is that we build bone by asking bone to be strong, which means having it hold a load. The byproduct of these bone-strengthening exercises is stronger ligaments, tendons, muscles, and joints.

When addressing bone loss, hormone optimization is also important. Growth hormone, IGF-1, testosterone, estrogen, and progesterone are all required to build bone. A few terms need to be defined:

- *Osteopenia* is a decrease in bone density.
- *Osteoporosis* is a dramatic decrease in bone density.
- A *T score* is a comparison of your bone density to a group of same-sex thirty-year-olds with a range of -3 t0 +3.
- A *Z score* is a comparison of your bone density to a group of age, sex, and weight, matched controls again from -3 to +3. -3 to +3 will take into account 99.7 percent of everyone in the group.

When you do a DEXA, you will get both a *T* score and a *Z* score. A *T* score of -1 or above is considered normal, with higher numbers indicating denser bones. A *T* score of -2.5 to -1 defines the degree of osteopenia, with lower numbers indicating less bone density. A *T* score below -2.5

defines osteoporosis, again, with lower numbers indicating lower bone density. If you haven't had a DEXA scan, I suggest you get one to see where you are because bone loss is silent, and you likely won't feel anything even as your bones get dangerously weak.

We have seen many people with osteopenia or osteoporosis who take supplements like calcium, Vitamin D, Vitamin K2, boron, etc., and they rarely ever *increase* their bone density by simply taking these supplements. The problem with medications—usually antiresorptive medications, which primarily include a class of drugs called bisphosphonates and are administered by injections—is that they may make a bone scan look better on a DEXA scan, but they are not building strong bones that will resist a fracture. Without hormone replacement therapy and weight-bearing exercise, we have found it very difficult to rebuild bone. We have repeatedly seen that with hormone replacement, coupled with the right weight-bearing exercises and the right supplements, can show a slow, steady increase in real bone density.

Two supplements that are major contributors to healthy bone structure are Vitamin D and Vitamin K2. We typically get enough calcium in our diet, along with adequate amounts of boron, but it's very common for many people to have Vitamin D deficiencies, and we do not get enough Vitamin K2. According to Intellxx DNA reporting, Vitamin K2 decreases bone resorption; ALA, EGCG, curcumin, ashwagandha, sulforaphane, and quercetin also positively affect this bone resorption pathway. This is achieved by reducing osteoclast numbers and, in the case of ashwagandha and ALA, also increasing osteoblasts.

When we do DEXA scans on clients, one of the most vulnerable areas is the neck of the femur. When someone falls and breaks a hip, the fracture is usually located directly outside the ball-and-socket joint at the neck. With the DEXA scan, we also find that some become hypercalcified in their lower spine, which can lead to immobility.

Measurement and Optimization

Understand you are not building any bone in spin class or on the elliptical. You need weight-bearing exercise, and yes, running is weight-bearing.

We have already mentioned that the DEXA scan is usually how bone density is measured and how T and Z scores are calculated. We also measure a blood test, N-terminal telopeptide of type 1 collagen, NTX, to indicate the degree of active bone resorption.

When you're looking to optimize bone density, exercise is a great way to build it. Note there are greater benefits if you expand your exercise beyond just walking. Walking has its benefits, but if that is your only form of exercise, then you're not loading the skeletal frame in a way that creates bone density. You need to be doing squats, preferably underneath a bar, where you push up with resistance and load the frame for about sixty seconds; push as hard as you can and load the frame. It doesn't even take many reps or sessions—maybe two or three reps twice a week.

Lifting weights, wearing a weight vest, or anything you can do to load the frame with extra weight will result in enhancement and bone density if you're hormonally replete. We think it's better to build bone by the techniques we have listed above—optimizing hormones and supplements and then optimizing your weight-bearing exercises rather than taking medication. As we mentioned above, OsteoStrong®

is a nice "biohack" consisting of pieces of gym equipment that, when used in a series of load-bearing exercises, safely simulate the loading of high-impact activity and have been shown to increase bone density.

Some additional items to consider:

- Vitamin D3 to optimize estrogen-receptor activity.
- Vitamin K2 will increase the bone-building process by causing calcium deposition in the bone and has a separate effect to decrease the bone-loss process by blocking bone resorption. It also keeps calcium out of your arteries.
- Alpha lipoic acid (ALA) reduces bone loss by lowering oxidative stress and inflammation, which slows osteoclastic bone-resorbing activity.
- Boron to enhance the duration of Vitamin D effects in your body.
- Ashwagandha helps with bone calcification and increases the number of osteoblasts that make bone.
- Green Tea, or EGCG, to inhibit Metallopeptidase Inhibitor 2 (MMP2). Higher MMP2 activity is associated with greater degradation of the extracellular matrix, which therefore increases osteoporosis and fracture risk.
- Sulforaphane with myrosinase in Avmacol to trigger osteoblast activity and bone growth.
- Hair-mineral analysis can be used to optimize your mineral levels with products from Upgraded Formulas®.
- Special Pro-resolving Mediators (SPMs), which are downstream metabolites of fish oil with over two-hundred times the anti-inflammatory effects of fish oil. Take twice a day to down-regulate the

Receptor Activator of Nuclear Factor Kappa B (RANKL), which is responsible for the inflammation that drives bone loss.

- One scoop of Perfect Amino daily to build your bone matrix.
- Optimize fish oil levels of DHA and EPA as they inhibit bone breakdown, increase calcium absorption from the diet, and enhance calcium deposition in bone.
- CJC1295/Ipamorelin, three or four nights a week, to increase growth hormone release, which builds bone.
- Work with a functional medicine doctor to optimize all your hormones.
- Curcumin as UltraCur to optimize estrogen-receptor activity.
- Intermittently eat high-phosphorus foods (if kidney function is good), such as organ meats, walleye, pollock or sardines, nuts, and seeds, which are especially high.

The presence of phosphate is crucial for bone growth and mineralization; if absent in sufficient amounts, rickets and osteomalacia will develop.

CHAPTER THIRTY-THREE

Muscle

Muscle mass has been called a currency of aging. We lose muscle as we age, and it is critical we maintain it. Myopenia is the medical term for muscle loss from any cause such as illness or aging. Losing muscle as we age is in part a function of decreasing energy from the loss of mitochondria, and reduced hormone levels like testosterone and growth hormone that both build muscle. Evidence suggests that skeletal muscle mass and skeletal muscle strength decline in a linear fashion, beginning as early as the fourth decade of life, i.e., our thirties. Up to 50 percent of muscle mass can be lost by the eighth decade of life, i.e., our seventies.

The term typically used for age-related muscle loss is sarcopenia. Sarcopenia and Myopenia, however, can be used interchangeably. The cause of sarcopenia are many, including not only reduced anabolic signaling from loss of anabolic hormones, but lack of resistance training, poor protein intake, insulin resistance, obesity, and other chronic diseases of aging like cellular senescence and inflammation. "Sarcopenia: Aging-Related Loss of Muscle Mass and Function," an article published in 2019 by the National Institute of Health National Library of Medicine's Institute for Biotechnology Information, states that muscle function ultimately progressively declines because of motoneuron loss. A motor neuron is a nerve that innervates a single muscle fiber and causes it to contract and relax. With aging, motor neuron loss is not adequately compensated for by reinnervation of the muscle fiber by the remaining motoneurons, and the muscle fiber atrophies. Therefore, muscle loss is not primarily a loss of the fibers but a loss of the nerves that innervate them.

It is fascinating to understand that the nervous system losing its neurons is causing the muscle loss. Ask any stroke or spinal cord injury victim; the muscle is nothing without the function of the nerves. A healthy nervous system enables a muscle to contract, relax, and keeps it viable.

With unaddressed aging, less muscle mass and fewer motor neurons mean greater weakness and less mobility. Add in poor balance, the increased risk of falls as well as reduced bone density, and you can see a rapidly evolving recipe for disaster. Decline begets decline, and recovery gets harder and harder.

You now understand that thinking of muscle only in terms of muscle is missing the point; the nervous system controls everything about the muscle. Just lifting weights or pushing against machines to hang meat on the bones is ultimately not very useful. Neuromuscular training is what we want!

Think of it this way. When we work out, we are training our nervous systems. Yes, we want muscle mass, but we really desire exquisite neuro-muscular control and coordination. Neuromuscular control creates all kinds of capabilities and opportunities. Neuromuscular control and coordination dramatically protect us from falls and injury from a fall. It provides us with the strength and coordination to enjoy life.

Measurement and Optimization

Muscle mass is measured at Gladden Longevity with both a DEXA scan and an InBody Scan. From these, we gain insight into the percentage of body fat, fat distribution, muscle mass, and muscle distribution. Hand-grip strength is a vital biological age metric, and we measure it routinely. Core strength is another key metric and is also measurable. The ability to get up off the floor from a seated position is also a good measure of neuromuscular strength, coordination, and flexibility. Ideally, it can be done without placing a hand on the floor. The more body parts that have to touch the floor to stand up the weaker the neuromuscular system is.

In order to optimize your neuromuscular training, it's important to conceptualize that you are training the nervous system and that the muscles come along for the ride. In addition, so do the tendons, ligaments, and bones. One of the best exercise categories is functional movement. We have a client, Steve Barkley, from the Austin area, who runs a martial arts studio called Rise Martial Arts. Martial arts can be great forms of functional movement training, yet he has now taken it to another level focusing on functional movements outside of sparring and to great effect. Jumping on elevated objects, rolling forward and standing, crawling on the floor without his knees touching, etc., are some of the best training to keep your nervous system young.

Personally, I have also found standup paddling in the ocean when there are 3–4 foot swells and a 20 mph headwind to be a fantastic full-body neuromuscular system workout. It requires balance, strength, core strength, and proprioception. Proprioception is the body's ability to know where it is in space and is foundational to having great balance. To understand proprioception think of vertigo. Vertigo results in a complete lack of proprioception. Dizziness, stumbling, and falling ensue because the body has lost its sense of what's up and what's down and where it is in space. When I get back from a standing paddle session in my ideal conditions, it feels like every neuromuscular bundle has been firing. This kind of functional training is incredibly invigorating and valuable to keeping my neuromuscular system young.

Optimizing sleep, diet, gut health, and hormones are critical prerequisites to getting optimal workout results at any age. (These are each addressed in other sections of the book.) Once these have been addressed, a routine of resistance training is the next step. Often, a physical therapy or sports chiropractic evaluation to look at old injuries is essential prior to initiating training to minimize the risk of injury and optimize the gains. Repairing asymmetries that have developed secondary to prior injuries is critical to avoiding repeat injuries. A primary goal of training is repairing those asymmetries because without doing so, you will never fully become balanced, coordinated, and strong.

Two things we've seen happen frequently:

- Trying to do too much too soon.
- Not doing enough to progress.

Working with a trainer can be beneficial, but we have seen that most trainers are married to their way of doing things and don't know how to work with clients across multiple decades. Many times, a one-size-fits-all approach is all they have to offer. I've heard many stories of elderly people being injured by working out with trainers who do not regress the exercises to meet the client's capabilities.

The other major—and fatal—error we see is the assumption that one is getting cardiovascular exercise during resistance training because heart rates are continuously or intermittently elevated. We have had clients join an interval training gym of one variety or another and come back and tell us, "My trainer wanted me to stop my cardio and focus on resistance training, but he or she says I'm getting plenty of cardio with the workouts we're doing."

Our response is, "Okay, we doubt it, but let's see."

When we do a CPET test, 100 percent of the time, their VO2 max and anaerobic thresholds are down compared to when they were doing isolated cardio. They are in worse cardiovascular shape and have an older biological heart age based on their lower VO2 max, a key metric of longevity. Once we get them back on a cardio regimen of four or five days a week and resistance training two or three times a week, their VO2 max increases, and their anaerobic threshold improves. Oh, and their strength is also better because they are taking an appropriate amount of time to recover from their resistance training sessions.

With resistance training, we are tearing down muscle during the workout. We build muscle during recovery. Resistance training two or three times a week is plenty to build and maintain muscle mass. That being said, doing a ten- to fourteen-day resistance training intensive can be useful, but this should not be the norm. As we age, there are tools and equipment to enhance muscle growth. Things we have found useful are:

1. Blood-flow restriction exercises. Think putting tourniquets on your extremities and then working out:

    - B Strong Bands
    - Kaatsu blood-flow restriction systems
    - Vasper blood-flow restriction interval training

    Blood flow resistance works by decreasing blood flow into and out of the muscle during training. It results in a greater anabolic stimulus, thereby building more muscle.

2. Electrical stimulation of the muscles. Think using electric current to force the muscle to contract:

    - NeuFit: for AC and DC stimulation and relaxation of the muscle
    - Compex: AC-only stimulation for muscle contraction

    These can be used alone or in conjunction with other exercises.

3. Optimizing anabolic stimulation to build muscle. Think activating growth hormone release, which activates the mTOR pathway we discussed earlier:

    - Hormones: Optimizing testosterone and its metabolite DHT
    - HMB, a metabolite of the amino acid Lysine increases muscle mass
    - Growth hormone-releasing peptides and hormones like CJC/Ipamorelin; a combination of a synthetic growth hormone-releasing hormone and growth

hormone-releasing peptide; or Tesamorelin, a synthetic growth hormone-releasing hormone
- A new product from BioProtein Technology, Bio-Pro+™, can also be used intermittently 3–4 days a week to get extra IGF1 and trophic factors. . Listen to the *Gladden Longevity Podcast* I did with Dustin Baker to learn more: GladdenLongevityPodcast.com

4. Selective Androgen Receptor Modulators (SARMS) also activate mTOR, but we don't use them, as it is illegal to sell them in pill or liquid form, and they have been associated with liver damage, heart attack, and stroke.
5. Myostatin inhibitors block the breakdown of muscle. Myostatin breaks down muscle when it is not being used because it is metabolically demanding to carry muscle around that you are not using:

- Physicians Muscle Health Formula containing Fortetropin made from fertilized egg yolks is a myostatin inhibitor. Please note that it may raise cholesterol levels. We use it only on days we are not able to work out to prevent muscle loss or it can be used daily to initially help build someone up.
- Follistatin, an injectable peptide, is used to reduce muscle loss from myostatin and induces bone formation as an activin-binding protein. We do not use it as it is not approved to be sold through compounding pharmacies.

A cautionary note: Continued use of myostatin inhibitors can be associated with an increased chance of tendon rupture, heart failure due to an inflamed cardiac muscle, and rhabdomyolysis, a breakdown of muscle fibers that may lead to kidney failure if it is severe enough. Therefore, we only use them intermittently and have not seen any side effects.

6. Rapamycin: An mTOR antagonist, discussed earlier, will cause muscle loss if used continually but used at the right dose intermittently. It protects aging muscles and protects against neuromotor and muscle fiber loss. We dose it every 2–3 weeks in a client-specific dose, usually between 8–12mg.

The good side of anabolic mTOR stimulation is that it will build muscle in the short term. However, too much mTOR stimulation results in muscle damage and loss as the body becomes insensitive to it. Use to excess, lifespan is shortened, cancer risk goes up, and the mTOR pathways are down-regulated.

Biology is truly an economy of balance. We believe replacing hormones is important, but that intermittently pulsing rapamycin is beneficial both for neuro muscle fiber preservation and longevity.

Muscle recovery is all about blood flow, relieving oxidative stress, replenishing the muscle's carbohydrate stores (glycogen stores), and supplying nutrients—such as electrolytes and amino acids—to enable optimal cell recovery and repair. Slow cardio after resistance training increases blood flow with little additional stress. The use of electrical muscle stimulation (e-stim) devices, like NueX or Compex, in a gentle fashion will also increase blood flow, wash out cellular waste, and minimize soreness. We drink hydrogen water to balance the oxidative stress, and take in carbs within thirty minutes of finishing the workout when the muscles are ready to replenish their glycogen stores. We take Perfect Amino and electrolytes to facilitate repair.

If you take the time to recover properly, you'll find it makes a huge difference in your performance the next day. The first time I noticed this was using a recovery product called Endurox. Normally after a hard cycling session, the next day I would be sore, and if I rode again, my muscles would be tired. Utilizing Endurox within 30 minutes of a workout changed all that and consecutive days of heavier exertion were not a problem.

For resistance training, we like the Adaptive Resistance Exercise (ARX) system. It is a safe, intense, complete workout—check it out at our Longevity gym or ARXFit.com. The Tonal® wall system approximates ARX and is quite a bit less expensive for home use.

These devices provide maximum resistance through the entire range of motion. During the concentric phase, as you push away from the body, and during the eccentric phase, as you resist, the machine pushes back toward your body. Weights are static and more difficult to get going, but easier to move once they have momentum and get further away from the body. That is not the case with the ARX or Tonal® systems; they are cable-driven and not a physical weight. If something doesn't feel right, you just let go or stop. There is nothing to fall or hurt you. These can provide wonderful, full-body workouts.

Interestingly, using ARX or Tonal®, if you can move one unit of weight in a concentric, pushing away exercise, we routinely generate 1.7–1.8 times that amount of force when we resist the machine pushing back against us during the eccentric phase. Think about the great effect that it has on safely building bone, tendon, ligament, muscle, and neuro-muscular strength!

In addition, we are fans of blood-flow restriction to add even more intensity to the muscle growth stimulus. B

Strong Bands, Kaatsu, and Vasper are all great blood-flow restriction systems. Blood-flow restriction bands can be added to a weight workout, ARX, or Tonal® workout or used with resistance bands or body-weight exercises.

Three to five grams of creatine can also increase muscle mass and workout energy. It also improves cardiovascular and brain performance. If you have kidney dysfunction, it will increase blood creatinine, but it has not been shown to be detrimental to kidney function.

Bodybuilders often advocate whey and other forms of protein. So is eating protein to build muscle a good idea? Yes . . . to a point. Data shows that high-protein diets in middle age are linked to a shorter life expectancy. In older age, generally speaking, more protein can be better; even here, however, there are caveats. Our approach is to use Perfect Amino post-workout because it contains a proprietary blend of amino acids, and 99 percent of them are incorporated into protein in your body. When you eat protein, less than half the protein you consume becomes protein in your body. The rest becomes carbohydrates or is stored as fat. If your kidneys are not perfect, too much protein can be hard on them.

Testosterone, growth hormone, or growth hormone-releasing peptides and hormones like CJ/Ipamorelin, sermorelin, and tesamorelin will also help grow muscle.

It is important to understand that the body perceives excess muscle as a metabolic liability because it requires extra calories to maintain it. Therefore, if a muscle is not being used, it atrophies. Myostatin is a protein that trims excess muscle and therefore limits muscle growth. As we age, inhibiting myostatin enables us to maintain muscle. Myostatin inhibitors will stop your body from breaking down muscle. Follistatin and Fortetropin are two myostatin inhibitors. We don't recommend Follistatin, as it can increase insulin resistance. Fortetropin has data to support its use in humans and animals, supported by a trial for twenty-one days in twenty older healthy individuals, that showed an 18 percent increase in muscle protein synthesis. Bottom line: Prioritize cardio for VO2 max optimization, but embrace smart resistance training to build muscle, bone, tendon, and ligaments. To build your nervous system, do functional fitness and balance training. There is no substitute!

CHAPTER THIRTY-FOUR

Detoxification

We live in a very toxic world, one that's full of natural and man-made pollutants—volcanoes, dust storms, mold, fossil fuels, wildfires, plastics, and so on. When you think about detoxification, it's typically spoken about as Phase Zero, Phase One, Phase Two, and Phase Three detoxification. But the way I like to think about detoxification is that it actually starts at the end, which is Phase Three, and works its way upstream from there.

What happens if you are living a toxic life? The symptoms are myriad—fatigue, headaches, reduced brain power, decreased athletic performance, muscle and joint aches, pains, increased inflammation, and even malignancies result—because you cannot get rid of these toxins. Breast cancer, for example, is associated with the build-up of heavy metals and estrogen metabolites improperly detoxed. Prostate cancers are also associated with estrogen metabolites not being detoxed appropriately. In fact, some of the most common cancers are related to an inability to rid ourselves of toxins.

In order to get a toxin out of the body, we must transform it into a non-toxin, or, in some cases, transform a toxin into another toxin before it can be transformed into a non-toxin.

The major ways that we eliminate toxins are through the urine, bile, intestine, and skin (think sweat). If you are unable to move things through the kidneys, the stool, or the skin, it doesn't matter what you're doing with phase one and phase two—you'll still have a problem with detoxification.

A healthy gut biome is very important in this process. An enzyme called beta-glucuronidase is secreted by several bacteria found in the colon: E coli, Bacteroides species, and Clostridium perfringens. These bacteria colonize the large intestine and then produce beta-glucuronidase. Beta Glucuronidase has the ability to take a toxin that's in the stool and liberate it from the glucose molecule that's been attached to it, marking it for elimination—such as the toxin gets reabsorbed back into our blood. Calcium D Gucarate can block beta-glucuronidase and is very helpful in the entire detox process.

Think about it like a sewer system. Things need to flush through and out. You have to make sure that toxins can get out first; as more trash comes through, Phases One and Two, you need to make sure it doesn't back up because of a faulty Phase Three.

Measurement and Optimization

Testing for beta-glucuronidase is one key to optimizing your body's detox system. It's possible to change the gut flora by using certain prebiotics, probiotics, and postbiotics, which can help decrease bacteria that produce b-glucuronidase. Lactobacillus and Bifidobacterium are especially helpful. As mentioned, Calcium-D-glucarate can neutralize beta-glucuronidase.

How do we optimize Phase Three? The first way to optimize Phase Three is to do something that enables you to sweat profusely. You'll recall from Part Two some of the longevity benefits of saunas, and a sauna is a great way to detox. Using a sauna, unlike IV chelation, doesn't put pressure on your liver or kidneys by exposing them to heavy metals or other toxins. Instead, toxins can simply move out through the skin. Other ways to detox include running, biking, or any other activity that allows you to break a good, protracted sweat.

The Phase Three pathway also involves the bowel itself. How many bowel movements do you have a day? If you're having one a day, that's good; two a day is better. Even three a day is great, as long as you're not having diarrhea. Frequent bowel movements are usually attributed to having fiber in your diet. A combination of raw and cooked vegetables will give you a lot of fiber, as can fiber supplements. You want your stools to be frequent, large, and bulky.

To have good bowel movements, eat six to eight servings of vegetables each day. Personally, I put a bunch of greens and vegetables into a pot, add a couple of inches of water, and cook it lightly until the volume collapses. Then I tamp all those vegetables down in the bottom of the pot and strain off the water. I lose some nutrients that way, but the "cooking" is only three or four minutes. I can eat a lot of greens without having to chew through a bushel of greens. It's also a very convenient way to get a high concentration of dietary nitrate used to make nitric oxide (NO). I put in multiple greens like kale, arugula—both high in dietary nitrate—and add others for bulk. I also add basal and sometimes parsley. Throw in a scoop of fiber and whatever else I want to add, and I get a lot of healthy dietary fiber.

I've recently discovered that pancakes are now the new smoothie as I can add all kinds of healthy things and fiber to a gluten-free pancake. Salads of course can be a great source of fiber. Soup is also the new salad. I can add virtually all of my salad ingredients into a bowl of soup. Try it and I'll bet it is the most delicious soup you've ever had!

Beans are also an excellent source of fiber and protein. Everyone worries about the lectins in beans, but if they are soaked and pressure-cooked, it neutralizes the lectins. Beans and rice together can make a complete protein and a good source of fiber. There are concerns about the blood sugar-raising effects of rice, but when it is combined with a protein source and healthy fats, its blood-sugar-raising potential is mitigated.

Prunes, apples, cherries, and berries can add to your fiber content as well. Another way to consume adequate fiber is to eat asparagus or resistant starches like green bananas or baked potatoes that have been cooked, refrigerated overnight, then eaten cold.

Likewise, you can sabotage Phase 3 by eating constipating foods, like too many dairy products. If you choose to consume dairy including cheese, understand that you are slowing down your intestinal transit times and will detox less effectively. When I eat it, I combine dairy with fiber to balance the effects.

The next Phase 3 pathway is the urine. Ideally, you should be well-hydrated and the urine should be dilute because the kidneys have to use a lot of energy to concentrate the urine. The toxins become much more concentrated also, causing additional stress to the kidneys. Interestingly, when I was growing up, my maternal grandmother constantly told me to drink more water and that my great-grandfather drank eight glasses of water daily. He lived what then would be considered a long healthy life and died at ninety-six after falling off a ladder and breaking a hip.

In early 2023, *eBiomedicine* published an article titled "Middle-age normal serum sodium as a risk factor for accelerated biological aging, chronic diseases, and premature mortality." The article states that those aged forty-five to sixty-four who kept their serum sodium between 138.5 and 142 by drinking an adequate amount of water each day (roughly eight glasses per day) lived longer and had fewer cardiovascular events. The study included over 14,000 people. Those with serum sodium levels greater than 142 were assumed to be more dehydrated and had a 50 percent increased risk of having a biological age that was older than their chronological age. In fact, the findings concluded that if you had serum sodium higher than 142 or lower than 138, it would make a negative impact on your longevity. Turns out you risked having an older biological age, and you risked having more age-related diseases, especially cardiovascular diseases. Here are the results.

- Serum sodium greater than 142 mmol/l was associated with a 39 percent increased risk of developing chronic diseases.
- Serum sodium greater than 144 mmol/l was associated with a 21 percent elevated risk of premature mortality.
- The ideal sodium concentration is 138.5–139.5, but up to 142 is acceptable.

Serum sodium was used as a proxy for hydration, but there is more to serum sodium than hydration. There are genetics at play. Some individuals are more avid in retaining sodium, and those same genetics can predispose to higher rates of hypertension and cardiovascular disease. That being said, it makes sense to be well-hydrated, but you *can* overdo it. A serum sodium of 135–136.5 mmol/l was associated with a 71 percent increased risk of all-cause mortality.

Remember, biology is an economy of balance.

Incorporating this information back into Phase Three, think about it this way: If you're trying to pass gasoline out of your blood through your kidneys, you don't want to poison the kidney in the process; you want to dilute it as much as possible. A big part of hydration's value is the ability it provides us to safely detox through the kidneys with minimal trauma to them.

Let's move further upstream to Phase Two Detox.

Phase two is what happens before elimination. It takes place primarily in the liver, but other tissues participate as well. There are five different ways for Phase Two detoxification to occur:

- Attaching a glucose molecule to the toxin
- Attaching a sulfate molecule to the toxin
- Attaching an acetyl group to the toxin
- Attaching an amino acid to the toxin
- Attaching a methyl group to the toxin

It's important to know that when things are handled by Phase One, some intermediates can be *more* toxic than the original toxin. Having a great working Phase One but a poor Phase Two is a potential disaster. Therefore, optimizing Phase Two becomes the next critical piece.

It is essential, then, to have enough sulfur-containing molecules in your diet, like N Acetyl cysteine, and sulfur-containing foods, like allium vegetables, garlic, onions, shallots, and leaks, and cruciferous vegetables like broccoli, cauliflower, kale, and arugula. Animal sources of sulfur are turkey, chicken, fish, beef, and eggs. Finally, nuts, seeds, and legumes also contribute.

Some individuals are very sensitive to sulfur and, therefore, will have to determine what works for them. However, eating some sulfur-containing foods is a great idea for most of us. You also want amino acids and enough protein in your diet but not too much because, as we've said, high protein diets in middle-aged people shorten life by over-activating mTOR. Proteins like egg whites, a biologically complete protein, will give you the amino acids you need for Phase Two.

From there, optimizing the methylation cycle, which typically is a function of getting molecules like TMG, folinic acid (5-formyl tetrahydrofolate), Vitamins B12, B6, and magnesium to help eliminate toxins. This is where some of those dietary and vitamin-mineral supplements come into play. Interestingly, the body uses a lot of its methylating capacity to make creatine, so taking creatine has the added benefit of improving your methylation cycle and detox as well as improving muscle and brain function.

In front of Phase Two is Phase One, which consists of a number of different enzymes that are coded by seven different families of genes. These families are responsible for breaking down many toxins, hormones, and medications. The first one is CYP1, it's responsible for metabolizing aromatic hydrocarbons and participates in the metabolism of steroid hormones like estrogen. However, it also has the ability to activate pro-carcinogens to full-blown carcinogens, hence making it critical that Phase Two works properly.

CYP1A2 is responsible for neutralizing xenobiotics, a chemical substance that is foreign to animal and human biology. It could come from plants. It could be a drug, a pesticide, a cosmetic, a flavoring, a fragrance, a food additive, an industrial chemical, or an environmental pollutant. CYP1A2 is also responsible for metabolizing caffeine and its configuration determines if you are a slow or fast caffeine metabolizer.

CYP2BK metabolizes nicotine and other drugs, including ketamine and methadone. It is one of our most polymorphic CYP genes. There are many different alleles, and they can have different configurations that work very well, pretty well, or not so well.

CYP2C6 metabolizes certain drugs like amiodarone, used to control abnormal heart rhythms, and the drug paclitaxel, used for diabetes.

CYP2C19 metabolizes proton pump inhibitors, commonly used for reducing stomach acid; certain antidepressants, such as tricyclic antidepressants like amitriptyline and SSRIs like Zoloft and Celexa. Certain antiplatelet drugs, like Plavix, are also metabolized through this pathway, along with antifungal in anti-cancer compounds, like cyclophosphamides.

CYP2D has been associated with Parkinson's and lung cancer. So if this snip is not working properly, it can increase the risk of both.

In cases where the Phase One genes are not working very well, they need to be supported. Upregulating these genes with sulforaphane, found in broccoli and with curcumin, chicory root, rosemary, and garlic, is helpful.

To reiterate, optimal health is an economy of balance; it's not about drinking green tea all day. Yes, green tea and cruciferous vegetables are good, but you need to balance it out with some of these other things, like garlic and other good sources of sulfur.

CYP2D6 processes are affected by multiple drugs like tricyclics, antidepressants, beta-blockers, and haloperidol (known as Haldol).

The first step will be working with someone to test your Phase One and Phase Two genetics. Doing a pharmacogenomic test can give you a good insight into your detox genetics as can doing an Intellxx DNA test.

Then, the primary detox strategy involves consuming the right foods and supplements that will specifically upregulate your genes while providing the needed detox cofactors to optimize your detox capabilities.

Measuring toxin levels in your body to determine your toxic burden is also helpful, but you will want to know your genetics to help you figure out where you focus your attention. Is it mold? Fungus? Glyphosate? A hormone metabolite that isn't being processed? Is it something related to the methylation cycle or not enough sulfur in your diet?

These are knots that have to be unraveled before they can be addressed. Testing is best done with a professional, but there are some things you can do at home. Start by optimizing Phase Three, elimination; eating a healthy, fiber-rich diet will help. Eating healthy herbs and broccoli seeds or sprouts will help with Phase Two, but optimizing Phase One requires a more critical examination of your genes and an understanding of how you will play those cards.

Finally, there's Phase Zero, which is doing everything possible to live in an environment free of toxins. While living in a toxin-free world is impossible, this is where you can look into your air and water quality and use air- and water-filtration systems. Consider buying organic foods to avoid pesticides—washing your fruits and vegetables with Dawn dishwashing soap removes pesticides—food additives, and cosmetics that can cause toxins to enter your system. It should be noted that antiperspirants containing aluminum have been associated with Alzheimer's disease and should be avoided.

Another common toxin is mercury. Something seemingly healthy, like fish, may contain mercury, but you may also be at risk of exposure if you live near any sort of coal-burning power plant. By understanding your environment, you can reduce the amount of pollutants that go into your system. This is particularly critical if you are genetically challenged because it's possible your system just can't process what's in your environment, and you simply won't feel well until you move to a better location.

Intellxx DNA reports on the genes used to detox metals and mercury and is particularly helpful. To avoid mercury in your fish, eat small cold-water fish like salmon, trout, sardines, herring, or anchovies. Mackerel, while rich in omega 3s, can be high in mercury.

Your friend's experience, my personal experience, or what you find on the internet or social media will not provide you with the answers you need. While I can offer you general advice in this book, you have to seek your specific answers because getting your answers will be critical to your success. When we talk about detoxification, it's important to understand that each person has their own system and that in order to do this properly, it's not enough to just read the generic information and think, *Well, if I do this and that, then I'll be fine.* It's important that you understand what cards *you* are holding, but you also need to understand the environment you live in and your specific toxic burden. Once you understand this, you can play the hand, but it is important to retest to measure the outcomes. Knowing what corrections to make along the way will make all the difference in optimizing your ability to detox.

CHAPTER THIRTY-FIVE

Digestive System–Stomach, Gallbladder, Pancreas, Intestines, and Metabolic Disease

D igestion starts in the mouth. We chew our food in order to break it down. As we chew, the enzyme amylase is released into the saliva. We can inherit between one and twenty copies of the amylase gene. The more redundant copies of the amylase gene, the better we adapt to eating carbs.

Agriculture is a recent invention. The earliest reports of agriculture were believed to be found in the areas now occupied by Iraq and Iran and southwestern Turkey twelve thousand years ago. Now, there is evidence of agriculture from 23000 years ago.

In that relatively brief period, many of us are still genetically hunter-gathers, with only one to four copies of the amylase gene. With more copies, we process carbs better, gain less weight from eating them and carry more weight without developing adult-onset diabetes. It definitely helps to know your amylase copy number to understand a basic component of your diet.

From the mouth, food travels through the esophagus across a valve that resides at the end of the esophagus and then opens into the acidic environment of the stomach. There, parietal cells release hydrochloric acid, which initiates the chemical process that breaks down, or denatures, proteins. We make Ceviche using the acidity of limes and lemons to denature the fish's proteins, and we cook meat to denature the protein. Denatured protein is easier to digest. The parietal cells also release an intrinsic factor, a molecule required for Vitamin B12 absorption.

As we age, parietal cell function can be lost, resulting in poor B12 absorption and less acid in the stomach, impairing protein breakdown and digestion. This can be partially remedied by taking Betaine (i.e., hydrochloric acid) or Betaine with the stomach enzyme pepsin with each meal. In order to get adequate B12, however, it may mean you will also need sublingual B12 or B12 shots. The acidic food is then passed to the small intestine.

For the small intestine to remain healthy, it's important that it experiences the now-acidic food from the stomach. This acidity restricts what kind of bacteria can grow in the small intestine. The natural flora of the small intestine can protect us by metabolizing carcinogens in our food. The natural flora of the small intestine also provides us with synthesized vitamins, such as biotin and folate, and helps produce Vitamin K, which we absorb and use. If the small intestine is not exposed to acidity from the stomach— because of loss of parietal cell function or gastric surgery—overgrowth with abnormal bacteria will occur, resulting in Small Intestinal Bacterial Overgrowth, also known as "SIBO." Yeast can also overgrow the small intestine (SIYO) and is potentiated by high-sugar diets and alcohol consumption. This overgrowth can lead to gas, bloating, malnutrition, weight loss, and diarrhea.

The small intestine is also where bile, which is made in the liver and concentrated in the gallbladder, is released to emulsify dietary fats, rendering them water-soluble. Not having a gallbladder is a liability when it comes to absorbing all fats, including healthy fats such as the omega3 like fish oil, and fat-soluble vitamins, like A, D, E, and K. If the gallbladder has been removed, taking bile-acid salts, in pill form, with each fat-containing meal can easily remedy this. Ideally, you would take your fat-soluble vitamins at the same time.

Pancreatic enzymes also weigh in and are released conjointly with the bile acids—including protease, lipase, and additional amylase—which contribute to the digestion of protein, fat, and carbohydrate, respectively. As we age, the pancreas can fail in its ability to supply these digestive enzymes, which may also need to be replaced with each meal.

The pancreas is also home to the islets of Langerhans, where alpha and beta cells reside. The beta cells secrete insulin in response to dietary carbohydrates and sugar to control rising blood sugar levels. The alpha cells secrete glucagon in response to low blood sugar in order to raise it. The balance between the two is responsible for maintaining a normal blood sugar level.

It is important to understand that genetics also plays a role in how quickly carbs and sugar entering the system are recognized; how aggressively insulin is released; the degree to which the insulin receptors on cells are sensitive to insulin; and how high blood sugars are likely to go in response to stress. All of these genetic issues can be addressed with proper interventions, but it is beyond the scope of this book to outline them. Intellxx DNA has a great panel of genes and recommendations to decode this for you. Other contributors to blood sugar and insulin levels are muscle mass, fat mass, and chromium levels needed for normal insulin receptor function.

This is an important knot to unravel because higher insulin and glucose levels are associated with accelerated aging through an increased rate of senescent cell formation, resulting in accelerated aging of blood vessels, nerves, and organs.

Measurement and Optimization

Amylase copy number is reported in many reports but is nicely decoded by the genetics company Fitgenes in Australia. Knowing your amylase copy number is useful in deciding how adapted to carbohydrates you will likely be. Wearing a continuous glucose monitor, however, is a great way to track your blood sugar levels throughout the day—unfed and fed, stressed and unstressed, and active and sedentary conditions will all have an impact. We have found many times that genes don't control blood sugar, weight, or hormone metabolites, for that matter, and it is important to unravel the knot in each of these instances beyond what your genetics might suggest. Unfortunately, glucose monitors cannot yet report corresponding insulin levels, which would be very helpful.

Stomach acidity can be measured directly by swallowing a pH probe to measure acidity. It is typically left in place for twenty-four to seventy-two hours. Hypochlorhydria, reduced stomach acid production, or achlorhydria (no stomach acid production) can be measured this way. In either case, taking HCL as betaine with meals will restore stomach acidity. Typically, you will take one capsule at each meal and increase the number until you feel heartburn. You will then know your ideal dose will be one or two capsules below where you had heartburn.

Gastroesophageal reflux, a major cause of heartburn, can also be diagnosed with the same type of probe and process. We like a supplement called Acid Calm™, a supplement with a number of soothing botanicals and zinc carnosine to modulate stomach acidity, and many times we can get people off their prescription or non-prescription medications by using it.

Gallbladder insufficiency can be diagnosed by having the stools examined for undigested and unabsorbed fat. If your gallbladder is inefficient, taking bile acids with meals and fat-soluble vitamins will compensate for this.

Pancreatic digestive enzyme insufficiency can also be diagnosed with a stool test, but this time, we are looking for undigested protein and meat fibers. If this is the case, complete replacement of pancreatic enzymes is usually recommended. Taken with meals, this replacement typically solves the problem.

When unraveling the incretin, insulin, and glucagon blood sugar knot, it takes genetic tests, micronutrient testing, a two-hour glucose tolerance test with an insulin curve, and wearing a continuous glucose monitor to sort it out. With this approach, we can define Type 1 juvenile diabetes, Type 2 adult-onset diabetes, insulin resistance, and adult-onset beta-cell failure. Therapy for diabetes used to consist of giving drugs called sulphonylureas to encourage the beta cells to produce more insulin, but this only led to accelerated beta-cell exhaustion.

Metformin and the supplement berberine lower blood sugar by altering intracellular energy production. They activate AMPK, a major longevity switch, which lowers ATP production. They increase insulin receptor sensitivity so that the available insulin works better to push glucose into the cells, provided adequate chromium exists. They also inhibit the liver's glucose production and decrease glucagon's blood sugar-raising effects. A full discussion of diabetes and insulin resistance is beyond the scope of this book; however, this is one of your most important knots to unravel and should be done with a functional medicine doctor who understands all the elements we have outlined above.

In terms of improving your digestion, eating more fiber is generally beneficial because it bulks up the stool and reduces constipation. It is also fermented in the gut, providing short-chain fatty acids, which serve as nutrients for good bacteria and help them out-compete harmful bacteria. Fiber that is fermented and the short-chain fatty acids it produces like butyrate, will also keep the intestinal enterocytes healthy and increase BDNF in the brain improving brain health.

Probiotics also play a role in digestive health. Regarding blood sugar control, we have been particularly impressed with the probiotic from Pendulum® called Metabolic Daily. The bacteria included in Metabolic Daily metabolize dietary fiber into the short-chain fatty acid butyrate. Butyrate feeds the enterocytes lining the intestine, making them healthier. Butyrate also promotes brain health and neuron regeneration by increasing the Brain-Derived Neurotrophic Factor (BDNF).

Another potentially helpful probiotic is Lactobacillus reuteri (L. reuteri), which decreases H Pylori, the bacteria associated with gastric ulcers.

Another often overlooked factor is the use of prebiotics. Prebiotics are like fertilizer for probiotics and other healthy bacteria already in the gut. Prebiotics are usually one or another form of fiber. (A lot of us don't eat enough raw vegetables or have enough fiber in our diet.) Taking a prebiotic gives you fiber, which feeds the good bacteria.

The bacteria in your gut respond to your diet. So if you eat lots of carbohydrates and sugar, you will grow that segment of bacteria that likes carbs and sugar. Have you ever tried to stop eating carbs, for example, and after about a day and a half, you give up? Interestingly enough, when you're not eating carbs, at least initially, you'll have a strong urge to eat them. Part of that urge is coming from the gut bacteria that want you to eat carbs. They are conspiring against you, and once you settle that group down by not feeding them for a few days, you'll find that urge starts to fade.

Postbiotics are also now available. They can restore the metabolites that a healthy microbiome produces, making the gut healthier and encouraging healthy bacteria to thrive even more. In essence, postbiotics are products created by a healthy microbiome and produced by using prebiotics and probiotics. Healthy postbiotics include nutrients such as vitamins B and K, amino acids, and short-chain fatty acids that help healthy bacteria flourish. Importantly they contain substances that inhibit harmful bacteria from growing. Synchronizing prebiotics, probiotics, and post-biotics can work remarkably well at healing the gut and impacting disorders linked to an unhealthy microbiome. They may prove to be effective in restoring a youthful microbiome which may, in turn, impact our ability to avoid elements of the aging process, stay young and live young for a lifetime. Remember, an altered gut biome is now a Hallmark of Aging.

In addition to taking probiotics, you can increase the number of useful postbiotics in your gut by increasing your intake of fermented foods, such as yogurt, kefir, tempeh, sauerkraut, and kimchi. Focusing on getting a variety of fiber-rich, probiotic-rich foods that promote a mix of healthy gut bacteria may help improve your overall health.

It is important to note that leaky gut is now considered one of the major contributors to inflammaging and, therefore, healing leaky gut is of the highest priority. Leaky gut can be understood as gaps that develop between enterocytes many times in the small bowel that allow particulate matter from the digestive process and bacterial products like LPS (lipo poly saccharide) to enter the bloodstream. When they do they can cause autoimmune reactions, food sensitivities, and systemic and neural inflammation.

In order to treat leaky gut, it is imperative to implement what we have previously outlined in this chapter, and will also likely require the use of peptides like oral BPC 157 and oral KPV. When this systematic approach is utilized the results can be dramatic.

It's beyond the scope of this book to talk about every gastrointestinal disorder, but testing along all the lines I've outlined above, will be a great start. It's difficult to do this alone, so working with a knowledgeable practitioner can be very helpful.

CHAPTER THIRTY-SIX

Thyroid

The thyroid is a master hormone because it regulates the *entire* body's metabolic rate. Metabolic rate is the rate at which chemical reactions happen in the cells or the rate at which oxygen is consumed to produce the energy required to perform those chemical reactions. An optimized metabolic rate is critical for health and longevity. Thyroid function, and its balancing of the metabolic rate, is essential for optimized brain, muscle, heart, hormones, digestion, sleep, and so on. *Everything* depends on the thyroid. In fact, it is so essential if you could only optimize a few hormones in your body, thyroid would have to be one of them.

For perspective: Those who have congestive heart failure have hearts with a diminished capacity to pump blood. In a healthy heart, the ventricles, or main pumping chambers, fill with blood before each contraction or heartbeat. Then, they pump out about 50–60 percent of that blood each time they contract. This percentage is referred to as the *ejection fraction*. Heart failure can occur for various reasons, but one of the most common is a weak heart muscle with a decreased ability to contract and pump or move blood forward into circulation.

If you have a failing heart and your ejection fraction is 20 percent, that is considered a severely damaged heart. Generally speaking, the weaker your heart, the shorter your life, so having a healthy ejection fraction is a big, big deal. But a heart failure patient low on thyroid (known as hypothyroidism), however, carries an even *bigger* risk of dying than someone with congestive heart failure with normal thyroid function.

Under normal conditions, the body signals the brain's hypothalamus that it wants more thyroid. The hypothalamus signals the pituitary gland with a thyroid-releasing hormone (TRH) to release thyroid-stimulating hormone (TSH). TSH then signals the thyroid gland to produce more thyroid hormone, which is predominantly metabolically inactive T4. The *4* in T4 indicates four iodine atoms attached to the thyroid molecule.

As inactive T4 circulates throughout the body, one of the iodine atoms is removed by an enzyme known as Deodinase (DIO). DIO1 is used in most of the body, and DIO2 is used in the brain to remove this iodine. Once the iodine atom is removed, the metabolically active form of thyroid T3 is generated and enters the nucleus of the cell, where it upregulates and down-regulates the expression of a wide variety of genes which, among other things, balance the metabolic rate.

Because T3 goes inside the cell nucleus and interacts with the DNA, it's very important to have enough T3 in the body and brain, meaning DIO1 and DIO2 must be working properly.

Genetically, approximately 25 percent of us have a partial or heterozygous deficit, and another 15 percent have a more profound homozygous deficit in our brain's DIO2 enzyme. The deficits have been shown to be clinically important.

Say you are feeling tired all the time, and your routine blood work shows your TSH, T3, and T4 to be "normal." What then?

You are told everything is normal, yet you have symptoms like lethargy, brain fog, weight gain, and poor sleep. Well, what's the problem? You're just a complainer, right?

At Gladden Longevity, we have heard this story many, many times. When we do more comprehensive blood work to look at Free T3, Free T4, Reverse T3, thyroid antibodies, and a resting metabolic rate (RMR), we can see if your body is getting the thyroid it needs. But even then, we must look at your brain's DIO2 genetics to understand what your brain wants.

If you are deficient in converting inactive T4 to active T3 in the brain, your blood work will look normal; even your resting metabolic rate will look normal. However, when we give you T3 or a T4/T3 combination, you will likely thank us profusely for waking up your brain.

We have seen this happen in concussion patients, also. They will come to us post-concussion, and despite working with first-tier university hospital concussion programs, they are making little or no progress in their recovery. We'll check their DIO2 genetics, obtain complete thyroid labs, perform a resting metabolic rate (RMR), and discover that the problem is that either they have undiagnosed hypothyroidism or have a deficit in their genetic ability to convert inactive T4 to active T3 in the brain. Once we address these issues, their brain wakes up, and they can recover their brain and their life.

Earlier in this book, I touched on my experience with having hidden, subclinical, undiagnosed hypothyroidism and how addressing this gave me my life back. If you are struggling, please get this addressed—it could be the answer you are looking for. When someone's T4 is low or even at a lower point of the "normal range," most doctors will prescribe Synthroid or levothyroxine, which is simple T4. But think about that; not everybody can metabolize T4 to T3 effectively, and many do not get a clinically optimal response to T4 alone. The doctor keeps raising the dose, the TSH looks normal, and they declare the patient is fine. If the patient still complains of not feeling well, at best, they may scratch their head and feel they have nothing left to offer; at worst, they blame the patient and tell them it's all in their head (which it is, but just not in the way they were thinking).

We strongly feel that everyone being evaluated with thyroid issues should have a resting metabolic rate and DIO2 genetics done.

One of our greatest delights in practice is seeing people who have been mismanaged elsewhere, and we get this right for them. All of a sudden, they feel great—and when our clients do well, that is always our greatest joy!

Measurement and Optimization

When we measure thyroid at Gladden Longevity, we measure TSH, T4, free T4, T3, free T3, Reverse T3, and antibodies to the thyroid. We also measure iodine, an RMR, and the DIO2 genetics.

The RMR is assessed through the same metabolic cart used to perform a cardiopulmonary exercise test, just minus the exercise and breathing tests. Essentially, you wear a mask over your nose and mouth, and we calculate your RMR by measuring how much carbon dioxide you are generating and exhaling and how much oxygen you are inhaling and utilizing. Patients often have normal blood levels of thyroid and TSH, but their resting metabolic rate is low. It's clearly not optimized; we know these individuals would benefit from thyroid. So we look at the brain genetics to see if they also need T3.

When you consider that so many of us with hypothyroidism evade detection using standard testing, it can become staggering. Based on what we see when the metabolic rate is optimized, the optimal range for TSH is close to one or a bit less, whereas labs record the optimal range between 0.5 and 5. Given that wide range, you can see that a simple TSH blood test would miss a lot of hypothyroidism. Recall a higher TSH is the brain's hypothalamus telling the thyroid gland to make more thyroid hormone.

Finally, the CDC reported in 2014 that a growing number of Americans are deficient in iodine; in the 1970s, it was 3 percent, and between 1988 and 1994, it was 12 percent. In our experience, it is the majority of people we test. Adequate iodine is critical for thyroid function; while many have stopped using iodized salt, we still need iodine. Seaweed, sea kelp, and other foods like cod, canned tuna, oysters, shrimp, milk, cheese, yogurt, eggs, and beef are good sources. Please note that if you plan to get pregnant, having enough iodine is crucial; it can raise your baby's IQ by seven points at age six.

CHAPTER THIRTY-SEVEN

Metabolic Balance, Insulin, Glucagon, Incretins, and Sugar

When we talk about metabolic health, we're talking specifically about insulin and glucose metabolism, but it's more complex than that. Regarding overall health and longevity, metabolic health isn't just a question of whether you have diabetes or will develop diabetes. Many do not have diabetes, yet genetically struggle with metabolizing carbohydrates—so metabolic health is vital to you.

And if you have diabetes or insulin resistance, you typically run high insulin levels and higher-than-normal blood sugars. Because elevated insulin and elevated glucose induce cellular senescence, you are aging at a faster rate.

In the section on digestive health, we looked at the amylase gene and the fact that there are up to twenty different redundant copies of this in each of us. You'll recall that amylase is an enzyme released in the saliva as soon as a carbohydrate hits your mouth. The amount of amylase you produce is based on the number of copies you have in your gene pool. So if you have one copy, you'll produce less amylase than if you have two copies; the more copies you have, the more amylase you make.

It's no secret that the Western diet is full of carbs, fat, salt, and sugar. It is nutrient-poor and calorie-rich. We are overfed and undernourished. Sometimes, you see people who are quite overweight, and they don't have any diabetes at all, or a thinner person who has Type 2 diabetes. The more copies of the amylase gene, the more carb-adapted you are and the more ability you have to process carbohydrates. In addition, the more copies you have, the more body weight you can carry without becoming diabetic.

Genetically, there are a number of genes that determine how quickly our body senses the presence of carbohydrates and how quickly it responds to releasing insulin to control it. There are a number of biochemical pathways involved, working together symphonically to control blood sugar. While I won't go into the details of those pathways, here is a quirky factoid: You can develop diabetes temporarily, even for just an hour or two, if you have genetics that does not detect the incoming carbs or sugar and signal the pancreas to release insulin in a timely manner. How does that happen? Your fasting blood sugar and HgbA1c can be perfect, yet you can still run a blood sugar close to 200 after ingesting a load of sugar.

I know this because this has happened to me. If I eat something sugary or drink seventy-five grams of glucose during a glucose-tolerance test, my fasting blood sugar may be eighty-nine but then will spike to 160 for an hour, putting me into a diabetic range. If you're eating a lot of sugary foods or drinking sugary drinks, even being diabetic for an hour can cause damage to your arteries by destroying the glycocalyx and overwhelming your cells. Once you get the signal that sugar is in the system, it becomes a three-alarm fire, and a lot of insulin is released to try to bring the sugar under control. Running high insulin levels ages us because it increases cellular senescence.

Knowing that you can have a normal hemoglobin A1C and a normal fasting blood sugar and still be intermittently "diabetic" for a period of time is one of the reasons we perform two-hour glucose tolerance tests with an insulin curve on all of our clients. By doing so, we detect many hidden issues they otherwise wouldn't have known about.

When we put on extra weight, we can develop Type 2 diabetes, but Type 2 diabetes is at the end of a long road . . . and that road is called insulin resistance.

Insulin resistance means that as you ingest carbohydrates, you cannot push the associated glucose into your cells with normal amounts of insulin. The cells have become resistant to insulin signaling. Consequently, the beta cells of the pancreas are forced to produce ever larger amounts of insulin to overcome the cells' resistance to taking up the additional glucose. In essence, the body is saying it doesn't need any more calories and doesn't want to take more calories into the cells. This conflict in agendas causes the beta cells of the pancreas to work extra hard, which exhausts them and eventually burns them out. When the beta cells have lost the capacity to produce insulin, a person is only left with the option to inject insulin.

Insulin resistance is often a result of carrying extra weight. Part of the reason obese individuals age more quickly and die sooner is because they run higher blood sugars and higher insulin levels. Another major consequence is increased inflammation and oxidative stress, accelerating aging.

It is the main reason to keep your weight under control. You hardly ever see an obese ninety-year-old and very few eighty-year-olds.

Measurement and Optimization

We can map how hard somebody is pushing their beta cells by doing a two-hour glucose tolerance test with an insulin curve. This test tells us how much insulin they need to release to control the incoming sugar. This sort of critical information cannot be captured by doing a fasting blood sugar and hemoglobin A1C test.

That's one of the tragedies of contemporary medicine. If your TSH is okay, they tell you that you're in a normal range, and if your hemoglobin A1C is fine, you are told you are not diabetic and, therefore, you have nothing to worry about. Traditional medicine is reassuring people that they are in a normal range for their age and that they're okay, when in fact, they may very well be suffering massive, long-term consequences from insulin resistance and subclinical hypothyroidism. They are *not* okay.

As a consumer and a patient, you need to have these things tested so that you have an idea of how well you are processing sugar. These are the tests you should have performed.

- Fasting glucose
- Fasting insulin levels
- HgbA1C (A 90-day running average of your blood sugar levels.)
- Fructosamine (A two-week look back at whether or not your glucose has been spiking.)
- A two-hour glucose tolerance test with an insulin curve

The glucose tolerance test (GTT) measures your blood sugar and insulin levels after a minimum eight-hour fast. Then you are given seventy-five grams of glucose to drink over a few minutes. Blood sugar and insulin levels are checked again at one hour and after two hours. The results come back in a few days, and the information is invaluable when it comes to your health and your aging.

Without this test, you may have a completely hidden problem that, over time, stresses your beta cells and potentially pushes them toward burnout. Once they are gone, they are difficult to rejuvenate, even with stem cells. At that point, to control your blood sugar, you become insulin-dependent. All those years you were silently and unknowingly running high insulin levels will impact your biological age and life expectancy.

Drugs like metformin and supplements like berberine or dihydro berberine, which is better absorbed than berberine, can help protect beta cells, modulate blood sugars, and increase insulin-receptor activity (because insulin receptor activity is also genetically determined). They can also assist with the body's response time to an incoming load of sugar and decrease the risk of cancer for those diagnosed with insulin resistance or diabetes. Yes, science has come a long way in the treatment and therapies available, but you need to know where you stand so you can modify your eating and never need therapy.

A new supplement we have started using is Sugar to Fiber. As previously mentioned, it can convert 50–90% of the incoming sugar to fiber and the rest to fructose. It can mitigate the load you are putting on your beta cells.

There is a category of medications called SGLT2 inhibitors that cause you to eliminate more sugar through the urine. One of the side effects is a bit higher incidence of urinary tract infections and yeast infections because more sugar means more bacteria or yeast growth. Initially, I was skeptical of them, but the data on diabetics have now shown that they are dramatically effective at decreasing cardiovascular events, like hospital admissions for congestive heart failure; they also improve arterial health by improving endothelial dysfunction, which, as you recall, is our first line of defense in fighting high blood pressure, heart attack, and stroke. They also improve and protect kidney function.

The same endothelial protection is true for GLP-1 agonists, which have also been shown to decrease the risk of heart attack, stroke, and hospital admissions for heart failure. In addition, GLP1 agonists—Semiglutide and Tirzepatide, in particular—partly decrease appetite by slowing the stomach's emptying. We use them to jumpstart weight loss but note they need to be started slowly, as they can cause nausea. In time, they should be tapered off, as leptin resistance can occur while you take them, leading to rebound eating if they are stopped abruptly.

Gladden Longevity has created a world class weight loss/body composition program that uses GLP-1 agonists and other drugs in this class but combines them with other interventions to reprogram the body and metabolic rate and enable you to taper off these drugs without a rebound weight gain.

A third class of newer diabetes Medicines—DPP-4 antagonists—work by blocking the action of DPP-4, an enzyme that destroys the hormone incretin. Incretins signal the pancreas to release insulin. DPP-4 inhibitors lower blood sugar by helping the body increase the level of incretins to signal the beta cells to release insulin after a meal. Interestingly there appears to be mounting evidence that these drugs may also improve some cardiovascular outcomes in diabetics but increase the risk of a non-life-threatening but serious arrhythmia Atrial Flutter. For now, SGLT2 inhibitors and GLP1 agonists and their analogs seem to have better data for protecting the cardiovascular system, and we lean toward using these. When it comes to blood-sugar control, Pendulum® Life has a probiotic called Glucose Control that we found to be incredibly helpful in controlling blood sugar. It requires refrigeration and is taken twice a day, but we've had very good success with lowering HbA1C by as much as one full point. Glucose Control increases GLP-1 signaling; it's also good for the integrity of the intestine and cellular health of the intestine, and it is associated with lower blood sugar. We have had a number of patients decrease their HbA1C by 0.6, on average.

If you struggle with insulin resistance, modifying your diet—low-carb, eating multiple small meals, eating complex carbohydrates instead of simple carbohydrates—is a good first step. There is no substitute for good cardiovascular exercise to get your heart rate to the point where you can't carry on a conversation while exercising. If you can carry on a conversation while exercising, you are not pushing hard enough to receive all the benefits of cardio exercise. Finally, you may want to consider some of the medications listed previously. Ultimately, you want to get into a state of good body composition and metabolic flexibility where you have good muscle mass and a good body fat percentage. For a man, a body fat percentage of 18 percent or less, and for a woman, that would be 22 percent or less, is considered good. What is ideal for you is another conversation. For men, a body fat percentage is around 12 percent; and for women, around 17 percent is seen in well-trained athletes not trying to get to single digits. We feel single-digit body fat is not particularly healthy and is not required for optimal health. Having a great diet and body composition with low body fat and good muscle mass is your best defense against metabolic disease.

There is a lot of buzz about fasting, particularly intermittent fasting, but how effective is this method from the standpoint of metabolic control for blood sugar, weight optimization, and longevity? When it comes to longevity, every trial ever performed has shown that eating less (calorie restriction) is beneficial; however, the cost is feeling hungry and cranky.

The benefits of fasting are as follows:

- Improved blood sugars
- Improved insulin sensitivity
- Lower LDL cholesterol
- Reduced blood pressure
- Lower resting heart rate
- Improved verbal memory
- Improved mental clarity
- Recalibrated appetite, so you eat less food and sugar
- Recalibrated your taste buds so you crave less
- Altered your gut biome and its function in a healthy way

- Increased ketone levels of beta-hydroxybutyrate
- Induced weight loss
- Reduced inflammation in joints, tendons, and ligaments
- Reduced protein crosslinking with sugar molecules, known as glycation
- Up-regulated T-Reg cells in the immune system and, consequently, reduced inflammation
- Lower neuroinflammation
- Down-regulated IGF1 and T3, associated with enhanced longevity
- Reduced cancer rates
- Decreasing Leptin-resistance

Dr. Valter Long0's work at USC led him to develop a product that mimics fasting while enabling some food consumption. It's called the ProLon® 5-Day Fast Mimicking Diet, and ProLon® sells the kit. We are fans of the Prolon® 5-Day Fast Mimicking diet as a way to jumpstart your health-optimization journey; repeating it monthly for three months and then quarterly seems to be an effective regimen, and we have seen excellent results using this strategy.

The issue with any fast is how to reintroduce food, which brings us to intermittent fasting.

The strategy of intermittent fasting, condensing caloric intake into a seven-to-ten-hour window during the day, has become very common in many circles—certainly, in health optimization and longevity circles. Dr. Yangbo Sun published a study that caused us to rethink intermittent fasting. The study looked at the self-reported eating habits of 24,011 people between 1999 and December 2015 and found the following.

- Those who ate one meal a day had a 30 percent increase in all-cause mortality and an 83 percent increase in cardiovascular mortality (in comparison with those who ate three meals per day).
- Those who skipped breakfast had a 40 percent increase in cardiovascular mortality (in comparison with those who ate three meals per day).
- Those who skipped lunch had a 12 percent increase in all-cause mortality (in comparison with those who ate three meals per day).
- Those who skipped dinner had a 16 percent increase in all-cause mortality (in comparison with those who ate three meals per day).

How do we make sense of this in a world where we are told that being keto most of the time is a good thing and that skipping meals is important? Calorie restriction has great data in lengthening lifespan in every animal model it has been tested in, and fasting has been shown to have so many health and longevity benefits.

Fasting is healthy in the same way that the right dose of any hormetic stress is healthy—exercise, saunas, cold plunges, and the like. I believe the problem with intermittent fasting is not the fasting itself but the eating that follows because we have mischaracterized eating as a restorative activity.

Eating in the right dose is also a hormetic metabolic stress, but the wrong dose is a very damaging, health-destroying stress. Consuming a large meal puts more metabolic stress on the body than many of us realize.

If we fast and then eat one meal a day, it has the potential to cause massive stress on the body, and all the good we thought we were doing by fasting has been undone.

We need to reframe how we think about food, meals, and fasting. If you are going to fast, then be very careful how you reintroduce food; small quantities, eaten more frequently, are less stressful and should be better. In the lay literature, intermittent fasting has been pitted against eating small meals more frequently as two competing theories on eating.

Combining intermittent fasting with eating smaller, more frequent meals during the feeding period may get us the benefits we are hoping for from intermittent fasting. More studies will need to be done to prove this, but this is currently our approach.

I'm more a fan of eating smaller quantities of nutrient-dense foods rather than eating full meals, eating more frequently within a certain time frame, and fasting the rest of the time. For example, maybe fast twelve to fourteen hours a day, then focus on eating five smaller, nutrient-dense meals in the next ten to twelve hours. This represents a smaller metabolic load and stress on the body. When I apply this strategy to my eating habits and select nutrient-dense, plant-based foods combined with healthy fats like olive oil, Omega 3s, and protein, I feel sated—but not overfed. If you ever feel tired after a meal, you've eaten too much. My advice is never to eat until you are full. A blue-zone staple is eating until you no longer feel hungry, but never until you are full.

Recently, we have also come across a company, Mimeo™, that appears to have unraveled the knot of fasting. They found that elevations in four molecules after a seventy-two-hour fast seem to provide most of the fasting's metabolic benefits. Two are cannabinoids and work on the endocannabinoid system: Palmitoylethanol amide Company (PEA) and Oleoylethanolamide (OEA). The other two are

Spermidine, good for autophagy and cardiac health, and Nicotinamide, important in NAD synthesis.

The bottom line is that we may be able to use their product and get the full benefits of fasting seventy-two hours without having to fast seventy-two hours. Fasting has other benefits beyond the metabolic, like resetting the gut biome, appetite, taste buds, and so on that are likely hard to replicate without actual fasting. Stay tuned—we are currently evaluating this and, so far, have been impressed with its ability to suppress appetite.

Hydrating avidly throughout the day also helps mitigate appetite and has its own longevity benefits.

This brings me to the effects of hydration on our metabolism and overall health. I previously described a study that looked at serum sodium as a surrogate marker for hydration and that people with a serum sodium between 138.5 and 142 had slower biological aging and a lower incidence of chronic disease and premature death.

Biology is an economy of balance. That being said, staying well-hydrated but not over-hydrated not only mitigates our appetite but appears to improve our health and longevity independently. It is also well-known that athletic performance suffers when we are dehydrated, so it is best to hydrate prophylactically instead of waiting until you are thirsty to drink something. Also, realize that caffeine and alcohol dehydrate us, so don't count them as hydration; we have to make up for drinking them by drinking more water.

CHAPTER THIRTY-EIGHT

Liver

The liver is fascinating, quite honestly, because it's one of the busiest and most complex organs in the body. This is easily understood when we realize it is also one of the biggest consumers of oxygen in the body.

The liver manages many aspects of metabolic health, digestion, and detoxification.

- Controls cholesterol
- Carbohydrate energy storage as glycogen
- Blood-sugar modulation
- Secretes bile to facilitate fat digestion
- Primary site of Phase 1 and Phase 2 detoxification

The liver is also involved with immune function. There's a reason it is a "vital organ." It is impossible to live without a liver.

It's widely known that alcohol consumption puts a lot of stress on the liver. It both metabolizes the alcohol and detoxifies the generated metabolites. Over time, the toxic load damages the liver. This can lead to fatty liver, followed by scarring of the liver, and ultimately cirrhosis and liver failure. During my internal medicine training, I saw people suffer and die from alcohol abuse, which is secondary to liver failure. I can tell you it's not a pretty picture: they are yellow with jaundice and have bloated abdomens, swollen extremities, and delirium.

Drinking some alcohol upregulates the enzyme alcohol dehydrogenase, which is linked to longevity. It has been known for many years that those who drink some alcohol live longer. Still, we see so many people who struggle to control their alcohol consumption that abstaining is likely more longevity-enhancing for them. An article was published in *Current Biology* showing improved longevity in a worm model, of longevity C. Elegans, associated with an increased ability to process glycerol, an age-accelerating alcohol. The elaborate mechanisms involved the down-regulation of mTOR and insulin signaling in conjunction with calorie restriction. Increased alcohol dehydrogenase has been shown in yeast and mice to improve longevity and is likely to do the same in calorie-restricted humans.

However, the most significant contemporary risk to the liver is not alcohol-related; it's non-alcoholic fatty liver disease. This disease has two stages: non-alcoholic fatty liver and non-alcoholic steatohepatitis—essentially fat-induced inflammation of the liver. Non-alcoholic fatty liver disease is diagnosed in the absence of alcohol abuse when the amount of fat that has accumulated exceeds 5 percent of the liver's weight. Non-alcoholic fatty liver disease occurs in approximately one- and two-thirds of those who have

Type 2 diabetes, but it occurs in 75 percent of people who are overweight (BMI >30) and in more than 90 percent of people who would have severe obesity (BMI > 35). It can be diagnosed with an ultrasound or MRI and has a constellation of findings that can be used to diagnose it clinically.

One key precursor to non-alcoholic fatty liver disease is metabolic syndrome, which consists of a cluster of five conditions. When three or more are present, it leads to a greater risk of heart disease, stroke, and diabetes. If you have three of the five following conditions, you will qualify as having metabolic syndrome:

- Large waist size: for women, greater than thirty-five inches; for men, greater than forty inches.
- Waist-to-hip ratio in inches greater than 0.8 for women; greater than 0.95 for men.
- High levels of triglycerides in the blood (raw fat in the blood).
- Low levels of HDL (good cholesterol).
- Increased blood pressure over 120/80mmHg.
- High blood sugar (fasting blood sugar over 100).

Abdominal obesity, a BMI over 25, increased blood clotting, and insulin resistance are also part of the picture. When you eat something fatty, like butter or a steak, the fat goes into your intestines. The bile acids emulsify the fats and the enzyme lipase from the pancreas, breaks it down into triglycerides. The triglycerides are absorbed across the intestinal wall into the bloodstream.

If you draw someone's blood shortly after they consume a fatty meal, their blood looks milky white because of the high volume of triglycerides in it. The blood is literally full of fat. That's one of the reasons you are asked to fast before you have blood drawn.

When triglycerides are high, HDL (good cholesterol) is low, and vice-versa. Low HDL is one of the markers of metabolic syndrome. HDL is important because when it is working properly, it is essential for the reverse cholesterol transport we touched on earlier in the section on cardiovascular health. Having a very high HDL used to be thought to be very protective but is now understood to be associated with HDL dysfunction and impaired reverse cholesterol transport. HDL dysfunction can be determined by measuring reverse cholesterol transport directly, which we do at Gladden Longevity.

People who carry extra weight are more prone to high blood pressure. Blood pressure is another diagnostic used to determine whether someone has metabolic syndrome, anything higher than 120/80 would qualify.

Having a higher-than-normal fasting glucose level (equal to or over 100) and not having a diagnosis of Type 2 diabetes is the fifth diagnostic criteria. In previous sections, we covered how important insulin and glucose levels are regarding other conditions, and they are also linked to non-alcoholic fatty liver disease. It stands to reason that if you have metabolic syndrome, you have a high probability of having non-alcoholic fatty liver disease. Any man or woman walking around with a protuberant abdomen likely has it.

Earlier, I mentioned two stages: non-alcoholic fatty liver and non-alcoholic steatohepatitis. While neither is optimal, non-alcoholic fatty liver is more benign. Steatohepatitis can lead to fibrosis in the liver, which can lead to cirrhosis and, ultimately, liver failure, which in many cases requires a liver transplant. Those with steatohepatitis also have a higher incidence of developing liver cancer.

We have a silent epidemic of non-alcoholic fatty liver disease because it's completely asymptomatic; people don't know they have it. This has to do with the physiologic reserve of an organ. The body's organs have a lot of redundant reserve capacity, up to ten times the capacity required to do its normal workload. When it's damaged, it can still carry out its function, making it possible for someone to have a very sick liver and not be aware of it.

Non-alcoholic fatty liver disease has also been associated with excessive calorie intake, high-fructose corn syrup, and poor physical activity. When you consider how many foods have high-fructose corn syrup, it's not surprising that non-alcoholic fatty liver disease has become an epidemic.

Genetics account for less than 10 percent of non-alcoholic fatty liver disease, which is incredibly reassuring because we can control it with lifestyle choices. You can control the status of your liver. You don't have to be a victim of non-alcoholic fatty liver disease; if you answer its wake-up call, you can take control and reverse it. Yes, it can be *reversed*.

Measurement and Optimization

Simple blood work can give you a good idea of the status of your liver and indicate whether it's inflamed, whether there is difficulty with gallbladder function, and whether there is significant oxidative stress. Checking your triglyceride and cholesterol levels will give you some insight into whether you might have non-alcoholic fatty liver disease (with the characteristic high triglycerides and low HDL). If your liver enzymes are off, you definitely want to pay attention and get follow-up testing with an ultrasound or MRI of the liver. Knowing your measurements, blood pressure, and fasting glucose levels are also important.

In our practice, we've had a number of patients who arrive with non-alcoholic fatty liver disease, and we have found several things that help reverse it. You can probably guess the first one: modifying the diet. The first step is moving away from high-fructose corn syrup and a diet laden with sugar, fat, and salt. We encourage our patients to embrace a plant-based diet—not to be confused with a vegetarian or vegan diet. Plant-based means plants play a major role, but animal protein is also consumed.

If you guessed the first one, then you likely already know what the second step is: exercise. Aerobic exercise, in particular, is not only good for your heart and your brain, but it's also good for your liver. It improves the fatty profile of the liver. Remember, the liver is central to the whole-health environment, so when you're exercising, virtually every organ system in your body receives massive benefits by virtue of the liver. That's why exercise will never go away as a foundational recommendation.

Once we clean up the diet and our client is exercising, we have had good success with activating their AMPK system. Earlier, we covered mTOR, which is related to a cell's growth and division, and its role in building muscle mass and bone density. You'll recall that if mTOR is activated all the time, it increases the risk of cancer, and people die sooner. So mTOR is important, but it's not something you want to be activating all day, every day. The counterpart to mTOR is AMPK, which is activated when we fast, exercise aerobically, and use a sauna.

Earlier, we covered the benefits of fasting. We are very intentional with people with alcoholic fatty liver disease taking up this practice. Usually, we start with a five-day fast-mimicking diet and then focus on eating smaller quantities of nutrient-dense foods more frequently within a designated portion of the day.

Some medications and supplements can assist in reversing non-alcoholic fatty liver disease, but I want to stress that cleaning up your diet and aerobic exercise are the foundation. Two agents that can assist in activating AMPK are Metformin, available by prescription, and Berberine, a supplement. I have also seen great results with tea containing Gynostemma pentaphyllum (also known as Jiaogulan or Southern Ginseng), which also activates AMPK.

I had a client who had advanced non-alcoholic fatty liver disease. His father had died with cirrhosis. He was a high-functioning individual who was overweight and had abdominal obesity and insulin resistance. Although he was a weight-lifter, he scored poorly on his cardiopulmonary exercise test (CPET), with a reduced VO2 Max and a low anaerobic threshold. He was not in the habit of regular cardiovascular, aerobic exercise, having been led to believe that weight-lifting was giving him the cardio he needed. To underscore the severity of his case: he had seen his gastroenterologist, who advised him that he would likely need to be put on a liver transplant list.

He had a liver biopsy and MRI of the liver. According to the results, he was one stage above needing the transplant. The natural history of this would be that it would progress to the point where the transplant was necessary, so we started him on the diet and exercise regimen and then had him drink the Jiaogulan tea.

He drank the tea two or three times a day, and a few months later, we retested him. His liver function had improved significantly. He went back to his gastroenterologist, who performed an ultrasound. The results concluded he no longer needed a transplant, and miraculously, his liver had minimal disease detected. We found that to be incredibly encouraging for others in similar situations.

Our practice is not devoted to taking care of people with non-alcoholic fatty liver disease, but this story goes to show you that when you get down to the root cause of what is happening and then go beyond the root cause by activating the levers of longevity, that it is possible to reverse things that traditional medicine cannot. We see this over and over again—it's possible to reverse things that are "irreversible." At the same time, you cannot cherry-pick the longevity strategies that appeal to you and expect optimal results.

CHAPTER THIRTY-NINE

Kidney

Most everyone understands that the kidneys act as very efficient filters for ridding the body of waste products and toxic substances. While filtering the blood of waste, the kidney returns certain vitamins, amino acids, glucose, a variety of hormones, and other vital substances to the bloodstream. The amount of blood the kidney can filter in a minute measures its overall health. This is called GFR. The higher the GFR, the healthier the kidneys are.

If you have kidney issues, be aware that high blood pressure can damage kidneys, as can insulin resistance and diabetes, the latter often resulting in dialysis later on. This is because the sugar is damaging the kidneys, and the high-insulin levels lead to cellular senescence in the blood vessels that feed the kidney, along with the kidney itself.

You are also probably aware that your urine is fairly clear when you're well-hydrated. Likewise, if you are dehydrated, your urine is more concentrated, with a darker color, stronger odor, and so on. If you have had your kidney function tested, you probably underwent two tests: the Blood Urea Nitrogen test (BUN) and a creatinine test (Cr). BUN measures the function of protein metabolism; if you're well-hydrated, the BUN goes down, and if it goes up, it indicates that you are either poorly hydrated or dehydrated. Creatinine is released from the muscles; the kidney filters it out of the blood, and it is excreted in the urine. If the kidney's filtration system is damaged, the creatinine levels will go up. It is important to note, however, that people with more muscle mass will have a higher creatinine.

If you're using the supplement creatine, it hasn't been shown to cause kidney damage but will contribute to higher blood creatinine levels.

Another critical test of kidney and blood vessel function is whether or not protein is being lost through the kidney. If you're losing protein this way, it indicates that there is underlying kidney damage and inflammation in the blood vessels that are bringing blood to the kidney. The inflammation causes the blood vessels to leak protein into the urine.

Kidney function declines with age. It is also a determinant of longevity so optimizing it and protecting it is crucial.

Measurement and Optimization

Another measure of kidney function involves measuring cystatin C, a protein produced by the cells in your body. This test takes things one step further to estimate your kidneys' filtration rates or GFR because it is not influenced by muscle mass like creatinine is.

People with higher muscle mass will have a higher serum creatinine. If muscle mass is not considered, it could be misinterpreted as reduced kidney function. Conversely, people with low muscle mass and low serum creatinine could be misinterpreted to have better kidney function than they do. Cystatin C bypasses this issue and gives a truer read of kidney function regardless of the person's muscle mass.

The gold standard to measure GFR, however, is to collect the urine for twenty-four hours and measure the amount of creatinine and protein in it, along with the volume of urine produced.

There are test strips you can buy over the counter that will provide limited insight into kidney function. They react chemically with various substances in the urine and give you a pH, detect whether or not any sugar is present, and grossly detect how much protein there is. The dipstick is quite crude when it comes to detecting protein and doesn't provide a lot of detail. In fact, you could receive "normal" results from these and still have protein in the urine. So even if you use these tests as a starting point, you would want to look at more sensitive and specific tests, like one that measures the microalbumin to creatinine ratio. This is not commonly tested, but it is a much more sensitive indicator of whether or not microscopic amounts of protein are being leaked into the urine, which is indicative of blood-vessel inflammation.

To optimize kidney function, it's important to minimize things that can damage the kidneys: high-salt/fat/sugar and non-steroidal anti-inflammatory drugs (like ibuprofen and naproxen) are two common culprits. If you have any kidney damage, it is very important that you not reach for these drugs for pain. They decrease the ability of the kidney to expand the blood vessels and keep you healthy and have been linked to stomach ulcers and heart attacks. Other drugs and procedures that stress the kidneys:

- Proton pump inhibitors to control stomach acid, like Prevacid, Prilosec, and Nexium, should be avoided. Pepcid, however, may be the safest choice if only used for a week or two.
- Aminoglycoside antibiotics are very hard on the kidneys and are typically used in hospital settings. The most toxic is neomycin, followed by gentamicin, tobramycin, and amikacin, in that order.
- High-dose statins used to lower cholesterol, like Lipitor, Zocor, and Crestor, can cause kidney damage.
- Radiographic contrast used in some X-ray-guided radiology and cardiology procedures is notoriously hard on kidneys, and there are hydration strategies to minimize the risk.
- Supplements can also be a problem, especially ones that act like a diuretic, like buchu leaves and juniper berries.
- Fat-soluble vitamins E, A, and K can build up to toxic levels in someone with reduced kidney function.

It's also vital to hydrate throughout the day so that your urine is clear. The kidney has to work harder when it has to concentrate the urine.

There is a trend toward eating high-protein diets, which can also be hard on the kidneys. As mentioned before, those in middle age who eat high-protein diets have a shorter life expectancy, as it puts tremendous stress on the kidney—and your entire system—to process all that protein. Remember, eating is a stressful activity, not necessarily a restorative one. Protein breaks down to amino acids, and amino acids also activate mTOR, driving cell growth and cell division, but at the expense of longevity.

The kidneys are very sensitive to oxidative stress. When I was actively working in the cardiac catheterization laboratory, we would use iodinated contrast to take pictures of people's arteries. We always had to be very cognizant of their kidney function because the kidney filtered the contrast, and it would increase oxidative stress in the vulnerable inner portion of the kidney. This could lead to kidney damage and, in extreme cases, kidney failure. We developed techniques for diagnostic and interventional cardiac catheterization procedures to spare the kidneys. For example, I innovated placing stents using intracoronary ultrasound and was able to use only 20cc of contrast instead of the usual 200–300cc. We got great results and alleviated stress on the kidneys. It has not been proven, but hydrogen should also relieve stress on the kidneys if used in conjunction with radiographic contrast procedures.

Optimizing kidney function is a particularly important topic for me. When I was five years old, I had strep throat, and the antibodies I developed to the bacteria attacked my kidneys. My urine turned very brown, and I wasn't making much of it. I went into kidney failure from post-streptococcal glomerulonephritis, which damaged my left kidney. So my kidney function has always been somewhat borderline, and it's something I pay a lot of attention to.

It's been shown that you can decrease the amount of protein in the urine by taking drugs like ACE inhibitors or angiotensin receptor blockers. They decrease pressure inside the kidneys' filtration units and decrease the leak to protein. Doing so decreases stress on the kidney and slows its degradation. These drugs have been shown to preserve kidney function. Remember, the diabetes drugs GLP-1 agonists and SGLT2 inhibitors have also been shown to preserve kidney function.

In my challenges with kidney damage, my creatinine had increased to over two, and I was leaking protein into the urine, which was concerning. I have some muscle mass, but not enough to account for that. I started doing several things to improve kidney function: drinking molecular hydrogen; taking Cordyceps, plus an ACE inhibitor; not eating a high-protein diet; and finally, activating AMPK and using a stem-cell procedure to help rebuild the kidneys. These steps have gotten my creatinine down to about 1.3–1.5.

Reversing chronic kidney disease is unheard of in traditional medicine. Typically, when the kidneys are not working, they will continue to progressively get worse. It's reassuring to know that you can take good care of your kidneys and improve function by doing the right things. For good measure, I don't drink much alcohol because too much alcohol damages the kidneys, too.

A probiotic called Renadyl has been shown to decrease inflammatory cytokines, TNF alpha, and IL-6, which are associated with inflammation in the kidney. Data suggests that the probiotic Renadyl can improve kidney function, even in patients with stage three or four kidney disease.

Additionally, the company Evergreen Herbs sells Chinese herbs that are particularly beneficial for kidney function. Their Kidney DTX product is excellent and highly recommended. In our practice, we have seen nice improvements in lowering creatinine and decreasing protein in the urine. Combining Renadyl and Kidney Detox is also a great strategy.

Finally, regenerative technologies like stem cell and exosome procedures have anecdotally shown great results. Dr.

Anthony Atala at Wake Forest is pioneering a technology where a biopsy is taken of your kidney. The cells are used to regrow your kidney outside the body, and then they will be used to replace your failing kidney surgically.

Technologies like these will offer people great hope in the near future.

CHAPTER FORTY

HPA Axis

The hypothalamic pituitary adrenal axis, known as the "HPA axis," comprises a good portion of the stress and hormone systems. We have come to know it as being directly related to the stress response and involved in the negative health effects of chronic stress. The *H*, which stands for *hypothalamus*, is a fascinating structure that releases signaling molecules in response to circulating blood hormone levels and stress in the system. These then signal the *P*—pituitary gland—which, in turn, releases its signaling molecules. These pituitary-signaling molecules then directly stimulate the thyroid gland, gonads, and adrenal glands (the *A* in HPA) to release their hormones.

The hypothalamus then monitors the circulating levels of the hormones, like thyroid T4 and T3; gonad-produced testosterone, estrogen, and progesterone; and adrenal-gland-produced adrenaline, cortisol, and mineralocorticoids. It adjusts the signaling to the pituitary to optimize hormone levels.

There are other hormones in this axis, but it is beyond the scope of this book to discuss them. The key point to understand is that the hypothalamus is also affected by the brain's perceived level of emotional and physical stress. When we are physically stressed or damaged, the hypothalamus will sense this from factors released by the stressed or damaged tissues and will rebuild us by signaling the release of more growth hormone from the pituitary; more testosterone and estrogen from the gonads; and the DHEA, cortisol, adrenaline, and mineralocorticoids from the adrenal glands, which control blood volume and blood pressure. These hormones then aid in the rebuilding of the stressed or damaged tissue.

In acute stress, this response of the HPA axis is exactly what we need to deal with the stress and recover. The problem comes when we are under *chronic* stress. Here, the HPA axis is activated, and we are exposed to the stress hormones cortisol, adrenaline, DHEA, and mineralocorticoids for too long. Under these circumstances, blood pressure and resting heart rate go up, and we sweat more easily, are nervous, retain fluid, and begin to tear down our bodies, resulting in ulcers, bone loss, and a weakened immune system.

These feedback loops are trying to compensate for emotional stress. They can be overstimulated, but they are so vital to our health and homeostasis we would die without them. Therefore, having an optimally functioning HPA axis is essential for health.

You have probably heard of the term *adrenal fatigue.* Adrenal fatigue is not only a problem of the adrenals, but a coping mechanism of the brain to turn down the stress response that the adrenals are mounting. High cortisol levels raise blood sugar, impair short-term memory, and sabotage sleep. The brain is trying to get the body back into equilibrium by shutting down the adrenals.

Supplements to support the adrenals are important, but dealing with chronic emotional or physical stress is the real key to recovery.

Measurement and Optimization

There are many ways to test the adrenal glands. I prefer a twenty-four-hour cortisol curve, where we can map cortisol production—total production for the day, then map the curve to see if it's low in the morning, then rises and drops appropriately for the rest of the day. If it doesn't, that gives us great insight into where somebody is—either they are highly stressed because their cortisol is high, or their adrenals have been shut down because their cortisol is low throughout the day. In either case, we can rehabilitate them.

A normal cortisol curve for an individual is at its lowest first thing in the morning when we wake up. It remains low until about thirty minutes later when their cortisol rises to its highest point to help us meet the stress of the day. Then it should be down to half the peak value a few hours later—mid-morning to mid-afternoon—half again by the evening, and then half again at bedtime, which, along with a rise in melatonin, enables us to sleep.

Some adaptogens, like rhodiola and ashwagandha, will "right the ship," raising or lowering the cortisol levels, depending on what's needed. Adaptogen brings things back into equilibrium. Other treatment options may include low doses of cortisol and adrenal extracts, which also help to modulate adrenal function.

Chronic stress is a major challenge to our health. There are many ways to deal with it, which were covered in Part One: Life Energy. They all come down to one thing: reprogramming the brain to perceive events differently. If we can do this through reflection, therapy, spiritual insight, and meditation as a means to spiritual insight and personal growth, we can break the cycle.

Brain Frequency, which we covered in the section on brain health, is an EEG-guided therapy that uses low-level electromagnetic energy in a precise format to reprogram the brain. Remarkable results are being achieved in a few centers using this technology, including Gladden Longevity. Anxiety, depression, PTSD, and even addiction can be addressed; it is not recommended, however, for anyone in the manic phase of bipolar disorder or for those with seizure disorders.

While BrainFrequency is beneficial, if we overlook the underlying problem of reframing how we see life, we will still be the victims of unnecessary stress. This brings us back to the Life Energy Circle and how important it is to optimize it. The Life Energy Circle is foundational and impacts the others: Health, Longevity, and Performance. If it isn't optimized, the others will never be, either. When the source of the anxiety can be identified and understood, it can be dealt with appropriately. Then, we can feel safe and loved. Remember, we are playing a symphony; the interrelationship among the circles cannot be ignored. Life Energy is not only the circle that binds them all, but it is critical to optimizing the HPA axis.

CHAPTER FORTY-ONE

Vision, Acuity, Presbyopia, Cataracts, Glaucoma, Retinal Issues, and Age-Related Macular Degeneration

When we are young, apart from myopia—a condition that usually originates in childhood, where the eyeball is elongated and doesn't focus light appropriately on the back of the retina, requiring us to wear glasses—we often take eye health for granted. Then, as we age, most of us encounter some form of presbyopia, which requires us to wear reading glasses. The lens of the eye loses its elasticity, and we can no longer read or view things that have fine detail or are up close. It turns out that presbyopia is related to shortened telomeres and is an indicator of the aging process itself.

At some point, cataracts also develop with age. Cataracts occur when proteins in the lens start to condense and produce a cloudy film. While cataracts are also associated with shorter telomeres, they are linked to diabetes and excessive exposure to sunlight.

As a cardiologist working in the cath lab, I wore leaded glasses to protect my eyes from the X-ray beams in the room. Nonetheless, cataracts in interventional radiologists and cardiologists remain quite common. The "usual suspects" we've encountered before also make cataracts worse: smoking, obesity, high blood pressure, and inflammation, along with previous eye injuries and surgeries.

Glaucoma is another issue characterized by increased pressure within the eye itself. You can be genetically predisposed to glaucoma, or it can be caused by trauma.

There are other age-related issues with the retina (the lining of the eyeball's interior). Rods and cones are located inside the retina, giving you visual acuity and the ability to see colors. As we age, we lose our night vision because we lose rod cells. Therefore, we are not able to detect light as well. An area on the back of a retina called the macula contains only cone cells, which provide sharp visual acuity and enable us to read fine print or see things in greater detail. Age-related macular degeneration (AMD) is a common disorder affecting women more than men, but it's a devastating disorder leading to visual loss and functional blindness. My mother suffered from it, and it was very demoralizing for her not to be able to drive or read in her final years.

AMD has two classifications: dry and wet. People with dry AMD will exhibit deposits of cholesterol and debris, collectively called drusen. Drusen accumulates in the cell layer underneath the retina and may damage the retina, particularly the macula itself. People with wet AMD may have fluid buildup around the retina as well as drusen around the macula. It is possible to have both wet and dry AMD. Many treatment options are available for wet AMD, but as of this writing, there is no way in traditional medicine to reverse the damage caused by dry AMD.

Measurement and Optimization

There are genes related to macular degeneration that can be tested for. If you find that you have some of these, particularly the HTRA-1 gene that carries nearly sixteen times increased risk of macular degeneration. There are some things you can do to improve those odds. Depending on what's found in the genetics, there may be certain supplements that are particularly advantageous to take—saffron, lutein, luteolin, fisetin, zeaxanthin, quercetin, berberine, sulforaphane, curcumin, pterostilbene or resveratrol can all be helpful.

If you have a family history of macular degeneration, it's important to either stop smoking or not take it up. Smoking is associated with an increased risk—up to fifteen times greater—of developing AMD. Increasing and maintaining adequate levels of Vitamin D and zinc will also help. Contrary to what many think, Vitamin A can make things worse for those with a genetic predisposition to AMD. It's beyond the scope of this book to delineate each of the different genes and how they work together, but understand that unless you know your genetics, you cannot develop a strategy for your eye health. IntellxxDNA does a great job of reporting these genes, and working with a certified practitioner will give you full insight into your risk and how to proceed.

Wet macular degeneration is more serious than dry; if left untreated, dry macular degeneration can progress to wet, resulting in loss of central vision.

There are anecdotal reports of an innovative new therapy that can assist in some cases to improve AMD. In our bodies, we carry very small embryonic stem cells in our blood that are dormant. Using a proprietary laser, they can be released and activated back into the bloodstream, with the laser "telling" them where to go. Reports have shown that some patients have had their vision restored using this method. In full disclosure, these are not FDA-approved procedures, and the results are *anecdotal*—there is no large-scale study to confirm these results, but it is encouraging. Telomere elongation may also be a viable strategy, but this is also in its early stages.

Whether genetically predisposed or not, you can do some general things to optimize your eye health. Certainly, wearing quality sunglasses is very important—I use polarized lenses all the time, or I won't go out during times when the sun will be directly in my eyes. Eyewear that blocks blue light—from television, computer, and cell phone screens— is beneficial for our eyes and reduces headaches from too much blue light. Blue light disrupts our circadian rhythms and may slightly increase our risk of macular degeneration, so reducing exposure is a good idea.

I find it fascinating that cataracts are another condition associated with shortened telomeres. We have patients who have taken a supplement to improve telomere lengths, and they have been able to get rid of their reading classes, which is remarkable!

With cataracts, we've found an eye drop called CanC containing L-Carnosine that, when applied, can either cause regression in the early stages of cataracts or at least stop the progression.

These age-associated deteriorations in eye function are associated with shortened telomeres, increasing senescent cells, and denatured proteins. What makes this fascinating is that if we are able to re-lengthen telomeres earlier in life, perhaps we can avoid some of these conditions. In addition, if we can prune senescent cells and decrease the pace at which senescent cells form, we may be improving our eyes as well.

And when you look at all the associated risks for eye disease—obesity, high blood pressure, smoking, high-protein diet, stress on the kidneys, increasing oxidative stress, and so on—all of these things accelerate cellular senescence. We're now seeing that many age-related disorders are a function of those drivers of aging working in the background. By manipulating those drivers and getting the symphony right, we increase our health *and* longevity and our ability to see.

CHAPTER FORTY-TWO

Cancer

I think most people fear cancer more than heart disease because at least a heart attack may take you quickly. Cancer is like heart disease in many respects—many times, it is self-inflicted.

Earlier, we covered a bit about the detox pathways and how important they are for optimizing health, but they are also critical for decreasing cancer risk. In part, cancer is caused by damage to the DNA through any number of different pathways: toxins, viruses, radiation damage, and so on. Dr. Otto Warburg first introduced a non-DNA damage cause of cancer back in the 1920s. He postulated that a decrease in mitochondrial function, which diminishes energy production, was a primary driver in causing a cell to activate other forms of energy production, ultimately activating the transformation to cancer. Weakening of the immune system, especially natural-killer cell function as we age, results in both senescent cells and malignant cells not being detected and destroyed. Finally, senescent-cell transformation from quiescent to senescence-associated secretory status, or SASP cells, is associated with cancer formation.

All of us are developing malignant cells in our bodies all the time, and the body has a way of detecting them and either shutting down their ability to divide or removing them. One way is to cause cellular senescence, taking a cell with damaged DNA and not allowing it to divide anymore so it cannot turn into a cancer cell. That's the good news about senescence.

When the senescent cells become secretory, however, they can potentiate the risk of cancer. As the natural-killer cells age, they become less effective at recognizing cancer, and cancer cells send signals telling the immune system: *There is no problem here. You don't need to be alarmed about us.* They evade the immune system.

In addition to cancer being a *function* of the aging process and a weakening immune system, there are a number of other things that play into our increasing risk. Lifestyle factors weigh heavily. We know that smokers have a much higher incidence of stomach, lung, throat, tongue, and bladder cancers. We also know that genetics play a role; BRCA 1, BRCA 2, and PALB 2 genes significantly increase the risk for breast cancer and pancreatic cancer in women (and, to a lesser extent, in men). BRCA1 and 2 also increase the risk of prostate cancer in men, particularly the presence of BRCA2.

There are other genetic disorders where the DNA simply cannot repair itself very effectively or the gene P-53 is underactive. P53 is one of the primary mechanisms by which we control cancer. If the DNA damage can be repaired,

P53 activates DNA repair genes; if the DNA cannot be repaired, P53 puts the cell into senescence or causes it to undergo self-death, i.e., apoptosis. Elephants have many copies of the P53 gene and rarely get cancer, despite having a massive number of cells and, therefore, opportunities for cancer to develop.

Environmental exposures can also contribute, along with some medical therapies themselves. High-dose chemotherapy and radiation therapy increase the risk of secondary cancers. If you have been diagnosed with cancer, your primary cancer might have gone into remission, but unfortunately, now you are at a higher risk for secondary cancer because of the trauma caused by the treatment.

Another cause can be Phase Two detox not working well. In this case, a carcinogen or a non-carcinogen may be processed by Phase One detox enzymes, creating an even stronger carcinogen. If Phase Two is not working well, this toxin can accumulate and cause real problems.

Measurement and Optimization

We can measure the relative senescence of the immune system using a test from UCLA. In addition, we know the thymus gland involutes as we age, removing our ability to produce T lymphocytes. In addition, shortening telomeres in the immune cells make them senescent and unable to respond to new challenges, like a virus or a malignant cell. Rehabbing the thymus gland and re-lengthening telomeres can have a rejuvenating effect on the immune system.

One of the problems with cancer is that it's always diagnosed too late—very few cancers seem to be caught at stage one or even stage two. We are more likely to hear something like, "He felt fine, didn't know anything about it, and now he has stage four prostate cancer." An effective preemptive approach to detecting and diagnosing cancer could eliminate these devastating surprises. A full-genome sequencing and germline genetics can give insight into what someone is predisposed to. Age- and gender-appropriate screenings are also useful. But what constitutes adequate screening?

Traditional cancer markers are, unfortunately, not very sensitive or specific. Traditional blood cancer markers are listed below, courtesy of the Cleveland Clinic:

- Alpha-fetoprotein (AFP) for liver cancer
- Beta 2-microglobulin (B2M) and lactate dehydrogenase (LDH) for blood cancers
- Calcitonin for thyroid cancer
- Cancer antigen 125 (CA 125) for ovarian cancer
- Cancer antigens 15-3 and 27-29 for breast cancer
- Carcinoembryonic antigen (CEA) for colorectal cancer, lung cancer, stomach cancer, pancreatic cancer, and others
- Human chorionic gonadotropin (HCG) for testicular cancer and ovarian cancer
- Prostate-specific antigen (PSA) and percent-free PSA for prostate cancer

While traditional blood cancer markers can be useful for following a known cancer, they lack the specificity and sensitivity to reliably diagnose cancer at an early stage. Other standard recommendations, like mammograms, have a risk of radiation to the breast. MRIs, breast ultrasounds, or breast thermography are much safer options. Digital prostate exams are very crude and unreliable for detecting disease, but a selective MRI of the prostate is useful in giving a sense of what is there.

Finding out whether someone is developing malignant cells before they develop cancer is the best opportunity to intervene—an actual cancer diagnosis with a scan is too late. The tumor is already much larger than we would like; the scans don't have the ability to see microscopic amounts of tumor cells, and neither do the blood tests.

More sophisticated testing that can look for even earlier signs of malignancy is also available. A lab in Greece, the RGCC-Group, can detect circulating tumor stem cells in the blood, even when the person does not have evidence of clinical cancer. This early detection can be very helpful as the tissue of origin can often be determined from the blood sample. In addition, DNA sequencing of the tumor calls can be done, and therapies are recommended specific to the cells found. This can result in an effective preemptive strategy. RGCC can build custom molecules to inhibit cancer cell division without harming normal cells and create vaccinations against your cancer.

Tzar Labs, a start-up in India, is on the cutting edge of pre-cancer detection. They claim to have the ability to look for circulating tumor cells and screen the blood for DNA fragments of different cancer cells. Using exosomes, DNA, and other markers, they have not been made public. They are getting ahead of cancer *before it becomes cancer* with even greater sensitivity and specificity than anything else currently available. We are awaiting more trials from them.

Another test called Galleri by GRAIL also uses exosomes to try to identify cancer. Exosomes are like mail sent from one cell to another inside the body. As previously described, an exosome has an "envelope" made from the cell membrane and has a content that consists of DNA,

RNA, protein, and lipids, and it has a signature that gives us an idea of which cell sent the mail in the first place. We currently use exosomes to screen for prostate cancer, and they are being used to try to diagnose other cancers as well.

The problem with Galleri is that it is not very sensitive or specific, which means it's not terribly helpful. A test that is 95 percent specific can reliably detect the presence of malignant cells, which would harbor the development of cancer before the person has clinical cancer. That is the point at which we want to intervene.

We also work with a company called NEO7BioScience which can sequence cancer-cell DNA and build custom peptides for a patient which they then take for a year. The peptides selectively poison only the cancer cells in the body. This approach can also be coupled with the approaches of RGCC, creating a very effective treatment strategy.

What can we do to avoid getting cancer?

Cleaning up your internal and external environment is a giant head start. We discussed detox in earlier sections, but controlling blood sugar is another key. Those with high blood sugars, high insulin levels, consistently high mTOR levels, and high growth hormone levels have a much higher incidence of developing cancer.

Making sure your pulses of testosterone and growth hormone-releasing peptides are cycled appropriately, having your telomeres appropriately re-lengthened, and testing your hormone plasma levels are other ways to get ahead of the cancer curve. Mitochondrial dysfunction is associated with the development of cancer, so optimizing mitochondrial function, as we have previously discussed, is critical.

Regular aerobic exercise, four days a week, has been shown to decrease cancer risk dramatically. Even those diagnosed with cancer will improve their longevity, so exercise is very important in mitigating the risk.

Certain peptides, like thymosin alpha-1, will boost your immune system but have been taken off the market. Other immune system-boosting peptides, like Thymulin and Thyamlin, are still available through compounding pharmacies. Neo7Bioscience makes a very potent form of Thymulin, which we use.

We also know that the diabetes drug Metformin will decrease the risk of developing cancer, likely due to its counterbalancing of mTOR by AMPK activation.

Rapamycin blocks mTOR expression and can reduce the incidence of cancer.

If you have a predisposition for skin cancer, a supplement called Heliocare® will significantly decrease basal and squamous cell carcinoma and even the risk of melanoma. Some supplements to consider for general prevention are listed below, but more specific recommendations need to be individualized:

- **HelioCare:** one-to-two pills for every four hours of sun exposure to minimize skin cancer, including basal-cell, squamous cell, and melanoma
- **Metformin SR:** 250-500 mg, one or two pills twice a day to kill malignant stem cells
- **Sulforaphane as Vitalica:** two pills twice a day to boost your Phase One and Phase Two detox
- **Boswellia:** one pill twice a day has some data
- **Ultra Cur Pro:** one pill twice a day; a highly bio-available form of curcumin
- **Kinoko Gold AHCC:** a mushroom-based product, one pill, twice a day
- **Cordyceps:** one to two pills twice a day

- **Anastrozole:** can be used weekly to balance estrogen and testosterone
- **DIM:** 100-150 mg, twice a day to decrease toxic estrogen metabolite formation
- **Resveratrol:** 250 mg, two pills twice a day
- **TocoTrienols:** one pill twice a day
- **Vitamin D3:** 5000 iu, one to three pills daily
- **5 FUNGI:** to boost immunity
- **Turkey Tail:** a mushroom used for breast cancer

As you review what I have suggested here and work on optimizing all of these different areas, you may encounter resistance from your traditionally trained healthcare providers. Because of my years as an interventional cardiologist, I can relate to their skepticism; once upon a time, I was the same way. If they don't know about it, understand it, or have any experience with it, they will dismiss and discourage it. They will call it experimental or quackery or do not believe in it because they have not seen the data.

You then have a choice: buy into traditional medicine's narrow frame of reference and dogma, or speak to a knowledgeable practitioner and get the information and data you need to feel confident in going down an alternative path. We occasionally come across traditionally trained colleagues who are open-minded, intrigued by what we do, and in many ways jealous that we can offer diagnostics and interventions they cannot.

That being said, I have given up trying to change the medical establishment because they are married to their answers and have an economic model they want to protect. If it hasn't had six double-blind, placebo-controlled trials with ten thousand people, then they are not going to believe it even though many of those trials are faulty in the first place. There is so much selection bias in trials, and those segments not included in the study have the results extrapolated and fed to them as a course of treatment. There are other problems with the medical literature being corrupted by economic, political, and relationship agendas that are beyond the scope of this book to discuss. Bottom line: don't believe every study you read.

Generally speaking, physicians have a mindset that they have superior training and, therefore, are very resistant to anything they were not specifically trained in. If you want to do something different, you will have to find a different practitioner.

That doesn't mean you should abandon your primary care physician; give them an opportunity. Some primary care physicians are understanding; they know they don't have all the answers, and they are sympathetic to and open to other integrative approaches. If you are fortunate enough to work with one of those, they will be happy to help you and won't feel threatened by the fact that you may want to talk to someone else.

30 Year Old Body

1. Resilient
2. Robust
3. Curious
4. Adventurous
5. Creative
6. Imaginative
7. Enthusiastic
8. Passionate
9. Fearless
10. Confident
11. Capable
12. Open Minded
13. Adaptable
14. Playful

Final Thoughts on Health

A common question may be circulating in your mind: *How long do I have to do all these things, take these supplements, make these lifestyle changes, to be the best version of myself?* The answer is issues with health, longevity, and performance fall into two general categories: short-term and long-term.

Typically, when a problem is new, it may seem that it will be of short duration. In our world of optimization, however, we understand that the problem has likely been developing for a long time. High-blood pressure, non-alcoholic fatty liver disease, a decline in kidney function, early cognitive decline, and diabetes do not appear overnight. Dealing with a new onset problem requires a short-term strategy to control the problem and a long-term strategy to unravel the knot of how it got there, how to fix it, and how to prevent its recurrence.

This is where longevity medicine provides a massive advantage over traditional or even functional medicine. As we referenced at the beginning of this section, the client receives what we believe to be the optimal approach by working on all three levels simultaneously. The most superficial level is responding to and treating symptoms—traditional medicine's approach. The second level is a root-cause approach, looking to see what is causing the symptoms in the first place—functional or integrative medicine's approach. Longevity medicine addresses levels one and two but also addresses the third and most foundational level: *the aging process*. Addressing the aging process enables us to address the root-cause of the root cause. Our go-forward strategy is to assess, treat, and construct a preventive environment to understand, fix, and keep you young. In essence, making you antifragile with greater resilience and robustness.

By focusing on the drivers of aging, our strategy is designed to not only reset your biological clock to a more youthful state but to provide you with what you want and need most: resilience, robustness, and adaptability. To that end, creating an environment that supports eating well, sleeping well, avoiding toxins, exercising, and optimizing life energy will always be part of a long-term strategy. In aggregate, addressing all four circles—life energy, longevity, health, and performance—to fix the past enables you to be a fully expressed human today and protect your future is an exponential strategy to an exponential problem. So, you see, every short-term issue must have a long-term solution.

Longevity medicine is the medicine of the future, and it is here today, available at Gladden Longevity outside and with our IRB-approved trial.

What's your strategy?

Health Notes

Carlos López-Otín and Guido Kroemer, "Hallmarks of Health," *Cell* 184, no. 1 (January 7, 2021): 33–63, https://doi.org/10.1016/j.cell.2020.11.034.

NES Health, "How NES Technology Works: NES Health," How NES Technology Works | NES Health, accessed July 14, 2023, https://www.neshealth.com/science/how-nes-works/.

Amirreza Sajjadieh et al., "The Association of Sleep Duration and Quality with Heart Rate Variability and Blood Pressure.," *Tanaffos* 19, no. 2 (November 2019): 135–43.

Shui Jiang et al., "Epigenetic Modifications in Stress Response Genes Associated with Childhood Trauma," *Frontiers in Psychiatry* 10 (November 8, 2019), https://doi.org/10.3389/fpsyt.2019.00808.

Cathy Spatz Widom and Linda M Brzustowicz, "Maoa and the 'Cycle of Violence:' Childhood Abuse and Neglect, MAOA Genotype, and Risk for Violent and Antisocial Behavior," *Biological Psychiatry* 60, no. 7 (October 1, 2006): 684–89, https://doi.org/10.1016/j.biopsych.2006.03.039.

Diana Armbruster et al., "Children under Stress – COMT Genotype and Stressful Life Events Predict Cortisol Increase in an Acute Social Stress Paradigm," *The International Journal of Neuropsychopharmacology* 15, no. 09 (October 12, 2011): 1229–39, https://doi.org/10.1017/s1461145711001763.

Joseph A Boscarino et al., "Higher FKBP5, COMT, CHRNA5, and CRHR1 Allele Burdens Are Associated with PTSD and Interact with Trauma Exposure: Implications for Neuropsychiatric Research and Treatment," *Neuropsychiatric Disease and Treatment*, February 11, 2012, 131, https://doi.org/10.2147/ndt.s29508.

Yuzhu Li et al., "The Brain Structure and Genetic Mechanisms Underlying the Nonlinear Association between Sleep Duration, Cognition and Mental Health," *Nature Aging* 2, no. 5 (April 28, 2022): 425–37, https://doi.org/10.1038/s43587-022-00210-2.

Jean-Philippe Chaput, Caroline Dutil, and Hugues Sampasa-Kanyinga, "Sleeping Hours: What Is the Ideal Number and How Does Age Impact This?," *Nature and Science of Sleep* Volume 10 (November 27, 2018): 421–30, https://doi.org/10.2147/nss.s163071.

Samara P. Silva et al., "Neuroprotective Effect of Taurine against Cell Death, Glial Changes, and Neuronal Loss in the Cerebellum of Rats Exposed to Chronic-Recurrent Neuroinflammation Induced by LPS," *Journal of Immunology Research* 2021 (July 5, 2021): 1–10, https://doi.org/10.1155/2021/7497185.

"NCI Dictionary of Cancer Terms," National Cancer Institute, accessed August 1, 2023, https://www.cancer.gov/publications/dictionaries/cancer-terms/def/pet-scan.

Jacques E Rossouw et al., "Risks and Benefits of Estrogen plus Progestin in Healthy Postmenopausal Women: Principal Results from the Women's Health Initiative Randomized Controlled Trial," *JAMA: The Journal of the American Medical Association* 288, no. 3 (July 17, 2002): 321–33, https://doi.org/10.1001/jama.288.3.321.

"What Is Pi-Rads and Why Should You Care?," THE "NEW" PROSTATE CANCER INFOLINK, September 24, 2014, https://prostatecancerinfolink.net/2014/09/24/what-is-pi-rads-and-why-should-you-care/.

Tomi S. Mikkola et al., "Reduced Risk of Breast Cancer Mortality in Women Using Postmenopausal Hormone Therapy: A Finnish Nationwide Comparative Study," *Menopause* 23, no. 11 (November 23, 2016): 1199–1203, https://doi.org/10.1097/gme.0000000000000698.

P. Stute, L. Wildt, and J. Neulen, "The Impact of Micronized Progesterone on Breast Cancer Risk: A Systematic Review," Climacteric 21, no. 2 (January 31, 2018): 111–22, https://doi.org/10.1080/13697137.2017.1421925.

Chiara Porro, Tarek Benameur, and MariaA Panaro, "The Antiaging Role of Oxytocin," *Neural Regeneration Research* 16, no. 12 (December 2021): 2413, https://doi.org/10.4103/1673-5374.313030.

Joseph Campbell, *The Hero with a Thousand Faces* (Los Angeles, CA: Joseph Campbell Foundation, 2020).

Natalie Guadiana and Taylor Okashima, *The Effects of Sleep Deprivation on College Students*, 2021, https://doi.org/10.33015/dominican.edu/2021. nurs.st.09.

Nikola Todorovic et al., "Hydrogen-rich Water and Caffeine for Alertness and Brain Metabolism in Sleep-deprived Habitual Coffee Drinkers," *Food Science & Nutrition* 9, no. 9 (July 19, 2021): 5139–45, https://doi.org/10.1002/fsn3.2480.

Roland R Griffiths et al., "Efficacy and Safety of Psilocybin-Assisted Treatment for Major Depressive Disorder: Prospective 12-Month Follow-Up," *Journal of Psychopharmacology* 36, no. 2 (February 15, 2022): 151–58, https://doi.org/10.1177/02698811211073759.

See also: https://www.hopkinsmedicine.org/psychiatry/research/ psychedelics-research.html

Dayan Goodenowe, *Breaking Alzheimer's: A 15-Year Crusade to Expose the Cause and Deliver the Cure*, 2021.

Eugenia Landolfo et al., "Effects of Palmitoylethanolamide on Neurodegenerative Diseases: A Review from Rodents to Humans," Biomolecules 12, no. 5 (May 5, 2022): 667, https://doi.org/10.3390/ biom12050667.

Dale E. Bredesen, *The End of Alzheimer's: The First Program to Prevent and Reverse Cognitive Decline* (Waterville, ME: Thorndike Press, 2021).

Anastasiya Volkova et al., "Selank Administration Affects the Expression of Some Genes Involved in GABAergic Neurotransmission," Frontiers in Pharmacology 7 (February 18, 2016), https://doi.org/10.3389/fphar.2016.00031.

Jill Rosen, "This Training Exercise Boosts Brain Power, Johns Hopkins Researchers Say," The Hub - Johns Hopkins University, October 17, 2017, https://hub.jhu.edu/2017/10/17/brain-training-exercise/.

Aki Vainionpää et al., "Effects of High-Impact Exercise on Bone Mineral Density: A Randomized Controlled Trial in Premenopausal Women," *Osteoporosis International* 16, no. 2 (June 17, 2004): 191–97, https://doi.org/10.1007/s00198-004-1659-5.

Lars Larsson et al., "Sarcopenia: Aging-Related Loss of Muscle Mass and Function," *Physiological Reviews* 99, no. 1 (January 1, 2019): 427–511, https://doi.org/10.1152/physrev.00061.2017.

William Evans et al., "Effects of Fortetropin on the Rate of Muscle Protein Synthesis in Older Men and Women: A Randomized, Double-Blinded, Placebo-Controlled Study," *The Journals of Gerontology: Series A* 76, no. 1 (June 29, 2020): 108–14, https://doi.org/10.1093/gerona/glaa162.

Sue C Bodine, "The Role of mTORC1 in the Regulation of Skeletal Muscle Mass," *Faculty Reviews* 11 (November 11, 2022), https://doi.org/10.12703/r/11-32.

Lars Larsson et al., "Sarcopenia: Aging-Related Loss of Muscle Mass and Function," Physiological Reviews 99, no. 1 (January 1, 2019): 427–511, https://doi.org/10.1152/physrev.00061.2017.

Natalia I. Dmitrieva et al., "Middle-Age High Normal Serum Sodium as a Risk Factor for Accelerated Biological Aging, Chronic Diseases, and Premature Mortality," *eBioMedicine* 87 (January 2, 2023): 104404, https://doi.org/10.1016/j.ebiom.2022.104404.

Lucija Tomljenovic, "Aluminum and Alzheimer's Disease: After a Century of Controversy, Is There a Plausible Link?," *Journal of Alzheimer's Disease* 23, no. 4 (March 21, 2011): 567–98, https://doi.org/10.3233/jad-2010-101494.

"First Evidence of Farming in Mideast 23,000 Years Ago," ScienceDaily, July 22, 2015, https://www.sciencedaily.com/releases/2015/07/150722144709.htm.

Hang-Yu Li et al., "Effects and Mechanisms of Probiotics, Prebiotics, Synbiotics, and Postbiotics on Metabolic Diseases Targeting Gut Microbiota: A Narrative Review," *Nutrients* 13, no. 9 (September 15, 2021): 3211, https://doi.org/10.3390/nu13093211.

Vijay Panicker et al., "Common Variation in the DIO2 Gene Predicts Baseline Psychological Well-Being and Response to Combination Thyroxine plus Triiodothyronine Therapy in Hypothyroid Patients," *The Journal of Clinical Endocrinology & Metabolism* 94, no. 5 (May 1, 2009): 1623–29, https://doi.org/10.1210/jc.2008-1301.

"Decrease of Iodine Intake Found in Americans," Centers for Disease Control and Prevention, May 20, 2014, https://www.cdc.gov/media/pressrel/ad981001.htm.

Sian M Robinson et al., "Preconception Maternal Iodine Status Is Positively Associated with IQ but Not with Measures of Executive Function in Childhood," *The Journal of Nutrition* 148, no. 6 (June 1, 2018): 959–66, https://doi.org/10.1093/jn/nxy054.

Mukul Bhattarai et al., "Association of Sodium-Glucose Cotransporter 2 Inhibitors with Cardiovascular Outcomes in Patients with Type 2 Diabetes and Other Risk Factors for Cardiovascular Disease," *JAMA Network Open* 5, no. 1 (January 5, 2022), https://doi.org/10.1001/jamanetworkopen.2021.42078.

Nikolaus Marx et al., "GLP-1 Receptor Agonists for the Reduction of Atherosclerotic Cardiovascular Risk in Patients with Type 2 Diabetes," *Circulation* 146, no. 24 (December 13, 2022): 1882–94, https://doi.org/10.1161/circulationaha.122.059595.

See https://prolonfast.com/products/prolon-offer-v1

Yangbo Sun et al., "Meal Skipping and Shorter Meal Intervals Are Associated with Increased Risk of All-Cause and Cardiovascular Disease Mortality among US Adults," *Journal of the Academy of Nutrition and Dietetics* 123, no. 3 (March 2023), https://doi.org/10.1016/j.jand.2022.08.119.

David A. Sinclair, "Toward a Unified Theory of Caloric Restriction and Longevity Regulation," *Mechanisms of Ageing and Development* 126, no. 9 (September 2005): 987–1002, https://doi.org/10.1016/j.mad.2005.03.019.

Shannon Miller, "Intermittent Fasting vs. Frequent Meals: What Does the Science Say?," Composition ID, December 12, 2019, https://www.compositionid.com/blog/nutrition/intermittent-fasting-vs-frequent-meals-what-does-the-science-say/.

Christopher H. Rhodes et al., "Human Fasting Modulates Macrophage Function and Upregulates Multiple Bioactive Metabolites That Extend Lifespan in Caenorhabditis Elegans: A Pilot Clinical Study," *The American Journal of Clinical Nutrition* 117, no. 2 (February 2023): 286–97, https://doi.org/10.1016/j.ajcnut.2022.10.015.

Abbas Ghaddar et al., "Increased Alcohol Dehydrogenase 1 Activity Promotes Longevity," *Current Biology* 33, no. 6 (March 2023), https://doi.org/10.1016/j.cub.2023.01.059.

Natalia I. Dmitrieva et al., "Middle-Age High Normal Serum Sodium as a Risk Factor for Accelerated Biological Aging, Chronic Diseases, and Premature Mortality," *eBioMedicine* 87 (January 2, 2023): 104404, https://doi.org/10.1016/j.ebiom.2022.104404.

Abbas Ghaddar et al., "Increased Alcohol Dehydrogenase 1 Activity Promotes Longevity," *Current Biology* 33, no. 6 (March 27, 2023), https://doi.org/10.1016/j.cub.2023.01.059.

Tasnim Momoniat, Duha Ilyas, and Sunil Bhandari, "ACE Inhibitors and Arbs: Managing Potassium and Renal Function," *Cleveland Clinic Journal of Medicine* 86, no. 9 (September 2019): 601–7, https://doi.org/10.3949/ccjm.86a.18024.

Ranganathan Natarajan et al., "Randomized Controlled Trial of Strain-Specific Probiotic Formulation (RENADYL) in Dialysis Patients," *BioMed Research International* 2014 (July 24, 2014): 1–9, https://doi.org/10.1155/2014/568571.

Christine Dunkel Schetter and Christyn Dolbier, "Resilience in the Context of Chronic Stress and Health in Adults," *Social and Personality Psychology Compass* 5, no. 9 (September 2011): 634–52, https://doi.org/10.1111/j.1751-9004.2011.00379.x.

Amber Snyder, "Restoring Lost Vision: New Stem Cell Treatment Developed for AMD," *NIH Record* 73, no. 15 (July 23, 2021).

Michelle Potter, Emma Newport, and Karl J. Morten, "The Warburg Effect: 80 Years On," *Biochemical Society Transactions* 44, no. 5 (October 15, 2016): 1499–1505, https://doi.org/10.1042/bst20160094.

"Blood Tests for Cancer: Diagnosis & Treatment," Cleveland Clinic, accessed April 20, 2023, https://my.clevelandclinic.org/health/diagnostics/22338-blood-tests-for-cancer.

Nasrien E. Ibrahim et al., "A Clinical, Proteomics, and Artificial Intelligence-Driven Model to Predict Acute Kidney Injury in Patients Undergoing Coronary Angiography," *Clinical Cardiology* 42, no. 2 (January 8, 2019): 292–98, https://doi.org/10.1002/clc.23143.

Ronald J. Jandacek, "Linoleic Acid: A Nutritional Quandary," *Healthcare* 5, no. 2 (May 20, 2017): 25, https://doi.org/10.3390/healthcare5020025.

Alexander A. Goldberg et al., "A Novel Function of Lipid Droplets in Regulating Longevity," *Biochemical Society Transactions* 37, no. 5 (September 21, 2009): 1050–55, https://doi.org/10.1042/bst0371050.

José Cipolla-Neto et al., "The Crosstalk between Melatonin and Sex Steroid Hormones," *Neuroendocrinology* 112, no. 2 (March 26, 2021): 115–29, https://doi.org/10.1159/000516148.

D. James Morré, Dorothy M. Morré, and Thomas B. Shelton, "Aging-Related Nicotinamide Adenine Dinucleotide Oxidase Response to Dietary Supplementation: The French Paradox Revisited," *Rejuvenation Research* 13, no. 2–3 (April 2010): 159–61, https://doi.org/10.1089/rej.2009.0918.

Kunihiro Tsuchida et al., "Activin Signaling as an Emerging Target for Therapeutic Interventions," *Cell Communication and Signaling* 7, no. 1 (June 18, 2009), https://doi.org/10.1186/1478-811x-7-15.

Cristina Planella-Farrugia et al., "Circulating Irisin and Myostatin as Markers of Muscle Strength and Physical Condition in Elderly Subjects," *Frontiers in Physiology* 10 (July 10, 2019), https://doi.org/10.3389/fphys.2019.00871.

H.Q. Han and William E. Mitch, "Targeting the Myostatin Signaling Pathway to Treat Muscle Wasting Diseases," *Current Opinion in Supportive & Palliative Care* 5, no. 4 (December 2011): 334–41, https://doi.org/10.1097/spc.0b013e32834bddf9.

Michela Campolo et al., "Pea-Oxa Mitigates Oxaliplatin-Induced Painful Neuropathy through NF-KB/NRF-2 Axis," *International Journal of Molecular Sciences* 22, no. 8 (April 10, 2021): 3927, https://doi.org/10.3390/ijms22083927.

Jun Kobayashi, Kazuo Ohtake, and Hiroyuki Uchida, "No-Rich Diet for Lifestyle-Related Diseases," *Nutrients* 7, no. 6 (June 17, 2015): 4911–37, https://doi.org/10.3390/nu7064911.

Ralph J. DeBerardinis, "Proliferating Cells Conserve Nitrogen to Support Growth," *Cell Metabolism* 23, no. 6 (June 2016): 957–58, https://doi.org/10.1016/j.cmet.2016.05.008.

Susan Amanda Lund, Cecilia M. Giachelli, and Marta Scatena, "The Role of Osteopontin in Inflammatory Processes," *Journal of Cell Communication and Signaling* 3, no. 3–4 (October 2, 2009): 311–22, https://doi.org/10.1007/s12079-009-0068-0.

Syed Faizan Mehdi et al., "Oxytocin and Related Peptide Hormones: Candidate Anti-Inflammatory Therapy in Early Stages of Sepsis," *Frontiers in Immunology* 13 (April 29, 2022), https://doi.org/10.3389/fimmu.2022.864007.

Jennie R. Stevenson et al., "Oxytocin Administration Prevents Cellular Aging Caused by Social Isolation," *Psychoneuroendocrinology* 103 (May 2019): 52–60, https://doi.org/10.1016/j.psyneuen.2019.01.006.

John Moffett, Nicole Kubat, and Linley Fray, "Effect of Pulsed Electromagnetic Field Treatment on Programmed Resolution of Inflammation Pathway Markers in Human Cells in Culture," *Journal of Inflammation Research*, February 2015, 59, https://doi.org/10.2147/jir.s78631.

Mary C. Stephenson et al., "Magnetic Field Therapy Enhances Muscle Mitochondrial Bioenergetics and Attenuates Systemic Ceramide Levels Following ACL Reconstruction: Southeast Asian Randomized-Controlled Pilot Trial," *Journal of Orthopaedic Translation* 35 (July 2022): 99–112, https://doi.org/10.1016/j.jot.2022.09.011.

Michael J Gonzalez et al., "Photobiomodulation, Energy and Cancer: A Quantum Notion.," *J Cancer Sci Res Ther* 1, no. 1 (2021): 1–10.

Samuel Abokyi, George Ghartey-Kwansah, and Dennis Yan-yin Tse, "TFEB Is a Central Regulator of the Aging Process and Age-Related Diseases," *Ageing Research Reviews* 89 (August 2023): 101985, https://doi.org/10.1016/j.arr.2023.101985.

Dr. Adam Tenforde, M.D., "Art of Shock Wave," CuraMedix, accessed July 16, 2023, https://www.curamedix.com/art-of-shock-wave-white-paper.

Low Tyramine Headache Diet* - National Headache Foundation, accessed July 16, 2023, https://headaches.org/wp-content/uploads/2021/05/TyramineDiet.pdf.

Tommaso Iannitti and Beniamino Palmieri, "Clinical and Experimental Applications of Sodium Phenylbutyrate," *Drugs in R&D* 11, no. 3 (September 2011): 227–49, https://doi.org/10.2165/11591280-000000000-00000.

Matthias H. Tschöp, Michael Stumvoll, and Michael Ristow, "Opposing Effects of Antidiabetic Interventions on Malignant Growth and Metastasis," *Cell Metabolism* 23, no. 6 (June 2016): 959–60, https://doi.org/10.1016/j.cmet.2016.05.017.

Jinumary Aji John and Revati Patel, Exacta Encyclopedic Liquid Biopsy Report, accessed July 16, 2023, https://datarpgx.com/.

Predrag Sikiric et al., "Stable Gastric Pentadecapeptide BPC 157, Robert's Stomach Cytoprotection/Adaptive Cytoprotection/Organoprotection, and Selye's Stress Coping Response: Progress, Achievements, and the Future," *Gut and Liver* 14, no. 2 (March 15, 2020): 153–67, https://doi.org/10.5009/gnl18490.

Hongxing Wang et al., "Potential Therapeutic Effects of Cyanidin-3-o-Glucoside on Rheumatoid Arthritis by Relieving Inhibition of CD38+ NK Cells on Treg Cell Differentiation," *Arthritis Research & Therapy* 21, no. 1 (October 28, 2019), https://doi.org/10.1186/s13075-019-2001-0.

Mariana G. Tarragó et al., "A Potent and Specific CD38 Inhibitor Ameliorates Age-Related Metabolic Dysfunction by Reversing Tissue NAD+ Decline," *Cell Metabolism* 27, no. 5 (May 2018), https://doi.org/10.1016/j.cmet.2018.03.016.

A M Wang et al., "Use of Carnosine as a Natural Anti-Senescence Drug for Human Beings," Biochemistry. Biokhimiia, July 2000, https://pubmed.ncbi.nlm.nih.gov/10951108/.

Ivana Jukić et al., "Carnosine, Small but Mighty—Prospect of Use as Functional Ingredient for Functional Food Formulation," *Antioxidants* 10, no. 7 (June 28, 2021): 1037, https://doi.org/10.3390/antiox10071037.

Steve Horvath et al., "The Cerebellum Ages Slowly According to the Epigenetic Clock," *Aging* 7, no. 5 (May 11, 2015): 294–306, https://doi.org/10.18632/aging.100742.

Suresh Patankar et al., "A Single Arm Trial in Treatment of CKD Patients with Sodium Copper Chlorophyllin Formulation," *American Journal of Food and Nutrition* 7, no. 3 (October 2019): 107–12, https://doi.org/10.12691/ajfn-7-3-5.

Er-Dan Luo et al., "Advancements in Lead Therapeutic Phytochemicals Polycystic Ovary Syndrome: A Review," *Frontiers in Pharmacology* 13 (January 9, 2023), https://doi.org/10.3389/fphar.2022.1065243.

Wei-hong Chen et al., "Therapeutic Potential of Exosomes/Mirnas in Polycystic Ovary Syndrome Induced by the Alteration of Circadian Rhythms," *Frontiers in Endocrinology* 13 (November 16, 2022), https://doi.org/10.3389/fendo.2022.918805.

Paul Clayton et al., "Palmitoylethanolamide: A Natural Compound for Health Management," *International Journal of Molecular Sciences* 22, no. 10 (May 18, 2021): 5305, https://doi.org/10.3390/ijms22105305.

Melissa V Yuen et al., "Phosphatidylcholine: Summary Report," The UMB Digital Archive, October 1, 2021, https://archive.hshsl.umaryland.edu/handle/10713/17690.

Wei Yin et al., "Melatonin for Premenstrual Syndrome: A Potential Remedy but Not Ready," *Frontiers in Endocrinology* 13 (January 9, 2023), https://doi.org/10.3389/fendo.2022.1084249.

JIN-SOO KIM et al., "Myokine Expression and Tumor-Suppressive Effect of Serum after 12 Wk of Exercise in Prostate Cancer Patients on ADT," *Medicine & Science in Sports & Exercise* 54, no. 2 (September 22, 2021): 197–205, https://doi.org/10.1249/mss.0000000000002783.

Suvarna Bhamre et al., "Temporal Changes in Gene Expression Induced by Sulforaphane in Human Prostate Cancer Cells," *The Prostate* 69, no. 2 (February 1, 2009): 181–90, https://doi.org/10.1002/pros.20869.

Daniel N. Costa et al., "Gleason Grade Group Concordance between Preoperative Targeted Biopsy and Radical Prostatectomy Histopathologic Analysis: A Comparison between in-Bore MRI-Guided and MRI–Transrectal US Fusion Prostate Biopsies," *Radiology: Imaging Cancer* 3, no. 2 (March 1, 2021), https://doi.org/10.1148/rycan.2021200123.

Daniel N. Costa et al., "Magnetic Resonance Imaging–Guided in-Bore and Magnetic Resonance Imaging-Transrectal Ultrasound Fusion Targeted Prostate Biopsies: An Adjusted Comparison of Clinically Significant Prostate Cancer Detection Rate," *European Urology Oncology* 2, no. 4 (July 2019): 397–404, https://doi.org/10.1016/j.euo.2018.08.022.

Robert U Newton et al., "Intense Exercise for Survival among Men with Metastatic Castrate-Resistant Prostate Cancer (Interval-GAP4): A Multicentre, Randomised, Controlled Phase III Study Protocol," *BMJ Open* 8, no. 5 (May 2018), https://doi.org/10.1136/bmjopen-2018-022899.

Hans C. Arora, Charis Eng, and Daniel A. Shoskes, "Gut Microbiome and Chronic Prostatitis/Chronic Pelvic Pain Syndrome," *Annals of Translational Medicine* 5 (January 2017): 30–30, https://doi.org/10.21037/atm.2016.12.32.

Eunse Park and Kimberly Castle. "The effect of an isometric trunk training during spinning in a child with Cerebral Palsy: A case report." (2021), https://digitalcommons.northgeorgia.edu/ijhr/vol1/iss1/4.

Katrine L. Rasmussen et al., "Associations of Alzheimer Disease–Protective *Apoe* Variants with Age-Related Macular Degeneration," *JAMA Ophthalmology* 141, no. 1 (January 1, 2023): 13, https://doi.org/10.1001/jamaophthalmol.2022.4602.

For more references, please visit GladdenLongevity.com/Book100.

Part Four

Performance

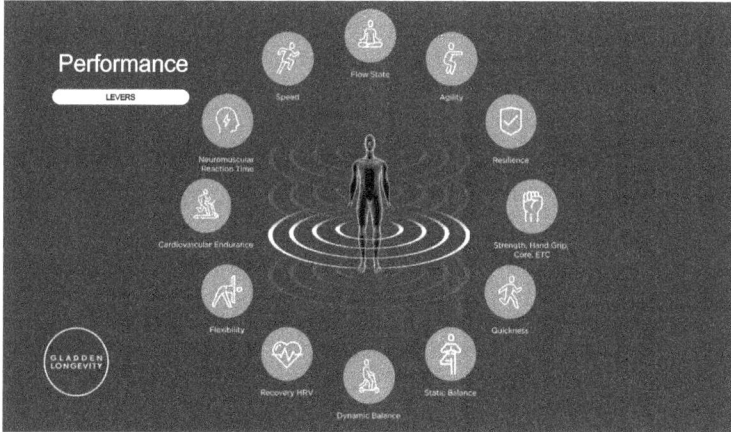

How Do We Live Young for a Lifetime?

What Is Performance?

I define great physical *performance* as being fast, agile, strong, quick, balanced, and flexible, with great cardiovascular capacity, endurance, and great recovery. If you want that kind of physical performance at age one hundred, you had better be sure you have it today; how close are you? When you think about a typical ninety-year-old's physical appearance and capabilities, you likely envision anything but what I've described above. So, where do we begin to reverse what we typically see and get young so we can live young?

When we're young and want to get in shape, all that's required is getting good sleep, doing various aerobic exercises, and resistance training with appropriate recovery and reasonable nutrition. If we need to master a skill, like playing tennis, golf, basketball, or skiing, we practice that particular skill to train the neuromuscular system to perform that task, but our general conditioning comes along quite easily. We don't have to think about the elements of *fast*, *agile*, *quick*, *balanced*, and *great recovery* in order to get them.

As we age, however, we lose important components of performance like agility, recovery, resilience, strength, quickness, flexibility, static balance, and dynamic balance.

We don't recover nearly as well. We don't have much in the way of cardiovascular capacity or endurance, lung capacity is reduced, neuromuscular reaction times slow down, and there is a loss of coordination.

I started noticing this when I hit my forties. Running, biking, calisthenics, balance training, and weightlifting got me back to a great level. When I hit my fifties, however, what I was doing was no longer working. This is not unusual, yet it is a critical concept often dismissed or overlooked: *What you did when you were younger will not get you where you want to be today. What you do today will not get you where you want to be tomorrow.*

It is critical to stay young by using advanced interventional protocols that stress timing, frequency, intensity, and duration, but it is also critical to continuously adapt your training to excel at all the facets of performance as we have defined them. In order to understand where you fall on the spectrum of performance, testing each of these capabilities is essential. Professional teams understand this. The NFL conducts a series of tests during the NFL Combine that measure an athlete's quickness, agility, speed, and strength. I've heard MLB trainers espouse that if they only had one test to assess an athlete, it would be a vertical jump. These tests the professionals use can be adapted to just about anyone who is reasonably fit and are very useful in evaluating athletic and not-so-athletic clients.

We incorporate similar testing into our Gladden Longevity performance assessments. When we do baseline testing to check these things, all of a sudden, it becomes very clear that, as they age, most people have lost much more than they think they have. They have settled into golf or tennis and can still play pretty well, so they may not be regularly reminded of their decline. They know that they can't run as fast, but they've lost not just speed but quickness and agility. When we lose capability, we lose confidence—confidence to push the envelope or try new activities or exercises. Ultimately, they have lost confidence in their neuromuscular system's ability to adapt and perform. That is a sad day.

But all is not lost!

In our world, the circle of performance is broken down into specific elements, and we test and train each of them. It is possible to train agility, flexibility, speed, balance, and so on. (Visit GladdenLongevity.com for videos that show you how.) With this in mind, let's work our way around the performance circle.

CHAPTER FORTY-THREE

Flow

The Performance Circle contains a lot of different physical performance checkpoints—neuromuscular reaction time, speed, balance, agility, quickness, and so on—but performance is not composed of those individual components. It's an integrated system that combines all those components to enable someone to perform at a high level. This is where *flow* comes in.

The godfather of flow physiology is Dr. Mihaly Csikszentmihalyi, a Hungarian-American psychologist. He was fascinated with understanding the *times* when people felt the very best in their lives; his research found that everyone's stories started to revolve around this one particular experience or feeling that he ultimately called *flow*.

Csikszentmihalyi defined *flow* as a state of being highly focused, fully present, committed to an outcome but not committed to a course of action; in essence, being highly adaptable. I would add that it has elements of being effortless and there is a lack of trying—there is only doing. When you are in flow, you are in a state of equilibrium and balance; in essence, you reside in an energetic field of all possibilities. Being in this state enables the effortless selection of action from the greatest number of available responses to best respond to the current challenge. People who are in flow are performing at a very high level, but they are not "trying" to do it; they are simply doing it. Things are happening, and they are both directing them *and* allowing them to happen. They are looking into the future, anticipating what's going to happen, but it is happening at the level of no thought—making good decisions requires no thinking. The brain's computer is free from thought and analysis and instead simply integrates the available information and responds with no judgment or emotional overtone. It is pure *doing pure flow!*

Being in flow gives us the ability to respond, adapt, create, and perform at the highest level. We've been trained to slow down and think things through, weigh the options, and think through the consequences, but there is no time to think in the rich data field of high-intensity activity. While it's possible to react by instinct, many times, instincts are clouded by emotion and preprogrammed software defining what's possible; this leads to suboptimal performance and outcome.

Being in flow means being in a headspace of being highly alert, calm in equilibrium, and doing without superimposed thought. I think of it as meditation in action. Learning to access flow—not only in athletics but in any life situation—is one of the ultimate skills for humans to achieve. Those in a state of flow are not under particular stress, even though flow states are generally precipitated by circumstances that could be considered stressful. Achieving a flow state is similar to building a meditation practice; with regular practice, you can find that place and get there, and once you have it, you can access it at will.

Author and journalist Steven Kotler explored the concept of flow by chronicling the achievements of extreme athletes in his book, *The Rise of Superman: Decoding the Science of Ultimate Human Performance.* He details the rate of progression in extreme sports compared to other sports, looking at the much higher rate of advancement in skills and abilities of extreme-sport athletes. Kotler discovered they could continually innovate and achieve exceptional results when in flow: the first backflip on a motorcycle; the first double backflip on skis; surfing incredibly large waves; kayaking Class 5 rivers, and so on. The athletes would only describe doing these things from within a state of flow.

To achieve a state of flow, there has to be enough external stimulation and enough internal awareness to trigger the body to move beyond thinking. Things have to be happening at a pace where thought can't keep up, anticipate, calculate, and try to solve the problem. One has to let go and rely on the innate ability of the brain to "do the math" and come up with the best solution. When you are in flow, it is like tapping into another part of greater consciousness and processing information that is beyond thought but not beyond joy.

When one can do that, all of a sudden, critical thinking is turned off. Yet, the ability to perceive, adapt, respond, and create is heightened and enhanced—primarily because there are no "overthinking" or preconditioned limitations placed on the situation. Just to expand the vernacular, you will often hear the flow state described as being "in the zone."

The beauty of being in flow is that the person is able to bring all their talents to bear. They transcend the frontal lobes, where overly critical, judgemental, and limiting thinking resides. Out of flow, we find ourselves worrying about the outcome, our technique, the consequences, etc. In doing so, our overthinking tends to paralyze or slow us down to the point where we can't effortlessly and fluidly perform the task.

When a person is in flow, however, they find themselves completely immersed in the moment—open, focused, and responding—in a fluid, trance-like state. According to both Csikszentmihalyi and Kotler, these are the moments when people feel the most alive and joyful. Again, it is analogous to an immersive loss of oneself in a meditative or enlightened state focused on being present and in a state of enhanced consciousness. This is why audiences loved the live Grateful Dead shows; they could feel when the band slipped into the flow, and they went along for the ride—the ultimate natural high.

When we think about why extreme athletes, musicians, or anyone else do what they do, everyone talks about adrenaline—the adrenaline high or adrenaline rush—and, in fact, adrenaline is a *driver*. Beyond adrenaline, however, is the massive draw to slip into flow. Based on my own experience, I think flow is what drives them. Even though the sport is extreme, it is not about being out of control or scaring themselves; it's about putting themselves into a context where there are enough external stimuli to exceed the capacity of their thinking minds to process all the data that pushes them into this flow state.

Maybe you're not doing extreme sports, an athlete, or a musician but you can also enter a flow state. Once you know that it is out there waiting for you, you'll start to ask, *How do I access flow?* It's possible to go into a flow state just about any time and anywhere—while writing, reading this book, looking out the window, driving your car, in a conversation, making love, in a business meeting, and so on. In fact, in Steven Kotler's book, he describes that when the participants are in flow, meetings have much higher productivity. Participants function at a much higher level, solve problems easily, and resolve conflict more effectively. This is because everyone is vibrating at a much higher level, resulting in better relationships and better outcomes.

According to Kotler, this can happen with a spouse, friend, or coworker. I'll add that it can also happen with yourself, particularly as you optimize the elements of the life energy circle, you can drop into a flow state relative to yourself, your life, purpose, relationships, etc. It is the experience of living your unencumbered life. Tying flow back to the Life Energy Circle also enables us to not be thrown off by unforeseen circumstances, typical stresses, or living in reaction to past trauma.

Flow is that sensation of letting go, connecting to a field of all possibilities, and allowing something beyond thought, to take the wheel. It's not closing your eyes; it's having your eyes wide open and you being unencumbered.

We spend so much time stressing about things and overanalyzing especially when it comes to health and longevity. We turn things over and over again in our minds and see all the potential positives and negatives of a given situation. Yet, our brains are incredibly capable of solving problems . . . if we just free them up and allow them to do it.

In my own journey, I find that being in flow is very nurturing. As we take on more and more responsibility, we experience less and less nurturing. All of us can probably count on one hand the number of people who truly nurtured us. Accessing flow is a way for us to nurture ourselves and be nurtured by the citations and experiences we find ourselves in.

Measurement and Optimization

When you achieve a flow state, you will know it. If you have to ask, *Am I there yet*, you likely aren't quite yet. Flow is an amazing, almost effortless, potent energy that you can feel ebbing and flowing not because of any specific thing you are doing; it's just "there," feeding you and simultaneously radiating from you and enabling you to effortlessly adapt and do what is called for in any situation.

Steven Kolter has been trying to teach others how to go into a flow state, and he has posted many videos online that are worth viewing. For someone trying to optimize their life energy, decrease stress, enhance performance and joy, and learn to achieve a flow state accomplishes all of those things in an instant. Understanding what flow is is the first step, and you are then on the road to experiencing it. The goal is not to play golf, ride your mountain bike, or attend a business meeting; the goal is to get into a flow state in anticipation of and during your participation in those activities. Doing so enables you to be your best self.

We hear that phrase a lot: "Be my best self." But what does it mean, what does it look like? For me, it is combining all the circles into one flow state, an integrated, durable state of flow.

I have flow experiences while riding my mountain bike, playing the guitar, snowboarding, sharing physical intimacy, and having deep conversations. I won't necessarily start in a flow state; I'm feeling out the equipment, getting my legs back under me, etc., but within the first fifteen to twenty minutes, everything will start to click. All of a sudden, I'm one with the bike, the board, the music, and my partner, and it is perfect. There is no past and no future; it's just *this moment*. I have a general direction, but the ability to make the best decisions without thinking about them is the most joyous thing!

Think of flow not as the "cherry on top" of working out physically, mentally, emotionally, and relationally, but the cake itself. When you work out in all these spaces—exercising, working new muscles, trying to learn new things—the goal is to be able to step into a flow state not only as a result of mastering them but while you are also learning and training. If you equate training with flow states, you will never miss a workout again. It's a reward unto itself and an amazing place to be and live. Your workouts and your life will transform.

When we talk about playing the Symphony of Longevity, it can look daunting. We might think, *I have all these things to do, all these different mosaics of ages, all these different elements of my life energy, health, longevity, and performance that I need to focus on.* It sounds overwhelming!

If you go into it understanding that one flow state is intertwined and holding all of them, you'll realize that flow enables you to play that symphony effortlessly.

When clients come to Gladden Longevity, we work to put them into a flow state as we work to turn back the clock. We do this with a well-orchestrated series of tests and treatments. Give us five days, we'll give you back ten years. A true flow state requires very little work and effort. By the time clients return home, they have been coached on how to access their flow state, enabling them to have the mindset, tools, and environment they need to succeed.

This is not about doing the same health routine every day. If you look at it from the perspective of *I want to access a flow state to navigate all these different opportunities,* it's suddenly a completely different world. Your ability to follow through will be much greater, and your enjoyment will be even more enhanced. You see, the reward isn't in the future, wrapped up in some lofty goal; the reward of a flow state is found right now, in real time, being present in this moment of living young.

Getting into a flow state can be therapeutic for things like anxiety and depression. It is the antithesis of being anxious; feeling anxious is a function of not feeling safe. In a flow state, you put yourself into a situation where more data is coming at you than you can process. So inherently, you're not going to feel safe, which will lead to anxiety.

But when you are in a flow state, you *do* feel safe, even though you are in a situation that is ostensibly very demanding and, from the outside looking in, appears overwhelming. You are allowing yourself to just be in that moment, and adapt within this energetic field of flow, this field of safety amidst the chaos.

When you feel incredibly safe and perform at a high level, it's the perfect antidote to anxiety and depression. People who are depressed have a difficult time taking action, yet *inaction* seems to compound depression, likely because they know and feel they are not making any progress. There is no light at the end of the tunnel.

If I find myself getting depressed, the first thing I do is take action. I may call a friend, find an activity, make my bed, strategize to solve a problem—anything that requires me to move and, therefore, *think* in a different direction. This helps me feel better—not necessarily because I've fixed whatever was bothering me, but rather because I took action. Ultimately, taking action enables me to reassess living in flow. The flow state is the place from which you want to live your life. If you are not living in that flow state, what's keeping you from getting there? How will you get back to it? What action do you need to take?

Simply put, flow is your official happy place. The flow state is where things will be effortless; your worries, cares, and fears will dissipate. If you struggle with depression, anxiety, or both, it's more challenging to get there. Understand that some intermediary steps may need to occur—perhaps therapy, supplements, medications, brain treatments, or a deeper understanding of what is driving your insecurity and lack of safety. But you can get there!

We have touched on the physiological benefits of being in a flow state, but to reiterate:

- Your stress levels will go down, which means your cortisol levels will ebb and flow the way they're supposed to;
- Your blood sugar will go down;
- Your brain is not being exposed to stress, which changes genetic expression;
- You are able to function from a place of joy;
- Your problem-solving skills will sharpen; and
- Your relationships will improve.

Flow has a profound impact on health and longevity. We know that telomeres shorten when we are under stress and that lower oxytocin levels will shorten telomeres. We also know that oxytocin is higher when joy is present; when connectivity is higher, you can optimize life energy, health, performance, and longevity by routinely accessing flow.

CHAPTER FORTY-FOUR

Static and Dynamic Balance

A few days ago in Colorado, I stepped on a piece of ice I didn't see. I would have hit the ground, except that I caught myself. It happened so fast that saving myself could have only happened instinctively; I could have easily broken a hip, rib, or wrist had I not been regularly incorporating static and dynamic balance training into my workouts.

I responded in a fraction of a second and did not fall or get hurt. This also happens when I mountain bike or snowboard; I can take a fall and walk away unharmed. While I do wear safety equipment, more importantly, my body knows how to fall. It knows how to instinctively protect itself as it is moving through space in an unrehearsed and unintended way.

As we age, we lose the neuromuscular reaction times and neuromuscular coordination to both avoid falls and fall safely. The number one greatest mistake I see in many workouts is that very little is in place to train a person's balance. Having great balance is one of the most fun and important aspects of fitness—fun because it allows you to do all kinds of activities confidently; important because it keeps you safe.

I discovered balance training during my forties—twenty-five years ago—through an introduction to a balance board called a Bongo Board®. Picture a skateboard deck sitting on top of a roller with a larger diameter in the middle of the roller and tapers as you move toward the edges of the roller, and that's pretty much the Bongo Board®. I could not balance on it without holding onto something or someone. I was hooked.

Determined to master it, it took me about three weeks to improve dramatically. At the same time, I noticed that I could run down the stairs faster and had a much greater sense of where my feet were and where I was in space. One evening, I was sitting at the dinner table, and a fork fell off the table. I simply reached out and grabbed it out of the air before it hit the ground. Everyone said, "Good catch," but I felt like it was effortless.

I felt like a ninja, and I loved that feeling.

Next came a Swiss ball, an inflatable plastic ball about two to three feet high. I wanted to see if I could kneel on top of it like I had seen others do in some videos. Of course, I couldn't—not at the time, anyway. Once again, I was hooked.

I placed the ball up against a wall to make it easier and learned how to roll onto it with my knees. Then, I was able to do it away from the wall all the time falling, falling, falling . . . except that I never hit the ground with anything but my feet! I was training myself on how to fall, how to react instinctively and quickly. Then I was able to stay on my knees on the ball as long as I wanted . . . with my eyes open. Could I balance on it with my eyes closed?

I couldn't—I was hooked. I started practicing getting up with my eyes open, then closing them for a second or two before I would have to catch myself. Three weeks later, practicing five to ten minutes each day, three days a week, I was able to do it consistently for thirty seconds with my eyes closed.

Balance training is one of the most underutilized techniques to maintain your health. Most of us take balance for granted until it starts to decline. Suddenly, we can no longer keep up with our grandkids or stumble and fall just stepping off a curb. We are less confident about our steps.

There are two types of balance: static and dynamic. *Static balance* refers to the control you have to hold your body in a specific position, like yoga poses. *Dynamic balance* is your ability to control your body while it's in motion or how quickly you can recover from a sudden shift in terrain, like on a balance device.

When it comes to using a balancing device, accept that at first, you won't be able to balance on it. Second, know that you will be able to if you practice. Then realize that:

- Just because you master one device doesn't mean you have mastered *all* the devices; each one presents a different challenge.
- Once you have mastered a device, you will find it three times more challenging with your eyes closed.
- When you can master six to seven devices with your eyes closed, you will be bulletproof when it comes to falling and getting hurt.

When I see older people holding onto the railing as they go down the stairs or feeling for the curb, they don't know where they are in space or where their feet are. They are worried about falling at every turn. Suddenly, balance becomes massively important.

As I mentioned previously, my mother died after a series of falls. First, she broke one hip and, a few years later, the next; then ribs, then ribs again; and then, her femur. She had no more reserve at ninety-three to recover. Falls and fractures later in life impair mobility and participation. She went from being an avid fast walker to barely being able to get around with a walker.

Static and dynamic balance are equally important, and balance doesn't just pertain to our ability to stand firmly on our feet and walk upright. When you start to work on your balance, you, too, can become like a ninja; if something falls off the table, you'll instinctively reach out and grab it. It becomes a reflex. People will wonder how you acted so quickly.

The scientific term for what we are doing is training our *proprioception*. Proprioception refers to our ability to know where we are in space, along with our torso, head, and limbs—relative to each other and the ground—and then place them where we would like them to be.

Measurement and Optimization

It is possible to measure balance. When a client stands on one leg, we can see how much muscle firing must occur to maintain alignment and static balance. We have a device that measures the amount of motion or wobble a person undergoes to maintain balance; the more wobble, the less balanced they are. The degree of wobble tells us how many muscles are firing for them to balance; the fewer, the better.

Dynamic balance refers to how quickly you "recover" your stability while moving or being displaced because the base of support keeps changing. As we age, it may look like how quickly you can respond to a stumble, a change in terrain, or being inadvertently pushed. We measure dynamic balance by having clients stand on an unstable surface, like a balance board, and measure the time they can balance before they have to step off.

Another way to measure neuromuscular reaction time is by using a device from a company called Senaptec that measures *visual* neuro-muscular reaction time; it is truly fascinating to measure and train this response. It benefits anyone looking to improve their vision and reaction times because it enhances balance.

Balance training doesn't require a lot of fancy equipment, either. In fact, you'll find that most devices are quite affordable. Variety is key. You may master one balance device, but that doesn't mean you've mastered them all; remember, each one presents its own challenge. Here is a good starter list of items in order of difficulty:

- Jumpsoles
- Swiss Ball
- Rocker Board
- Circular Boards
- Extreme Balance Board
- Indo Board®
- Bongo Board®

It's essential to have a variety of these things to keep you challenged and ninja-ready. It is also important to approach this with a learner's mindset, not a competence mindset. If your identity is tied up in only what you can do well, you will avoid this training altogether. Or, you will master one or two boards and call it good.

If you have a 100 is the new 30 mindset, a learner's mindset, you will keep challenging yourself in other ways, too. For example, if you master a balance board with your eyes open, then, as we mentioned, try mastering it again with your eyes closed. Or, open and close them intermittently to see how quickly you can balance. Eventually, you will get to a point where you can keep your eyes closed for extended periods. Then, go to the next device—but don't forget to practice the old one, or you will lose your competence. If you do this, you will be stunned at how it changes your whole perception of where you are in space, your confidence, and your joy of being in motion.

Apart from joy, you are training your neuromuscular system to be safe. If you have been doing some balance training and lose your balance, your body will instinctively know how to fall; you will not get hurt like someone who has no sense of balance. Not to mention it's just fun to be able to skip down the stairs.

I try to do balance training two or three times a week for five to ten minutes. You can do it while you're on a phone call, brushing your teeth, standing at your desk—really, just about anywhere. Put the balance devices in places where you bump into them frequently. Make them a part of your life. You will not regret improving your balance; it's probably the most enjoyable form of exercise out there because it makes you feel like a kid again.

CHAPTER FORTY-FIVE

Agility

Agility is a combination of balance and quickness. In order to be agile, it is critical to train balance, as we described in the previous chapter, and it is also important to train quickness, as described here. Putting the two together creates the capability of changing direction left, right, forward, backward, and up and down quickly while maintaining a sense of balance and equilibrium. Think of a running back like Barry Sanders, cutting in and out of tacklers and blockers. Think of a slalom skier moving from gate to gate, transferring weight and speed while maintaining dynamic control and equilibrium.

Measurement and Optimization

We measure agility as part of our Gladden Longevity physical assessment and quantify it based on how quickly and accurately someone can perform a predetermined task. We can also train agility by training balance first, then quickness, and then putting the two together by doing step-overs on a raised platform or using an agility ladder or cones. Agility is also trained as a form of interval training because it requires good aerobic capacity. Being agile will greatly enhance any activity you engage in, from shopping in the grocery store to hiking challenging trails, especially on the descent. If you are agile, it's a great way to ensure that your balance training and quickness training have been adequate.

CHAPTER FORTY-SIX

Quickness and Speed

Quickness and speed are linked but a bit different. One can be fast but also "not quick." Let's say you run one hundred meters, and you can get up to a good top speed, but you may not be quick about doing so; quickness gives you a good reaction time and start.

Whereas quickness is more about the neuromuscular connection than the muscle itself, speed is more dependent on the structure of the actual muscle. As a frame of reference, fast-twitch muscle fibers give us explosive speed or power with less endurance. Slow-twitch muscle fibers give us more endurance but less explosive speed or power.

Some of us are born with more Type 2 fast-twitch muscle fibers, and others are born with more Type 1 endurance muscle fibers. As we age, we lose type 2, fast-twitch muscle fibers. Fast-twitch muscle fibers can contract and relax at a faster rate, leading to more explosive and quickly repeated bursts of power.

This distribution of fast- and slow-twitch muscle fibers occurs on a continuum and has a strong genetic link to the ACTIN3 gene configuration. Studies have found that most elite power athletes have a specific genetic variant in a gene related to muscle composition, the RR configuration of the ACTN3 gene, as opposed to the XX configuration or RX configuration. This variant causes muscle cells to produce alpha-actinin-3, a protein found in fast-twitch muscle fibers. Approximately 20–30 percent of the population (over 1 billion people worldwide) have the X/X genotype. A variant in this gene called R577X, the X variant, leads to the production of an abnormally short α-actinin-3 protein that is quickly broken down.

Roughly speaking, the more copies of the R variant you have, as opposed to the X variant, the more likely you are to excel at sports requiring power or speed. (You can be RR, RX, or XX.) Persons of West African heritage have the highest preponderance of the RR configuration. The RR configuration leads to quickness, speed, and explosive jumping performance.

Measurement and Optimization

We measure speed by how fast someone can run forty yards, and we measure quickness using an NFL Combine test to see how quickly one can complete a roundtrip on a course of cones set up at predetermined distances around which one is weaving in and out.

Genetics aside, anyone can train quickness and speed by training Type 2 muscle fibers. This is critical whether you are RR or XX because, over time, you lose Type 2 fast-twitch muscle fibers. We like to train fast-twitch muscle fibers with resistance bands and isometric exercises, holding for no more than fifteen to twenty seconds to focus on the Type 2 fibers. Agility training consists of cross-stepping on and over an elevated flat plank. Other techniques are plyometric exercises, like box jumps, or with electrical stimulation, like Compex or NuX. Suffice it to say, we can help you build a program that is safe and effective to build up your fast-twitch muscle fibers and increase both your quickness, agility, and speed.

When it comes to speed, not only is the muscle fiber type important, but the neuromuscular reaction times can also be rate-limiting. To train the neuromuscular system, we like clients to run on a treadmill and ramp it up to a high speed to train the nervous system to be able to move the legs faster. Combining muscle training to increase Type 2 fibers with nervous system training to increase your turnover rate and focus on the muscle groups that build speed—like the glutes and hamstrings—will lead to your best results. We like Ben Patrick's program of Knees over Toes and the use of Nordic curls to enhance glute and hamstring strength. It is possible to transform a genetically slow person into a fast and quick athlete using these techniques. You can find more information on Ben Patrick's program by searching "Knees Over Toes" on YouTube.

A final thought on speed. Using the Supplement L-Carnosine, previously discussed in section two, selectively supports fast twitch muscle fibers and prevents age-related neuromuscular fiber loss, known as sarcopenia.

CHAPTER FORTY-SEVEN

Strength

W hen we think about working out or going to the gym, the first thing most of us think about is strength training. We think of bodybuilders as men and women getting jacked up on steroids. I hear all the time, "I don't want to get big. I just want to tone," or "I lift light weights to avoid injury."

Let's dispel a few myths.

Having good muscle mass and bone density is critical in the face of age-related sarcopenia, muscle loss, osteoporosis, and bone loss. Most people could lift heavy weights five days a week and not get "big" because only certain body types respond to resistance training in this way. Now the question becomes, *How do I train efficiently to get the most bang for the time I spend strength training and not get hurt?*

Measurement and Optimization

In our population, we are not measuring one rep max to evaluate strength. Hand-grip strength is a standard measure of strength we perform for all our clients. In addition, we evaluate how many times someone can sit and stand up from a chair in one minute, how many pushups they can do in a minute, or how long they can hold a plank. Another good test is having someone sit on the floor and see how many points of contact they need to stand up.

The answer is not to train with an athletic trainer in their twenties who knows exactly what you need to do to get ripped. The first order of business is to understand how you can proceed safely and what your goals are, so the answer is, in fact, working with someone who has taken the time to evaluate your prior injuries and concerns by conducting a physical therapy and chiropractic exam, plus comprehensive cardiovascular testing—and by that, I don't mean simply a Cleerly CTA. I'm referring to a cardiopulmonary exercise test.

Once you have those assessments, we can build you a program that gets you further than you thought possible while helping you to avoid injury. When building muscle and bone, weights work but are old-school. We have found that using resistance bands combined with blood-flow restriction bands or a Tonal® or ARX—with or without blood-flow restriction bands—can be more effective and safer than lifting weights. We like programs like OsteoStrong® for bone density, which focuses on isometric exercises. ARX and Tonal® resistance training emphasize the push and pull components of the exercise—the concentric and eccentric motions of the exercise. We also love

Vasper™ blood flow restriction interval training for building strength and endurance.

It is beyond the scope of this book to map out workout programs for you, but the elements you need to focus on are all included in this section. We use even more sophisticated technologies to train in the office, like Senaptec and AllCor, if you'd like to check them out.

Some final thoughts on fatigue and strength. Why do muscles fatigue? It has been shown that when an animal or a person stops for fatigue, the muscle can still be contracted using electrical stimulation, so why do we stop?

It has to do with one of two things: Either we are out of fuel, fat, or glucose, or we have increased the metabolic rate to the point the acidity of the environment is now high, and there are many oxygen-free radicals to deal with. To combat fatigue, we train with blood-flow restriction to train the muscles to adapt to more harsh conditions.

This can also be done with sustained or interval training using the Kaatsu® system, B® Strong Bands, or Vasper™. In addition, training with an elevation training mask, not to simulate low ambient oxygen conditions, but to increase the work of breathing, is very helpful. In addition, training in actual low-oxygen environments using a Hypoxico or LIVEO2™ system. These all can be excellent hormetic stresses that up-regulate the body's capabilities. We find the use of hydrogen to be critical here, along with eating a diet high in nitrates and using a supplement like Neo40® Pro to boost NO production to enhance blood flow. H2 is critical because it helps to balance oxidative stress.

Using creatine just prior to your workout and carnosine at night in conjunction with hormone replacement works very well to increase strength and mitigate sarcopenia and strength loss. As mentioned in previous chapters, the product from BioProtein Technology called BioPro+™ also builds strength and muscle by adding IGF-1 and other trophic or growth factors. We are not fans of using this all the time, as we like to oscillate between activating mTOR and then lowering mTOR activation with rapamycin and carnosine.

It's important to note that while shutting down mTOR, rapamycin has been shown to protect against muscle wasting; too much mTOR stimulation can down-regulate muscle growth. Truly, this biology is an economy of balance, and you want to work with a professional to get this right and be sure you are optimizing the good being done and not moving into an unhealthful area.

CHAPTER FORTY-EIGHT

Endurance

To build endurance, mixing protracted, lower-heart activities with shorter, higher-intensity activities is essential. It is also critical to work on both the muscle portion of endurance, the cardiovascular portion of endurance, and the breathing associated with endurance.

Measurement and Optimization

To work on the breathing component, we like to train with an Elevation Training Mask or Airofit—not because they simulate elevation, but because they increase the work of breathing. When you increase the work of breathing, the diaphragm and intercostal muscles (the muscles between the ribs) are trained and strengthened. These devices force you to inhale deeper and exhale more completely.

I have found that training my breathing makes a marked difference in my ability to perform on a mountain bike, running, or on a snowboard. You simply don't get as winded, and when you do, your improved lung capacity and training help you breathe deeper and more completely; you can also clear the breathlessness in a few breaths.

To train my endurance, I do sustained cardiovascular exercises for 45 to 90 minutes in zone, two or three twice a week. I also do sustained cardio for 45 to 90 minutes in zone four and five twice a week. In addition, I do interval training on my Vasper for twenty-one minutes with sprints in zone four or five. I have found that, for me, this combination yields the best results and has given me a VO2 max that is excellent for someone in their twenties.

Ultimately, one of the real joys of being thirty at any age is our capacity to do things and enjoy them confidently.

CHAPTER FORTY-NINE

Recovery, Resilience, and Robustness

When it comes to performance, I have had several genetically gifted clients. The challenge was getting them to mix up their training to minimize the wear and tear. For example, one woman was a gifted runner; as a middle schooler, she was already competing against high-school upperclassmen and beating them. However, genetically she lacked sturdiness. As she aged, she continued to run but was more prone to injuries. In her case, it was possible to take something you're really good at and just run the wheels right off it. It wasn't because she wasn't a great runner but because she ran so much that she literally ran the wheels right off her body and was crippled with debilitating musculoskeletal and joint pain.

We tend to think of golf as a leisurely sport when it's actually very violent. The swing alone can take out your lower back—ask Tiger Woods how many back surgeries he's had. If you do the same thing over and over again, you're going to run the wheels off yourself, no matter how talented you are.

Recovery is the ability to return to a state of being replete after depleting yourself during a customary activity. For example, I was tired after I hiked the Grand Canyon rim to rim in eleven hours, covering twenty-two miles and traversing eleven thousand vertical feet. But two days later, I felt great and was ready to go again.

Beyond recovery, however, is resilience and robustness. Building *resilience* means you can encounter unexpected, extraordinary stress and recover from them. *Robustness*, on the other hand, involves being minimally affected by unexpected, extraordinary stresses. Consider someone who had COVID-19; perhaps they were resilient and recovered quickly from a hospitalization. However, in contrast, consider someone who was robust and, therefore, minimally affected by COVID-19.

Youth is characterized by faster recovery, resilience, and robustness. As we age chronologically, we want all three. Therefore, when you are training, you want to build all three. The first step is to build them by taking time to recover.

When the body is chronically stressed, it breaks down. This is why athletes can age faster than their peers if they overdo it. Interestingly, they also use up their reserve of stem cells faster and may be unable to recover later in life. A flame that burns twice as bright burns half as long. When it comes to building resilience and robustness, training with recovery is king; it enables us to maintain our capabilities for decades to come.

Measurement and Optimization

As I stated previously, I'm a big fan of rotating activities. I love running, but I won't run more than probably twice a week because I don't want to over-stress that portion of my body, plus I want to take time to recover. I also love mountain biking but typically don't mountain bike more than twice a week. I could body surf every day, but I don't, and I usually only snowboard every other day or two days out of three. I love all of these activities so much, but I make a point not to overdo them.

Rather than saying, "It's Tuesday. Last week I did this; I'll try to beat it this week," one of the best ways to stay fit and healthy is to do something active every day but tailor what you do to match your recovery. In the spirit of not overtraining, paying attention to your recovery score and strain score on your Whoop®, Oura®, Apple Watch®, Garmin®, BioStrap®, or any other device that computes this is critical. The "no pain, no gain" mindset will not serve you as you strive to make 100 the new 30. But the "I'll do something every day and tailor it to my recovery score" mindset will serve you very well.

You've probably figured out that I love being outdoors, even if only for a few minutes; I find it quite therapeutic, nurturing, and centering. I always run outside, and on other days, I will hop on my mountain bike. If it's not a running or mountain-biking day, I ride an ElliptiGo®, which is like an elliptical on wheels. I can get a nice workout, and it's time-efficient. Sometimes, I'll wear the elevation training mask on the ElliptiGo®, and I'm not beating myself up; I'm just making myself stronger, more robust, and more resilient.

The one piece of equipment I use indoors, besides some resistance training, is the Vasper™. It combines blood-flow restriction with interval training, electrical grounding, and cooling in a twenty-one-minute protocol. It is an incredibly efficient piece of technology for maintaining muscle mass, strength, and aerobic capacity—it can be done as either a strength-building or a recovery exercise. I will hit the Vasper™ two or three times a week, and the intensity is a function of my recovery score on my Whoop®.

It's important to have a quiver of activities you enjoy; otherwise, you're putting tremendous stress on yourself by just doing one or two things. You are in danger of running the wheels off. If you love tennis, for example, don't join five teams so that you can play every day. Mix them up so you are not doing the same activity every day. Doing so decreases your chances of running the wheels off and not being able to enjoy it. If you need to find some new activities to balance things out, do it.

To recover, it's important to prioritize sleep, saunas, and use Perfect Amino to rebuild protein post-workout, collagen, and electrolytes are also required. Products like Endurox® combine glucose and protein in a 4:1 ratio to restore glycogen stores after endurance activities. This has been a game-changer for back-to-back days of heavier endurance activity.

Peptides are also useful. BPC 157 and GHK-Cu, used in combination, aid body repair. CJC/Ipamorelin or Tesamorelin to boost growth-hormone release will aid in recovery, rebuilding, and repair.

These peptide combinations are compatible with Rapamycin, which would be used every second to third week. In addition, red light, massage, and cold plunges are also helpful in boosting recovery.

CHAPTER FIFTY

Flexibility

Have you ever indulged in dessert at dinner and woke up the next morning feeling stiff? Part of the reason flexibility diminishes with aging is that dietary sugars start to attach to proteins and stiffen them up. This is protein cross-linking or glycation. Pro tip: Healthy fats, like coconut, avocado, and fish oil, loosen muscles, tendons, and ligaments, and carnosine will decrease protein glycation.

Another reason that we get stiffer is that we don't know how to stretch or strengthen properly. We sit in chairs all the time, which creates bad posture and tightens hamstrings. As we get old and stiff, we have less agility, less speed, poorer balance, and become more injury-prone.

Measurement and Optimization

Strategies that help us maintain flexibility and strengthen our full range of motion are incredibly important. At Gladden Longevity, we have become enamored with Ben Patrick's system of exercise called Knees Over Toes. Having endured multiple knee surgeries, he was told he would face yet another. Ben decided to rehabilitate his knees himself. He went from having an eighteen-inch vertical jump to a thirty-inch vertical using the training techniques that ultimately became his signature method. His flexibility and strength dramatically improved. The Knees Over Toes method is predominantly body weight-based, although over time, as someone gets stronger, they can add some extra weight. Regardless of fitness level, anyone can do the exercises, which is another bonus.

Remember: In addition to doing the Knees Over Toes program, avoiding sugar, taking the dipeptide carnosine, and consuming healthy fats like olive oil, fish oil, and MCT will help keep you limber.

CHAPTER FIFTY-ONE

Cardiovascular Endurance

Ultimately, all endurance is a function of cardiovascular endurance. If you can't pump enough blood to supply oxygen and remove waste from the muscles and brain, it doesn't matter how strong you are—you will be as weak as a kitten in sixty seconds. Too many people focus on what they can see in the mirror and don't focus on what makes it all work: cardiovascular endurance.

Measurement and Optimization

At Gladden Longevity, we conduct cardiopulmonary exercise tests on everyone to measure a number of variables: VO2 max, anaerobic threshold, and something called the heart rate work rate slope. We do this to understand heart-pumping capacity, physical fitness, and the status of the arteries, respectively. We also look at lung capacity, the ability to move air, and the ability to exchange oxygen and carbon dioxide. Without this information, you have no idea where you are in your fitness program or if what you are doing is safe for you. With it, however, you are empowered and confident in what you are doing and the gains you are making.

Building cardiovascular endurance requires protracted cardio. Ten minutes on the treadmill before you lift weights does not do it. You need forty-five to sixty minutes, three days a week, plus interval training for twenty minutes on two separate days to build actual endurance. The key is to do this within the parameters of what is safe and what your recovery score is and to utilize a variety of exercises to be sure you are not wearing out any one part of yourself. If you do this, along with what I have outlined above, you will outperform most thirty-year-olds you come in contact with—now, isn't that fun?

CHAPTER FIFTY-TWO

Neuromuscular Reaction Time

A mong our clients, we have a number of athletes—golfers, tennis pros, race car drivers, and so on. They all want to keep their edge, particularly when they reach an age when the competition is much younger. They know that younger drivers, for example, have quicker reflexes than theirs, so they are trying to optimize their strengths.

Training the brain to process information more quickly means a quicker response from the neuromuscular system—your hands move quicker, your back moves quicker, you get the idea. I love that it is possible to train this because we tend to think of these sorts of responses as mere reflexes—we'll determine whether we have either good or poor reflexes instead of considering how to achieve a better response. It's quite fun to think that this is trainable, particularly for us as we age.

We talk a lot about cardiovascular exercise, but when it comes to raw strength, resistance training is essential. The problem with most strength training is that it consists of weights, which we think is an archaic way to train; if you pick up a weight, you have to hold it, sometimes over your head, which puts you at risk of dropping it or hurting yourself in some other way. And if you're just lifting weights, all you're doing is increasing your slow-twitch muscle fibers, yet we know that we lose our quickness with age. We need to be exercising the fast-twitch muscle fibers, as we described above. We're not huge fans of weights, per se, when there are much better options.

Measurement and Optimization

A company I've mentioned previously, Senaptec, has developed a set of glasses that will close off your visual field. In other words, they become opaque for a fraction of a second, and then they become transparent again for a fraction of a second. They oscillate like this, causing your brain to have less information to make decisions with. It's a similar technique that baseball players use to be able to hit a fastball. They improve their batting average this way because even though the ball is moving faster and they see less of it, their brains have been trained to process the information more quickly. The fact that a pair of glasses can help us, in the same way, makes this a very exciting technology.

Final Thoughts on Performance

We want to be healthy but in a way that positively impacts performance. While we talk a lot about longevity and health, it's the performance we're after. If we can perform like we are thirty years old—intellectually, physically, and sexually—we are happy campers. We feel great about our lives. We know we can tell *when* we're aging because we don't look like we did, don't feel like we did, and can't do what we did. Being able to perform on all those levels and look younger, feel younger, and perform younger, is when we're ultimately at our best. That's why performance is such an important metric in this whole process.

Performance Notes

Mihaly Csikszentmihalyi, *Flow: The Psychology of Optimal Experience* (Harper, 1991).

Steven Kotler, *The Rise of Superman: Decoding the Science of Ultimate Human Performance* (Seattle, WA: Amazon Publishing, 2021).

Nan Yang et al., "ACTN3 Genotype Is Associated with Human Elite Athletic Performance," *The American Journal of Human Genetics* 73, no. 3 (September 2003): 627–31, https://doi.org/10.1086/377590.

Huibin Tang, Joseph B. Shrager, and Daniel Goldman, "Rapamycin Protects Aging Muscle," *Aging* 11, no. 16 (August 27, 2019): 5868–70, https://doi.org/10.18632/aging.102176.

Hirofumi Tanaka and Douglas R. Seals, "Endurance Exercise Performance in Masters Athletes: Age-Associated Changes and Underlying Physiological Mechanisms," The Journal of Physiology 586, no. 1 (January 1, 2008): 55–63, https://doi.org/10.1113/jphysiol.2007.141879.

Adam R. Konopka et al., "Metformin Inhibits Mitochondrial Adaptations to Aerobic Exercise Training in Older Adults," Aging Cell 18, no. 1 (December 11, 2018), https://doi.org/10.1111/acel.12880.

Eunse Park and Kimberly Castle, "The Effect of an Isometric Trunk Training during Spinning in a Child with Cerebral Palsy: A Case Report," Interprofessional Journal of Healthcare and Research, 4, 1, no. 1 (2021): 1–10.

Why everyone should be doing it and how ARX stacks up against the ..., accessed August 21, 2023, https://uploads-ssl.webflow. com/63615a046fa44d99b190efa9/638f95f11800442e39a2a171_ ARX%20Ebook_4-15-2021_V6.pdf.

Ivana Jukić et al., "Carnosine, Small but Mighty—Prospect of Use as Functional Ingredient for Functional Food Formulation," Antioxidants 10, no. 7 (June 28, 2021): 1037, https://doi.org/10.3390/antiox10071037.

Frank W. Booth, Gregory N. Ruegsegger, and T. Dylan Olver, "Exercise Has a Bone to Pick with Skeletal Muscle," Cell Metabolism 23, no. 6 (June 2016): 961–62, https://doi.org/10.1016/j.cmet.2016.05.016.

Caio dos Trettel et al., "Irisin: An Anti-Inflammatory Exerkine in Aging and Redox-Mediated Comorbidities," Frontiers in Endocrinology 14 (February 10, 2023), https://doi.org/10.3389/fendo.2023.1106529.

William Evans et al., "Effects of Fortetropin on the Rate of Muscle Protein Synthesis in Older Men and Women: A Randomized, Double-Blinded, Placebo-Controlled Study," The Journals of Gerontology: Series A 76, no. 1 (June 29, 2020): 108–14, https://doi.org/10.1093/gerona/glaa162.

Karla J. Oldknow et al., "Follistatin-like 3 (FSTL3) Mediated Silencing of Transforming Growth Factor β (Tgfβ) Signaling Is Essential for Testicular Aging and Regulating Testis Size," Endocrinology 154, no. 3 (March 1, 2013): 1310–20, https://doi.org/10.1210/en.2012-1886.

James Jermey McCormick, "The Effect of Acute Aerobic Exercise and Rapamycin Treatment on Autophagy and the Heat Shock Response in Peripheral Blood Mononuclear Cells of Prediabetics," UNM Digital Repository, July 2018, https://digitalrepository.unm.edu/educ_hess_etds/98.

Giuseppina Rose et al., "Further Support to the Uncoupling-to-Survive Theory: The Genetic Variation of Human UCP Genes Is Associated with Longevity," PLoS ONE 6, no. 12 (December 27, 2011), https://doi.org/10.1371/journal.pone.0029650.

For more references, please visit GladdenLongevity.com/Book100.

Conclusion

By now, I think you can clearly see that our current "health-care system" is anything but—it is a sick-care system designed to take care of people who get sick or injured. It can be wonderful if you need that type of care, but if you are looking to optimize your health and longevity, it will never be capable of helping you.

Optimizing your health, longevity, performance, and life energy is a quest that becomes your hero's journey, one that you will be traveling by yourself and occasionally with like-minded medical experts and friends. It is your hero's journey to reclaim your birthright of robust health, longevity, performance, and life energy.

When it comes to life energy, it is your right to live an unencumbered life devoid of fear and full of love and purpose. Look for, and partner up with, practitioners and friends who are on the same page as you. Ask yourself what your current circle of people is focused on; if they are not interested in joining you on your journey, maintain loving contact, but look for people who will energize you and collaborate with you on your quest. Gladden Longevity can fill this key role for you; beyond scientific insights, we can energize and encourage you on your journey.

We are also able to architect your home and office environments to support your mission and enable you to succeed at living young for a lifetime.

We have entered into a new era. Your birthday has very little to do with your true age. Age is a function of both mindset and physiology. In many ways, the key drivers of aging and the key expressions of aging are found in the sixteen Hallmarks of Aging. We are now fortunate to have evidence-based strategies that, when symphonically linked together, have the possibility to slow, arrest, and even reverse our functional age. We believe this can be done across the entire Mosaic of Ages across all four circles. We are so excited to have the tools now to be able to measure whether this is happening for you. It's quite a thrill to remain on the cutting edge of this sort of healthcare, and even more thrilling for our clients who reap the benefits. It's now possible for each of us to do the impossible!

Doing the Impossible

By addressing all four circles—Life Energy, Longevity, Health, and Performance—while using new diagnostic and regenerative therapeutic tools and applying them across all three layers of medicine—symptom-driven, root cause, and longevity, the true drivers of aging—we have created an exponential strategy. This exponential strategy addresses the exponential problem we all face: aging and decline.

To do the impossible, we must devote time, attention, and resources to ensure we know how old we are, understand what cards we are holding, have the right interventions, and live in the right environment. We need all of these to succeed. Identifying just the right therapies isn't enough, however; if we're going to play a symphony correctly. The right therapies must also have the right timing, sequence, frequency, intensity, and duration. This is how we'll optimize our youthfulness.

In addition, it is essential that you organize your environments, home, office, and travel to support your ability to implement what you need to do. If the environment— physical things and people—is not supporting you, you will fail. Willpower will never be enough; you must create an environment where doing what you need to do becomes effortless and free of distraction. Gladden Longevity can help you think this through and build it.

I hope I have provided enough evidence to prove that the Life Energy Circle is foundational to everything—including your longevity, health, and performance. If that circle is not optimized, none of the other circles will be able to function effectively. Take time to cultivate this side of yourself and reflect on the elements I've outlined on the Life Energy Circle. Master that circle, and you will master life.

In time, we may get to a point where we have gene-editing technology or ways to reboot ourselves to a youthful age, but those processes are still undergoing development. For now, we feel we can help push you back in time, but you must understand just how critical the environment you reside in is to your success.

As we have learned from the Mosaic of Ages, you are only as strong as your weakest link, only as young as your oldest age. It's great to be excited about your progress, watching yourself "grow younger," but it's also important to understand that you want to bring along that area that is still lagging behind. Be eternally vigilant about this. At

Gladden Longevity, our vision is to continue to be empowered by our four questions:

- *How good can you be?*
- *How do we make 100 the new 30?*
- *How do we live well beyond 120?*
- *How do we live young for a lifetime?*

If better questions come along, we will rapidly embrace them. These questions serve as fuel for me every day. They get me up in the morning, constantly working to improve my twenty-seven-year-old self and improve the quality of services we can bring to our clients. We truly want to crack the code on aging and then democratize that information so everyone can benefit from it!

When space travel began, it was an incredibly expensive journey. Now we have learned how to go to space much more economically. Cracking the code on aging is a similar process; it is more expensive right now. Remember in the Introduction how I compared the Symphony of Longevity to traveling to Mars? The first people who "go to Mars" are in for an expensive journey, and there are certainly people willing to write the check. They understand the value of it and recognize that their health is their greatest asset. To them, money is a resource, not an asset. And to that end, they are the pioneers, and we should all be thankful for them—they will help us make it more available and more accessible. The information will become democratized, and it will become less expensive. It will still take time, attention, and resources to push back against this very strong current of aging and likely will never be cheap.

Playing this symphony is how we will stay young for a lifetime. This is how we get the freedom to live life on our own terms and the opportunity to make a massive, positive, even exponential impact on our families, our communities, mankind, and the planet.

Wanna join?

What's Now and What's Next

We have created a study, our first symphony of longevity, entitled LIFE RAFT, which is the Institutional Review Board's (IRB) approved trial to see how far we can push ourselves and our clients back in time. Over the course of a year, we believe this symphonic approach will ultimately be the right one; we are convinced that we will make significant progress in the lives of all who participate. We also know that there will be continued refinement, additions, and other tweaks, to continue to improve. Staying open-minded, curious, and relentless are the mindsets that will ultimately make it successful.

The LIFE RAFT protocol also has sub-studies that we refer to as "Life Jackets." The Life Jackets focus on a specific issue someone might have. For example, for brain optimization, we can use our technologies to help those who have experienced traumatic brain injury, concussions, or struggle with anxiety, depression, or ADHD. Another Life Jacket is focused on cardiovascular health—improving cardiac function, both from the standpoint of pumping function and smoothing out arrhythmias (we do not have the ability to correct mechanical issues like valve disease).

The possibilities are endless: Rejuvenating the lungs to improve respiratory function; the kidneys to improve kidney function; the liver to treat non-alcoholic fatty liver disease; enhance immune system function; rejuvenating sexual function; and reverse musculoskeletal and joint issues.

Life Raft™

Playing the "Symphony" of Longevity

IRB Approved Clinical Trial

Life **E**nergy, **R**esilience **A**nti-**F**ragility **T**rial

The Life Jackets can also deal with post-infection and post-vaccination issues like those with COVID long-haul. We can improve gut function and cosmetic issues, like breast sagging, without requiring any surgical procedure. This is where the Life Jackets stand today but be assured more will come and more areas will be able to be addressed.

There is a second IRB-approved trial for a telomerase product, which is extremely potent. In fact, the younger the individual, the more potent the anti-aging effects. Our preliminary data has demonstrated it numerous times from the standpoint of muscle rejuvenation, cosmetic rejuvenation, energy, libido, sexual performance, and brain function. This is a six-month protocol, and participants would consume the telomerase for two days every ninety days. Those in their thirties and forties who aren't interested in our more advanced programs might be interested in the benefits of this trial.

In the meantime, Gladden Longevity has expanded our current program offerings to simply answer the question, *How old am I?*

One of the reasons we are so excited about these developments is that even just two short years ago, we didn't have effective strategies for the nine hallmarks of aging. Now, we are playing this symphony of longevity, across all sixteen hallmarks; we believe the LIFE RAFT trial will blow the doors right open!

I'm cheering for each of you!

Let's Live Young!

Jeff

How Do I Live Young?

How Do I Make Progress?

If you would like to Live Young for a Lifetime™,
you can contact us at Info@GladdenLongevity.com
or call 972.310.8916.

We'll be happy to get to know you and help you select
the right program.

How Do I Live Young for a Lifetime?

I Want to Be 30 Year Old

Glossary of Terms

Acetyl groups: Acetyl groups are chemical groups consisting of a methyl group (CH3) connected to a carboxyl group (COOH). In biochemistry, the acetyl group is often added to lysine residues in the DNA's histones by a process called acetylation. Acetylation of the DNA's histone proteins, like the methylation of DNA, is involved in the up-regulation and down-regulation of gene expression. The patterns of acetylation and methylation change with age and are believed to be both a result of aging and a cause of aging. Reprogramming the cell to youthfulness, as with Yamanaka factors (see below), is reflected in younger patterns of histone acetylation and DNA methylation.

Adenosine triphosphates (ATPs): Adenosine triphosphate (ATP) is a molecule that serves as the currency of energy for cells in all animal life. ATP is produced in the cell in two locations by two different means. In the mitochondria, the Krebs cycle combined with Oxidative Phosphorylation can ultimately utilize food from any source, such as glucose, protein, or fat, which, once broken down to acetyl-Co-A, can enter the mitochondrial process. The other location is in the cell but outside the mitochondria and utilizes the glycolytic pathway, which only utilizes glucose as a food source. In either case, ATP is produced, and it is then used to fuel cell activities such as muscle contraction, protein synthesis, DNA synthesis, cell division, messenger molecule production, and maintenance activities like autophagy (see below).

Adipocytes: Adipocytes (also known as fat cells) are specialized cells that store and release energy in the form of lipids (fats). They are responsible for regulating energy homeostasis and play an important role in various metabolic processes and insulin resistance.

Allele: An allele is one-half of a gene inherited either from the mother or the father. Variants in alleles are the basis of genetic variation exp., eye color, height, etc. Alleles can be dominant, recessive, or co-dominant.

Amino acid: Amino acids are the building blocks of proteins and are essential for all living organisms.

Amiodarone: Amiodarone is an anti-arrhythmic drug used to treat irregular heartbeats and other heart rhythm disorders, including atrial fibrillation, atrial flutter, ventricular tachycardia, and ventricular fibrillation. It works by slowing the conduction of electrical impulses in the heart, which helps to regulate the heart rate.

Adenosine monophosphate (AMP): It is an important component of the energy-carrying molecule adenosine triphosphate (ATP). AMP helps to transfer energy within cells and is involved in a variety of biochemical reactions.

It also serves as a signaling molecule in the body and is involved in the regulation of various metabolic processes.

AMPK: Adenosine Monophosphate-Activated Protein Kinase (AMPK) is an enzyme that plays a crucial role in the regulation of energy homeostasis in the cell. It is activated when the cell's energy stores are low, such as when the cell is under stress, exp fasting, or exercise. AMPK works by increasing the production of ATP while simultaneously decreasing the production of other molecules that require energy. It also triggers conservation and regeneration activities in the cell. Its activation is associated with longevity.

Amylase: Amylase is an enzyme found in saliva, pancreatic juice, and intestinal juice that helps break down carbohydrates for the absorption of carbohydrate-based nutrients. The number of redundant copies, one to twenty copies are possible, affects how we process carbs and correlates to our susceptibility to diabetes in response to excess weight.

Amyloid Alpha/Beta: Amyloid Alpha/Beta (Aβ) is a protein that is found in the brains of individuals with Alzheimer's disease. It forms deposits in the brain known as senile plaques. The protein is formed when an enzyme known as β-secretase cleaves the amyloid precursor protein (APP), which is then further cleaved by a second enzyme, γ-secretase. Amyloid β is a peptide thought to play a role in the pathogenesis of Alzheimer's disease.

Anaerobic: Anaerobic is a type of exercise or activity that is performed at a high intensity where the energy demand exceeds the available oxygen supply. It necessitates the body making ATP for energy through a more ancient pathway that does not require oxygen. It typically involves short bursts of activity such as sprinting, weightlifting, and plyometrics. Examples of anaerobic exercises include burpees, sprints, and HIIT workouts, which are accompanied by feelings of breathlessness.

Andropause: Andropause is a term used to describe the various physical and psychological symptoms experienced by men as their hormones decline with age. These symptoms are often associated with declining levels of testosterone and its metabolites. These hormones are responsible for sexual desire, muscle strength, and bone mass. Symptoms of andropause can include fatigue, depression, reduced libido, decreased muscle mass, and increased body fat. Treatment typically involves lifestyle changes and hormone-boosting activities, supplements, medications, and peptides, or hormone replacement therapy.

Apoptosis: Apoptosis is a type of programmed cell death that occurs in multicellular organisms. It is a regulated process that is essential in the normal development, growth, and maintenance of healthy cells and tissues as it enables damaged cells to be removed and recycled. Apoptosis is triggered by a variety of signals and leads to the rapid breakdown of the cell, resulting in cell death. Senescent cells and cancer cells resist apoptosis, and pruning them in part is focused on inducing them to undergo apoptosis.

arNOX: Aging-related cell-surface NADH oxidase (arNOX) Dr. Morre demonstrated that arNOX increases with age between age 30 and ages 50–65. Activity in the blood correlates with a number of aging-related disorders, including arterial plaque formation from oxidized LDL cholesterol and oxidation of collagen and elastin in the skin. arNOX inhibitors are found in the herbs typically used in French cooking, such as summer savory, basil, tarragon, and rosemary. Their regular use may contribute to an understanding of the nutritional basis for the French Paradox, whereby the French eat seemingly unhealthy foods and yet have less heart disease.

Ashwagandha: Ashwagandha is an adaptogenic herb that is native to India, Pakistan, and Sri Lanka. It is a member of the nightshade family and is used in Ayurvedic medicine. Ashwagandha has traditionally been used for a variety of health conditions, including stress, anxiety, fatigue, depression, and insomnia. As an adaptogen, it will lower the stress hormone cortisol if it is high and raise it if it is low. It is also believed to have anti-inflammatory and antioxidant properties important for brain health.

Autophagy: Autophagy is the natural, regulated mechanism of the cell that removes unnecessary or dysfunctional components. It allows the orderly degradation and recycling of cellular components. Autophagy is essential for normal cellular homeostasis and plays a key role in many physiological processes, such as adaptation to fasting, exercise, development, differentiation, and stress response.

Basal medial hypothalamus (BMH): Basal medial hypothalamus (BMH) is an area of the hypothalamus, a region of the brain that plays a major role in controlling various aspects of behavior and physiology, such as hunger, thirst, sleep, body temperature, and hormones. The BMH is located in the center of the hypothalamus and is involved in the regulation of food intake, energy balance, and body weight. It also plays a role in the regulation of emotions and motivation. Stem cells that reside there are believed to be a controlling factor in the aging process. Protecting and rejuvenating those stem cells with exosomes or endogenous very small embryonic-like stem cells is being studied as a way to reverse aging.

Berberine: Berberine is a natural plant alkaloid found in several different plant species, including goldenseal, barberry, and Oregon grape. It has been used for centuries in traditional Chinese medicine to treat a variety of conditions, including infections, digestive disorders, and inflammation. Recent research has shown that berberine has antioxidant, anti-inflammatory, and antimicrobial properties. It is as effective as metformin in controlling blood sugar and also activates AMPK, thereby balancing the effects of mTOR to enhance longevity.

Beta-blockers: Beta-blockers (or beta-adrenergic blocking agents) are a type of medication prescribed to treat a variety of conditions, such as high blood pressure, chest pain, anxiety, and migraine headaches. These drugs work by blocking the effects of certain hormones called epinephrine (adrenaline) and norepinephrine (noradrenaline) on the body. By blocking these hormones, beta-blockers can reduce heart rate and blood pressure and relax smooth muscle in the airways. In the brain, blocking the action of adrenaline and noradrenaline can reduce anxiety.

Biome: A biome is a large-scale community of plants and animals that share a common environment and interact with each other. Biomes are typically classified according to the type of climate, vegetation, and animal life present in the area. In medicine, the Gut Biome is a major player in health, digestion, brain function, and mood. Because the gut biome changes as we age it is now considered a Hallmark of Aging.

Blood Urea Nitrogen (BUN) test: A Blood Urea Nitrogen (BUN) test is a test that measures the amount of nitrogen in the urea that is present in your blood. Urea is a waste product that is created when proteins are broken down. The BUN test can help to determine how well your kidneys are working. It is typically used to diagnose dehydration and kidney problems.

Brain-derived neurotrophic factor: Brain-derived neurotrophic factor (BDNF) is a growth factor that helps to promote the survival, growth, and differentiation of neurons in the brain. It plays a key role in the development and maintenance of the central nervous system, and its lack is thought to be involved in a number of neurological disorders. It is also involved in the regulation of synaptic plasticity, which is essential for learning and memory. One of the major goals of protecting and recovering brain health is to increase BDNF with food choices that contain or increase butyrate in the gut. It can be upregulated with various peptides and anaerobic exercise.

BRCA1/BRCA2: BRCA1 and BRCA2 are genes that are responsible for the repair of damaged DNA. In women, mutations in these genes can lead to an increased risk of breast, ovarian, pancreatic, and other cancers. In men, mutations can lead to an increased risk of breast, ovarian, pancreatic, and other cancers.

BUBR1: BUBR1 (budding uninhibited by benzimidazole-related protein 1) is a protein involved in the proper attachment and maintenance of chromosomes during cell division. It plays a role in the regulation of the spindle assembly checkpoint, which ensures that the correct number of chromosomes are segregated into daughter cells during cell division. Mutations in the BUBR1 gene can lead to an increased risk of cancer, impacting longevity. Optimal genetic expression is associated with longevity and is unregulated by SIRT2. Lower expression is associated with increased cancer risk and increased mortality.

Carbohydrates: Carbohydrates are nutrients made up of sugars, starches, and fibers and are the body's main source of energy. Carbohydrates are found naturally in plant-based foods such as grains, fruits, vegetables, and legumes and are also added to processed foods like breakfast cereals and snack bars.

Carboxyl: Carboxyl is an organic functional group consisting of a carbonyl group (C=O) bonded to a hydroxyl group (O-H). The group is often referred to as a carboxylic acid group and is commonly found in organic molecules such as proteins, carbohydrates, and fats. Carboxyl groups are polar, making them water soluble, highly reactive, and important in various biochemical processes.

Catalase: Catalase is an enzyme found in most living organisms that helps to break down hydrogen peroxide into oxygen and water. It is a powerful antioxidant that helps to protect cells from oxidative damage. It can also help to prevent cellular damage from free radicals that can cause diseases like cancer. It is part of a triad of enzymes, superoxide dismutase, glutathione peroxidase, and catalase that function as an assembly line to neutralize oxygen free radicals. Oxygen free radicals are also referred to as reactive oxygen species.

Cholesterol: Cholesterol is a type of fat molecule found in our diet and made in the body. It is found in all of the body's cells and is a critical molecule for health. It is used to make hormones, Vit D, and is concentrated in cell membranes. Cholesterol in food is especially abundant in animal products such as eggs, dairy, and organ meats such as liver and heart. The body needs some cholesterol, but too much can be associated with an increased risk of heart disease and Alzheimer's in those who are genetically inclined.

Cortisol: Cortisol is a hormone produced by the adrenal glands. It is involved in many processes in the body, including metabolism, the immune response, and stress. It is often referred to as the "stress hormone" because it helps the body respond to and manage stress. High levels of cortisol can have negative health effects, including an increased risk of obesity, diabetes, heart disease, and depression. Optimizing cortisol is the mainstay of optimizing psychological and metabolic health.

Creatinine: Creatinine is a waste product that is produced as a result of normal muscle breakdown. It is normally removed from the body by the kidneys and is commonly used as a marker for kidney function. High levels of creatinine in the blood can be an indication of a reduced capacity of the kidney to remove it. This is typically related to kidney disease or damage.

Curcumin: Curcumin is a compound found in turmeric, a spice commonly used in Indian and Southeast Asian cooking. It has powerful antioxidant and anti-inflammatory properties and is used in many traditional medicines. It is believed to have a wide range of health benefits, including reducing inflammation, and neuro-inflammation in the brain, improving digestion, optimizing gut health, and even helping to prevent certain cancers.

Cyclophosphamide: Cyclophosphamide is a chemotherapy drug used to treat certain types of cancer. It is a type of alkylating agent, which means that it works by interfering with the growth of cancer cells and preventing them from multiplying. Cyclophosphamide is used to treat many types of cancer, including lymphomas, leukemias, multiple myeloma, and other solid tumors.

DAMP: Damage Associated Molecular Patterns (DAMPs) are cellular components that are released from damaged or dying cells. They activate the immune system, promoting inflammation while also initiating the healing process. Examples of DAMPs include ATP, heat shock proteins, and high mobility group box 1 protein.

DEXA scan: A DEXA (Dual-Energy X-ray Absorptiometry) scan is a type of imaging test used to measure bone mineral density. It can be used to diagnose osteoporosis, detect bone loss, and monitor the effectiveness of treatments for bone-related conditions. It is also used to measure body fat, muscle, and other tissue composition.

DHEA: Dehydroepiandrosterone (DHEA) is a hormone produced by the adrenal glands. It is a precursor to other hormones, including testosterone and estrogen, which are important for regulating sexual development, metabolism, and brain function. DHEA levels peak in the body during the late 20s and then gradually decline with age. It is commonly optimized as a supplement to help boost energy levels, improve cognitive function, and slow the effects of aging.

Dihydrotestosterone: Dihydrotestosterone (DHT) is an androgen steroid hormone produced from testosterone. It is responsible for the development of male sexual characteristics, such as facial and body hair, a deep voice, and increased muscle mass. DHT is also involved in the development of male-pattern baldness and prostate enlargement and can increase the risk of prostate cancer in genetically predisposed men. It is more prevalent with topical testosterone as the skin converts testosterone to DHT at a higher rate. It can also lead to penile or clitoral enlargement.

DNA: DNA (Deoxyribonucleic acid) is a molecule that contains the biological instructions that make each species unique. It is made up of four chemical bases (adenine, thymine, guanine, and cytosine) that are paired together. Adenine pairs with Thymine, and Cytosine pairs with Guanine. It is found in nearly all living organisms. DNA is responsible for the genetic code in organisms, which determines everything from physical appearance to health.

Double-stranded DNA: Double-stranded DNA is a type of DNA molecule that consists of two strands of nucleotide bases held together by hydrogen bonds. It is the most common form of DNA found in nature, and it is essential for the replication and transmission of genetic information.

Double-stranded DNA consists of two complementary strands of nucleotides, which are the building blocks of DNA. The two strands are held together by hydrogen bonds between the complementary bases of each strand. The base pairs in double-stranded DNA are Adenine with Thymine and Cytosine with Guanine.

Embryogenesis: Embryogenesis is the process of cell division and differentiation that results in the formation of an embryo after the sperm and egg have united. It occurs involves the growth of cells and tissues that form the body of the organism. Embryogenesis is a complex process that involves the interaction of various genetic, epigenetic, and environmental factors resulting in pluripotent stem cells becoming differentiated into the tissues that comprise every organ in the body.

Endogenous: Endogenous is a term used to describe something that is generated from within. It is often used to refer to processes that occur within an organism or system, such as hormones or rejuvenation factors like stem cells, PRP, or exosomes.

Endogenous sugars: Endogenous sugars are sugars that are naturally produced within the body. These sugars are used to modify the structure and function of proteins to enhance our structure and function. They can promote health or disease depending on what they are attached to Examples are: xylitol, mannitol, galactose, inositol, sialic acid, fructose, etc.

Endothelium: Endothelium is a layer of cells that lines the inside of blood vessels and lymphatic vessels. It plays an important role in controlling the expansion and contraction of the vessel exp. blood pressure. It also impacts clotting and inflammation. Endothelial cells also produce a number of hormones and chemical messengers such as nitric oxide (NO) that regulate blood flow and coordinate the body's response to stress. Covid 19 attached the endothelium increasing clotting.

Epigenetics: Epigenetics is the study of how the physical and psychological environment and lifestyle choices can influence gene expression without changing the underlying DNA sequence. It is the study of changes in gene activity that do not involve changes to the DNA sequence, but still get passed down to at least one successive generation. These epigenetic changes can be caused by environmental factors such as psychological abuse, physical abuse, stress, diet, temperature, and exposure to toxins, as well as happiness, joy, and exercise. Methyl groups are attached and removed from the DNA in the epigenetic process of storing information, and there are predictable patterns of DNA methylation that serve as a clock relative to aging. DNA methylation is one measure of biological age. Reprogramming cells to be young has been shown to change the DNA methylation patterns to younger patterns.

Estrogen: Estrogen is a hormone found in the body that is responsible for the development and regulation of female sexual characteristics and reproduction. It is released in higher levels in females than males and is one of the main hormones involved in the menstrual cycle. Estrogen dominance can lead to heightened emotions, irritability, and premenstrual symptoms (PMS).

Extrinsic age: Extrinsic age is the age of a material or object based on factors other than its actual age. Examples of extrinsic age include the amount of wear and tear an item has experienced.

Exosome: Exosomes are a type of extracellular vesicle, which are small membrane-bound particles that are released from cells and contain proteins, lipids, and genetic material such as mRNA and microRNA. Exosomes are involved in intercellular communication and can transfer genetic material from one cell to another, which can alter the behavior of the receiving cell. They have been studied extensively for their potential use in diagnostics such as cancer and in therapeutics such as rejuvenation and regeneration technologies. They can be added to stem cells' PRP and Peptides to enhance rejuvenation.

Fed state: Fed state is a term used to describe the state of the body when it is received nutrients recently as in eating a meal. It is the opposite of a fasted or low-calorie state. When in this state, the body is better able to build and support cell division and growth.

Fibrinolysis: Fibrinolysis is a process in which the body breaks down a blood clot. Clots restrict or stop blood flow and can cause heart attacks or strokes. Fibrin is a protein that helps form blood clots, were as plasmin is a protein that breaks them down. This balanced process is important for maintaining healthy blood flow and preventing bleeding should a blood vessel be cut. These enzymes protect us from blood loss while breaking down into smaller components to allow the blood to flow freely.

Fisetin: Fisetin is a dietary flavonoid found in fruits and vegetables such as strawberries, apples, persimmons, onions, and cucumbers. It has health benefits, including anti-aging and anti-inflammatory properties. It may also have anti-oxidant, anti-cancer, and neuroprotective properties. It has gained notoriety as being as effective as the combination of dasatinib and quercetin in pruning senescent cells.

Flavonoid: Flavonoids are a type of phytonutrient, or plant nutrient, found in fruits and vegetables. They are a class of polyphenolic compounds that possess antioxidant and anti-inflammatory properties. Flavonoids provide health benefits, such as protection against cardiovascular disease, cancer, and other chronic diseases.

Flow/Flow State: Flow, also known as "the flow state" or "being in the zone," is a mental state in which a person is fully immersed in an activity, to the point of being completely unaware of their surroundings and the passage of time. It is a state of intense presence and focus, during which a person is completely absorbed in what they are doing. Flow is often associated with peak performance and creativity, as it allows people to access their full potential. It is analogous to a meditative state in action that enables creative responses to situations as opposed to reactions. Being in Flow can happen in any activity.

Fox-O: Fox-O is a family of four transcription factors (FOXO1, FOXO3, FOXO4, and FOXO6) that are involved in the regulation of many cellular processes including cell cycle arrest, DNA repair, apoptosis, and metabolism. They are regulated by various signaling pathways, including the

PI3K/AKT pathway and the mTOR pathway. The actions of FOXO3 are especially associated with health and longevity.

Growth Hormone, GH: Growth Hormone, also known as somatotropin. It is a peptide hormone produced by the anterior pituitary gland that stimulates growth, cell reproduction, and cell regeneration in humans and other animals. It is converted to IGF1 which mediates most of the actions through the mTOR pathway. It is critical for life, but too much of it increases health risks and shortens life expectancy.

Glomerular filtration rate (GFR): Glomerular filtration rate, GFR is an important indicator of kidney function and is used to diagnose and monitor kidney disease. GFR is a measure of how many milliliters of blood the kidney is able to filter each minute. It is ideally calculated by collecting urine for 24hrs and measuring the volume of urine and the amount of a certain protein (creatinine) in a blood sample and the collected urine. GFR can also be estimated by measuring the blood level of creatinine or more accurately the blood level of Cystatin C and using an equation to estimate the GFR.

Glucose: Glucose is a simple sugar molecule found in many foods such as fruits, vegetables, grains, and dairy products. It is the main source of energy for the body and is essential for normal functioning. When "blood sugar" is measured, it is blood glucose levels that are monitored. Continuous Glucose Monitors or CGMs can give real-time readings on "blood sugar levels" This is important as excess glucose and subsequent insulin release increase senescent cell formation.

Glutathione: Glutathione is a naturally occurring compound found in the cells. It is a tripeptide consisting of three amino acids: cysteine, glutamic acid, and glycine. Glutathione plays an important role in many biochemical processes, including protecting cells from oxidative stress, metabolizing toxins and carcinogens, and maintaining the integrity of DNA. In addition, it is essential for the proper functioning of the immune system and may help protect against certain diseases. Having optimal levels is important for health and longevity. N-acetyl cysteine is taken to support its production.

Glycans: Glycans are complex carbohydrates composed of a chain of monosaccharides (simple sugars) linked together by glycosidic bonds. They are found added to many different base molecules to modify the base molecule's behavior or create new behaviors. They appear in many different forms, including glycoproteins, glycolipids, proteoglycans, and mucopolysaccharides. Glycans play important roles in many biological processes, such as cell adhesion, signaling, and inflammation.

Glycemic Index: Glycemic Index (GI) is one measure of how a food affects your blood sugar level. It is a measure of how quickly a food will raise your blood sugar level after it is eaten. Foods with a high glycemic index (GI) will cause your blood sugar to rise quickly, while those with a low GI will not cause such a large and sudden spike in blood sugar.

Glycemic Load: Glycemic Load (GL) is another measure of how a food affects your blood sugar level. It denotes how much sugar is in the food you are eating, which is independent of how quickly the sugar is released. Both metrics (GI) and (GL) are important in optimizing carbohydrate intake.

Glycocalyx: Glycocalyx is a slimy and sticky substance that covers the surface of many types of cells, such as those found in the digestive and respiratory systems. It has especially been found to be important for arterial health. It is composed of glycoproteins and polysaccharides, and its purpose is to protect the endothelium from damage, regulate nitric oxide release, and enable protect the arteries from clotting and plaque formation.

Glycoproteins: Glycoproteins are a type of protein that contain carbohydrates, or sugar molecules, attached to them. They can be found in the membranes of cells, in the extracellular matrix, and in the bloodstream. These proteins play important roles in cell recognition, cell adhesion, and the regulation of hormones and enzymes.

Glymphatic system: The Glymphatic system is a recently discovered neurological waste removal system responsible for the clearance of metabolic waste from the brain. It works by pumping cerebrospinal fluid (CSF) through the brain's interstitial space in order to clear away waste products, such as amyloid plaque, that can accumulate in the brain and cause neurological diseases. The system is active primarily during deep sleep, optimizing the brain's ability to clear away waste products during this period. It is enhanced when we sleep with our right cheek on the pillow.

Growth Hormone: Growth hormone, also known as somatotropin, is a hormone produced by the pituitary gland. It is responsible for stimulating growth and cell reproduction, and regeneration in humans and other animals. Growth hormone is important for growth, development, and metabolism. Excess growth hormone can potentiate premature aging and cancer formation.

Gynostemma pentaphyllum: Gynostemma pentaphyllum, commonly known as jiaogulan, is a climbing vine native to parts of China and Japan. It is known for its medicinal properties and has been used in traditional Chinese medicine for centuries. The leaves are used to make teas and tonics, and extracts of the plant are used to treat a variety of conditions, such as fatigue, stress, digestive issues, and immune system disorders. It is especially good at activating the AMPK system to improve healing, autophagy, and, we believe, longevity.

Hemoglobin: Hemoglobin is a protein found in red blood cells that carries oxygen throughout the body. It is oxygenated Hemoglobin is responsible for the red color of blood. Levels are controlled by the kidneys as well as by the environment. We have seen Testosterone and altitude training raise hemoglobin concentration significantly to levels over 50%. This is not necessarily dangerous, but as the cell percentage increases, the blood gets thicker and is more prone to clot and harder for the heart to pump through the vasculature.

Heterozygous: Heterozygous is when an organism has two different alleles for a given genetic trait. This can occur in both plants and animals, and it is responsible for the variation in physical characteristics that we observe between individuals, as the allele expression can be nuanced. An example would be eye hazel eye color.

Hippocampus: The hippocampus is a part of the brain located within the temporal lobe. It is involved in the formation of memories and is believed to play a role in spatial navigation. It is targeted by the processes of dementia that result in memory loss.

Homozygous: Homozygous is a term used in genetics to describe an organism that has two identical alleles of a gene for a particular trait. This means that the organism has identical copies of a gene located on both chromosomes of a particular pair. An organism that is homozygous for a gene will always express the trait associated with that gene.

Hormetic stress: Hormetic stress is a type of stress that is beneficial to the body as it induces the body to get stronger, more robust, and more resilient. It is caused by exposure to a variety of mild stressors such as heat, cold, exercise, and certain nutrients. This type of stress has been shown to cause beneficial physiological responses such as increased alertness, improved cognitive function, increased muscle mass, and increased endurance. It can also help the body to become more resilient to future stressors.

Hydrocarbon: A hydrocarbon is a compound made up of only hydrogen and carbon atoms. Carbon atoms can form up to four bonds. An example is a methyl group. A methyl group is a carbon with three attached hydrogens that uses its remaining fourth bond to attach to DNA to modify the expression of the DNA by either silencing or upregulating gene expression.

Hypothalamic pituitary adrenal axis: The hypothalamic pituitary adrenal (HPA) axis is a complex set of interactions between the hypothalamus, pituitary gland, and adrenal glands. The HPA axis is responsible for the body's response to physical and psychological stress. It is responsible for the release of hormones such as cortisol and adrenaline, which help the body cope with stress. Dysregulation of the HPA axis has been linked to a number of mental health disorders, such as depression and anxiety, as well as chronic stress reactions.

Hypothalamus: The hypothalamus is a region of the brain located just above the brain stem. It is responsible for regulating many essential processes in the body, such as appetite, sleep, body temperature, and hormones. It is also involved in emotions, motivation, and reward processing. In addition, it monitors the body and balances our hormones by signaling the pituitary gland to release its hormones when needed. In addition, the third ventricle contains stem cells that are believed to control the aging process.

Immunosenescence: Immunosenescence is the age-related decline in the function of the immune system. It is characterized by an increased susceptibility to infections and a decreased response to vaccination. It is also associated with increased inflammation and a higher risk of autoimmune diseases. It is related to a loss of natural killer cell function and loss of adaptability to cope with new challenges, be they infections or malignant cells.

In silico: In silico is a term used to refer to experiments or other analyses that are performed using computer models and simulations, as opposed to being done in a laboratory or on an actual organism. It is commonly used in fields such as biology and medicine to study the behavior of cells, proteins, and other biological systems.

Insulin: Insulin is a peptide hormone produced by the pancreas that helps the body use glucose for energy by causing cells to take glucose in. It regulates blood sugar levels by allowing glucose to enter the body's cells, where it can be used for energy. It also helps store excess glucose in the liver and muscles for later use. Without insulin, the body cannot properly use glucose, leading to high levels of sugar in the blood, which can cause a wide range of health problems, as seen in diabetes.

Insulin-resistant: Insulin resistance is a condition in which the body does not respond properly to the hormone insulin. This can cause glucose to build up in the bloodstream instead of being absorbed by the cells, leading to high blood sugar levels. Insulin resistance is a key factor in the development of type 2 diabetes. Running higher than normal insulin levels overworks the pancreatic beta cells and causes them to burn out, leaving a person dependent on insulin injections. High insulin levels also increase senescent cell formation and accelerate aging.

Intrinsic age: Intrinsic age is a term used to describe a person's physical age as opposed to their chronological age. It is based on the idea that a person's physical health and wellness can vary widely from their chronological age and that age is not always an accurate indicator of a person's overall health. Intrinsic age is determined by assessing factors such as lifestyle, physical activity, diet, and other health indicators. In essence, we are all a mosaic of intrinsic ages.

IRB: An Institutional Review Board (IRB) is an independent body that reviews research involving human subjects as part of an ethical and regulatory process. The IRB is responsible for protecting the rights and welfare of research participants, ensuring that the research is conducted in an ethical manner and meets all applicable laws and regulations.

Isometric exercise: An isometric exercise is any type of exercise where the muscle length and joint angle do not change during contraction. It involves the static contraction of a muscle without any visible movement in the angle of the joint. Examples of isometric exercises include wall sits, planks, and bridges. Any resistance exercise can be made to be isometric.

Isotonic exercise: An isotonic exercise is any type of exercise where the muscle length and joint angle change through a range of motion during contraction. It involves resistance as the body part moves closer to the body, eccentric motion, and as it moves away from the body concentric motion.

Ketamine: Ketamine is a dissociative anesthetic used in both human and veterinary medicine. It is a Schedule III controlled substance in the U.S. and is used as a general anesthetic. It is also used for the treatment of pain and depression. It has a rapid onset of action and produces a trance-like state in which users feel disconnected from reality. Ketamine can produce feelings of relaxation, confusion, and euphoria and can also lead to hallucinations. Ketamine centers are scattered across the US and treat resistant depression and PTSD.

Knees Over Toes method: The Knees Over Toes (KOT) method is a physical therapy technique developed by Ben

Patrick used to improve knee and ankle mobility, strength, and stability. It involves positioning the knee in a slightly bent position, above the toes, and then activating the muscles around that joint to create stability. This technique can help to reduce pain associated with knee and ankle instability and improve overall posture, movement, and athletic capability.

Krebs cycle or tricarboxylic acid (TCA): The Krebs cycle (also known as the citric acid cycle or the tricarboxylic acid cycle) is a series of chemical reactions that take place in the mitochondria of cells and comprises the initial chemical steps required to produce energy. The cycle involves a series of enzyme-catalyzed reactions in which acetyl-CoA is oxidized to produce carbon dioxide, water, and energy in the form of ATP and reduced coenzymes. Mitochondrial energy is the primary source of energy produced in the cell.

LIFE RAFT: Life Energy Resilience Anti-Fragility Trial. A Gladden Longevity IRB-approved trial designed to play the symphony of longevity. It is designed to teach us the best ways to reverse our mosaic of biological clocks.

Ligand: Ligands are molecules that bind to other molecules, forming a chemical bond. They are often found in biological systems, such as proteins, and can be used to alter biochemical pathways or activate or inhibit specific processes. They can also be used in chemical reactions to create new compounds or to increase the reactivity of existing ones.

Lipids: Lipids are a type of fat molecules, fatty acids, glycerol, cholesterol, etc. They are an important part of the cell membrane and are also used as an energy source and provide the structural backbone for the production of sex hormones.

Lymphatic system: The lymphatic system is a network of tissues and organs that help rid the body of toxins, waste, and other unwanted materials. It is composed of a system of lymph nodes, lymph vessels, the spleen, thymus, and bone marrow. The lymphatic system helps fight infection and other diseases by producing and transporting lymph, a clear fluid that contains white blood cells. It also helps maintain fluid balance and absorbs fats from the digestive system.

Melatonin: Melatonin is a hormone naturally produced by the pineal gland in the brain. It helps to regulate other hormones and maintain the body's circadian rhythm, which is the body's internal clock that tells it when to sleep and wake. Melatonin is often used as a supplement to help people reset their circadian rhythm. It has also been studied for its potential as an antioxidant and for its ability to help protect against certain types of cancer. It is also known to modulate inflammation.

Menopause: Menopause is the natural biological transition in a woman's life when she stops having menstrual periods and is no longer able to become pregnant. The average age for menopause is 51 years old, although it can vary from woman to woman. Menopause is considered a part of the normal aging process for women. It is marked by a decrease in the production of the hormones estrogen and progesterone. During menopause, women may experience a variety of physical, psychological, and emotional symptoms such as hot flashes, irritability, poor sleep, and weight gain. Symptoms can be reduced with bioidentical hormones.

Metformin: Metformin is a prescription medication used to treat type 2 diabetes. It belongs to a class of drugs known as biguanides and works by decreasing the amount of glucose produced by the liver, slowing the release of liver glucose stores, and helping the cells to respond better to insulin. Metformin is usually taken orally and can be used in combination with lifestyle changes such as diet and exercise. Metformin has been shown to decrease cancer and improve longevity in diabetics. The Targeting Aging with Metformin (TAME) Trial is a trial looking to see if metformin can improve longevity in non-diabetics. One of the longevity actions is the activation of AMPK.

Methyl groups: Methyl groups are organic chemical groups composed of one carbon atom bonded to three hydrogen atoms. They are found in a wide variety of compounds, including amino acids, nucleic acids, lipids, and some hormones. Their pattern of attachment to DNA is a reliable clock of an organism's age.

Microglial system: A microglial system is a network of specialized immune cells found in the brain and spinal cord. Microglia are responsible for monitoring the brain and spinal cord for any potential damage or infection and clearing away damaged cells and debris. They also play a role in the development and maintenance of the central nervous system. When they are activated inappropriately, they can cause neuroinflammation and brain damage and contribute to brain fog and dementia. Microglial exposure to pathogen-associated molecular patterns (PAMPs) and/or endogenous damage-associated molecular patterns (DAMPs) can trigger their activation. Likewise, the removal of the immune-suppressive signals can lead to their activation. Short-term activation can be healthy, while long-term activation is detrimental.

Mitochondria: Mitochondria are organelles that are found in all of our cells. They are the powerhouses of the cell, providing energy through the process of cellular respiration involving the Krebs cycle and the Electron transport chain. Mitochondria not only produce ATP aerobically, i.e. with oxygen, but they are important for a wide variety of cellular processes, including metabolism, calcium homeostasis, the cellular defense response to infections, and apoptosis. Long-haul symptoms and chronic fatigue are many times related to a reduction in mitochondrial activity. Rebooting the mitochondria is a strategy to deal with these low-energy conditions.

Mitophagy: Mitophagy is a process of selective autophagy that involves the degradation of damaged or unnecessary mitochondria. It is an important process for maintaining the quality of the mitochondria and for keeping the cell healthy. It can be encouraged with a supplement of Urolithin A.

Molecular hydrogen: Molecular hydrogen (H2) is a colorless, odorless, tasteless, and non-toxic gas made up of two hydrogen atoms bound together. It is a remarkable molecule. It balances oxidative stress in the cell and has been shown in unpublished Insilico testing to modulate pain as well.

mRNA: mRNA (messenger ribonucleic acid) is a type of RNA molecule that carries genetic information from DNA to the ribosome, where it is translated into proteins. It is composed of a single strand of nucleotides, which are the building blocks of DNA and RNA. Transcriptomic testing looks at mRNA as well as proteins to determine which genes are being expressed. Knowing this is critical in decoding the aging process and measuring progress.

mTOR: mTOR (mechanistic Target of Rapamycin) is a protein kinase that acts as an important regulator of cell growth and metabolism. It is a key mediator of the cell's response to changes in environmental conditions, such as nutrient availability, and is involved in a wide range of important cellular processes, including protein synthesis, cell growth, metabolism, and survival. It decreases autophagy and, if overstimulated, has been linked to an increased risk of cancer and shortened survival. Rapamycin is used inside the IRB-approved trial Life Raft to modulate mTOR expression. AMPK is the alter ego to mTOR. When AMPK activity is up, mTOR is down. When mTOR activity is up, AMPK is down.

Myeloperoxidase: Myeloperoxidase (MPO) is an enzyme found in neutrophils, a type of white blood cell, where it helps protect the body against infection by breaking down harmful compounds. MPO is also found in other tissues, where it is involved in processes such as wound healing, tissue repair, and the production of hormones. It is a major component of the inflammatory response and can be used as a biomarker of inflammation. It has been shown that when levels are increased in the blood, it increases the risk of plaque rupture, which can lead to heart attack or stroke.

Myopia: Myopia, also known as nearsightedness, is a common vision condition in which objects that are far away appear blurry, while objects that are close up appear clear. People with myopia can often see well for activities such as reading and computer work but have difficulty seeing distant objects clearly. The condition is typically caused by the shape of the eye, which causes light entering the eye to be focused in front of the retina instead of directly on it. Myopia can be treated with eyeglasses, contact lenses, or refractive surgery. It can also be used to describe being short-sighted in your perspective.

NAD/NADH: NAD (Nicotinamide adenine dinucleotide) and NADH (Nicotinamide adenine dinucleotide - hydrogen) are coenzymes involved in many metabolic processes. NAD is an electron acceptor for oxidation-reduction reactions, while NADH is an electron donor. NADH is involved in the production of energy through the electron transport chain and is a critical component of cellular respiration. Optimizing the NAD to NADH ratio can be done with NAD precursors such as Nicotinamide Mono Nucleotide (NMN), Nicotinamide Riboside (NR), and Niacin. Exposure to ozone will oxidize NADH to NAD, boosting energy. As we age, CD38 released from senescent cells utilizes NAD and causes a loss of energy. CD38 can be blocked with apigenin found in parsley.

Neurons: Neurons are specialized cells that transmit information throughout the body. They are the basic building blocks of the nervous system, which can be conceptualized as the building infrastructure of the body. Neurons are responsible for sending, receiving, and processing information from the brain and spinal cord to the rest of the body.

Nitrate: Nitrate is an inorganic compound and salt of nitric acid, consisting of one nitrogen atom and three oxygen atoms (NO_3). Industrial nitrate is a common component of fertilizers, explosives, and food preservatives. Dietary nitrate is a necessary precursor to the production of nitric oxide.

Nitric oxide: Nitric oxide (NO) is a gas molecule produced naturally in the body that helps regulate blood flow, immune response, and other important physiological functions. It is also an important signaling molecule in the nervous system and has been studied for its role in a variety of diseases. (NO) causes arterial dilation important for sexual function, athletic function as well as blood pressure lowering.

Oligopeptide or peptide: Oligopeptides and peptides are short chains of amino acids connected by peptide bonds. Oligopeptides are made up of two to twenty amino acids, while peptides are made up of more than twenty amino acids. They are used in various biological processes, such as forming proteins, controlling cell activities, and delivering hormones. Peptides can also be signaling molecules that set off cascades of regenerative processes in the body.

Oxidative stress: Oxidative stress is an imbalance between the production of free radicals and the body's ability to detoxify and eliminate them. Sources are mitochondria as they use oxygen to make ATP as well as inflammatory and immune processes. It is caused by an excess of reactive oxygen species (ROS) in the body, which can damage cells, proteins, and other molecules. Oxidative stress is thought to play a role in the development of many diseases, including cancer, diabetes, cardiovascular disease, and neurological disorders. Hydrogen is used to balance oxidative stress.

Oxytocin: Oxytocin is a hormone and neuropeptide produced in the brain. It is often referred to as the "love hormone" or "cuddle hormone" because it is involved in social bonding, sexual reproduction, and childbirth. It is released during hugging for twenty seconds, kissing for eight seconds, breastfeeding, touching, and other positive social interactions. Oxytocin also plays a role in regulating body temperature, appetite, and stress. It has been shown to increase telomere lengths.

Paclitaxel glitazone: Paclitaxel glitazone is a combination drug used for the treatment of advanced or metastatic non-small cell lung cancer (NSCLC). It is a combination of paclitaxel, a chemotherapy drug, and glitazone, a type 2 diabetes medication. The combination helps to increase the effectiveness of paclitaxel in treating NSCLC.

PAMP: Pathogen-associated molecular patterns (PAMPs). PAMPs are a set of molecules that are present on the surface of various classes of microbes. So, they trigger the innate immune system to recognize pathogens and, thus, protect the host from infection. Exposure to them can lead to chronic inflammatory states when after exposure to PAMPs, the innate immune system does not turn off its inflammatory response appropriately.

Parasympathetic nervous system: The parasympathetic nervous system is a division of the autonomic nervous system that acts to slow down the heart rate, increase intestinal and gland activity, and relax the sphincter muscles. Think of it as the brake pedal, rest and repair, and being Zen. It functions in opposition to the sympathetic nervous system, which is the gas pedal, anxious, excited, and energized.

Peptides: Peptides are short chains of amino acids. They are commonly used in research and in medicine and can be found in many cosmetics and dietary supplements. Peptides like BPC 157 and Thymosin Alpha can be used to treat a variety of medical conditions, including cancer, heart disease, diabetes, and gut disorders. They are also used as building blocks for proteins and hormones and can be used to augment the regenerative effects of stem cells and exosomes.

Peroxidase: Peroxidase is an enzyme that catalyzes the oxidation of various substances by hydrogen peroxide. It is used by the immune system to kill bacteria.

PET scan: A PET scan (Positron Emission Tomography) is a type of imaging test that uses a radioactive substance called a tracer to look for disease in the body. The tracer is injected into a vein, and then a special camera is used to track its location in the body. The camera detects the radiation from the tracer and creates detailed 3-dimensional images of the inside of the body. PET scans are used to diagnose and monitor a variety of conditions, such as cancer, heart disease, and brain disorders.

Pituitary gland: The pituitary gland is a small, pea-sized organ located at the base of the brain that is responsible for producing hormones to regulate vital body functions. It is under the control of the hypothalamus, that anatomically sits above it. The hormones it produces affect growth (growth hormone, GH), and sexual development (luteinizing hormone, LH, & follicular stimulating hormone, FSH), metabolism (thyroid stimulating hormone, TSH), and the body's response to stress (adrenocorticotropic hormone, ACTH).

Plasmapheresis: Plasmapheresis is a medical procedure that involves removing blood from the body, separating out the plasma, and then returning the remaining components back to the body along with albumin. It is used to treat certain conditions that have excess inflammation, like autoimmune diseases, where the plasma contains high levels of antibodies or other proteins that are attacking the body's own tissues. It is now also used to treat aging by removing inflammatory cytokines that are part of inflammaging. In addition, Young plasma from a sex-matched donor between the ages of 18 and 25 can be sued to replace the removed plasma.

Plasmalogens: Plasmalogens are a type of phospholipid found in cell membranes. They are composed of a fatty acid linked to a glycerol backbone, with a phosphoethanolamine group attached. Plasmalogens are involved in a wide range of biological processes, including cell signaling, energy metabolism, and gene expression. In addition, they play a role in health and disease, as they are important components of cell membranes and are involved in the development of several chronic diseases like Alzheimer's, heart disease, and cancer. They can now be tested for and treated.

Pluripotent: Pluripotent is a term used to describe cells that have the potential to develop into any cell type in the body. Pluripotent stem cells are stem cells that are able to differentiate into any type of cell in the body, including those found in the heart, brain, muscles, and other organs and tissues. Very Small Embryonic Like Stem Cells are pluripotent.

Polypeptide: A polypeptide is a chain of amino acids bonded together by peptide bonds. Polypeptides are the building blocks of proteins and have a wide range of functions in the body, including acting as enzymes, hormones, and signaling molecules.

Polyphenols: Polyphenols are compounds found in many plant-based foods, including fruits, vegetables, grains, and legumes. They are also found in tea, coffee, chocolate, and red wine. Polyphenols are antioxidants, which means they help protect cells from damage caused by free radicals. They may also help reduce inflammation and improve heart health.

Prebiotic: Prebiotics are dietary fibers that are not digested by the body but are used as fuel by beneficial bacteria in the digestive system. Think of them as fertilizer for the gut biome. They help to support a healthy balance of good bacteria in the gut, which is essential for overall health, digestion, and immunity.

Probiotics: Probiotics are living or dead microorganisms (usually bacteria) that modulate the gut biome to provide health benefits when consumed. They are found in various fermented foods like sauerkraut, yogurt, and pickles, as well as in supplements. Especially when combined with pre-biotics and can help to balance the bacteria in the gut, improve digestion, decrease gut inflammation, improve mood, lower blood sugar, and support the immune system.

Progesterone: Progesterone is a hormone that is produced by the ovaries, the adrenal glands, and the placenta during pregnancy. It plays a role in regulating the menstrual cycle, preparing the uterus for pregnancy by thickening the endometrial lining, and maintaining that thickness during pregnancy. Progesterone also helps to regulate the development of the breasts, uterus, and other reproductive organs in both men and women. It has a calming effect on most women and counteracts the irritability and emotional lability experienced as pre-menstrual symptoms. It is typically given orally.

Proprioception: Proprioception is the sense of where we are in space relative to gravity, the environment, and relative to the position of our own body parts. It also enables us to perceive the strength of effort being employed in movement. It is sometimes referred to as the "special sense." Proprioception is what enables us to know where we are in space even with our eyes closed.

Prostate-specific antigen (PSA) test: The Prostate-specific antigen (PSA) test is a blood test used to measure the level of PSA in the blood. PSA is a protein produced exclusively by the cells of the prostate gland. Elevated levels of PSA may indicate the presence of prostate cancer, although it can be elevated due to other benign conditions such as after sexual activity, riding a bike, or with inflammation of the prostate known as prostatitis. The PSA test is a poor metric to reliably diagnose cancer but can be improved by adding a % free PSA measurement to it from the same blood sample. In the case of known prostate cancer, PSA levels are helpful to monitor prostate cancer, as well as monitor the effectiveness of prostate cancer treatments.

Protein: Proteins are large molecules made up of amino acids. They are essential for life and are involved in virtually every process within cells. Proteins are the building blocks of the body and play a vital role in the structure and function of cells, tissues, and organs. They also provide energy, transport molecules, and regulate metabolic activity. The body can produce some but not all the amino acids required to make proteins, and hence "essential amino acids" can only be obtained from the diet.

Proteoglycans: Proteoglycans are a type of large molecule composed of a protein core and one or more attached glycosaminoglycan (GAG) chains. They are found in the extracellular matrix of cells and in the ground substance of the connective tissues of animals. Proteoglycans are involved in many biological processes, including cell adhesion, migration, signaling, and tissue morphogenesis. They are also part of the blood vessel's glycocalyx, which coats the inner lining of the blood vessel and is essential for maintaining arterial health.

Proteomics: Proteomics is the large-scale study of proteins, including their structure, function, and interactions. It is a rapidly growing field of bioscience research that seeks to understand the structure and function of proteins in a cell, tissue, or organism. Proteomics is used to identify, quantify, and characterize proteins, as well as to understand how these proteins interact with each other and how they are regulated by environmental factors. Proteomics techniques are now also used to assess age and to assess the effects of drugs, supplements, and other interventions on the aging process. Proteomics couples with transcriptomics and DNA sequencing to give an even more comprehensive view of an individual's status.

Proteostasis: Proteostasis is the regulation of proteins within the cell. This includes the transcribing, folding, assembly, trafficking, and degradation of proteins, as well as the maintenance of their correct conformation and activity. Proteins are three-dimensional structures, and Proteostasis is essential for ensuring their integrity enabling the proper functioning of all cells. Proteostasis is a Hallmark of Aging and is particularly important for a healthy aging process.

Psychedelics: Psychedelics are a class of psychoactive substances that produce changes in perception, mood, and cognitive processes through the agonism of serotonin receptors. They produce their effects by modulating neural circuits in the brain and creating new neural connections. Psychedelics are used for a variety of medical purposes because of their ability to enable a person stuck in a particular thought pattern, perception, or mental state to see and experience an alternate way to be. Research is now underway at Johns Hopkins and other institutions for the treatment of mental health disorders and spiritual exploration.

Rapamycin: Rapamycin is a drug used in high doses to prevent organ rejection in transplant patients. It is also used as an adjunct to treat certain types of cancer. It is being studied as a potential treatment for aging as it counteracts mTOR activity. Using it episodically can lead to immune system rejuvenation, reduce muscle loss, protect brain function, and decrease cancer risk. It has also been shown to decrease senescent cell formation and protect against age-related diseases.

Redox: Redox (short for reduction-oxidation) is a type of chemical reaction in which the oxidation states of atoms are changed by gaining or losing an electron. This reaction involves the transfer of electrons between two reacting molecules or ions. Redox reactions are important in many areas of biology, as they are used to make energy as ATP but can also be involved in propagating damage in the cell if not modulated appropriately.

Resting Metabolic Rate (RMR): Resting metabolic rate (RMR) is the amount of energy (measured in calories) that your body uses to sustain itself when at rest. RMR is influenced by your body composition, age, gender, level of physical activity, and thyroid hormone levels. It is an important indicator of overall health and can be used to diagnose subclinical hypothyroidism and assess the effectiveness of thyroid replacement as well as diet and exercise programs.

Rhodiola: Rhodiola is an adaptogenic herb that has been used for centuries as a natural remedy for a variety of health issues. It is believed to help boost energy, reduce stress and anxiety, improve cognitive function, and protect the body from environmental toxins. Rhodiola is also thought to have anti-inflammatory and antioxidant properties, making it a popular supplement for those looking to improve their overall health and well-being. It is many times given in the morning coupled with ashwagandha taken in the afternoon.

RNA: RNA (ribonucleic acid) is a type of biological molecule that plays an important role in the process of gene expression. It is single-stranded and made up of nucleotides that contain ribose sugar and phosphate groups. RNA is involved in the transfer of genetic information from DNA to the ribosome, where it is used to produce proteins. Transcriptomics looks at RNA molecules as well as proteins to understand which genes are being expressed and to what extent. RNA has other signaling functions in the cell that modulate cellular functions.

Senolytics: Senolytics are drugs or compounds that target and eliminate senescent cells from the body. Senescent cells are aged cells that accumulate in the body over time and contribute to the aging process in several ways. They take up space, and they can become a secretory known as senescence-associated secretory phenotype (SASP). SASP cells add to the inflammation that occurs with aging. By removing these cells, senolytics may help reduce the effects of aging and improve overall health.

Senomorphics: Senomorphics are drugs or compounds that focus on reducing the formation of senescent cells in the body, senostasis, or preventing them from becoming senescence-associated secretory phenotype (SASP). Senomorphics, by attenuating the pro-inflammatory secretory phenotype, cause senostasis, which is believed to slow the expression and experience of aging.

Serine: Serine is an amino acid that is found in proteins and is important for many physiological processes. It is a non-essential amino acid, meaning that the body can produce it from other compounds. It plays a role in many biological processes, including metabolism, muscle growth, immune system function, and the production of neurotransmitters. It is of particular interest in its ability to chaperone protein folding to enhance the proteostasis process.

SIRTs: Sirtuins (SIRTs) are a class of proteins numbered 1-6, exp. SIRT2. They play a role in a range of metabolic processes such as metabolic control, apoptosis, cell survival, development, inflammation, and DNA repair. They use NAD as a cofactor and therefore boosting NAD levels has been shown to boost Sirtuin activity. They have multiple anti-aging effects and have been linked to lifespan extension in animals. They are also thought to be involved in stress resistance, energy metabolism, and gene silencing.

Spermidine: Spermidine is a naturally occurring polyamine found in all living cells. It is involved in a variety of cellular processes such as DNA repair, gene expression, and regulation of cell growth and death. It is of interest as a driver of autophagy. Spermidine has been studied for its potential benefits in extending lifespan and preventing heart disease. It is also being studied for its potential to improve cognitive function and protect against neurological disorders.

Subclinical: Subclinical refers to a condition or symptom that is present within an individual but is either not causing symptoms or is causing symptoms but an abnormality is not picked up with traditional medical testing. These conditions can be detected through more advanced laboratory tests or other medical tests such as biometric testing. An example of biometric testing would be measuring the resting metabolic rate to diagnose subclinical hypothyroidism.

Superoxide dismutase: Superoxide dismutase (SOD) is an enzyme that acts as an antioxidant and helps protect cells from oxidative damage caused by superoxide radicals. It is the rate-limiting step in neutralizing neutralize free radicals, which can damage DNA and other cellular components. SOD activity can be upregulated by exercise, hydrogen water, supplements such as Glisodin, and foods such as broccoli, and spinach. Optimizing SOD activity plays an important role in fighting the aging process.

Sympathetic nervous system: The sympathetic nervous system is part of the autonomic nervous system, which controls unconscious bodily functions such as digestion, respiration, and heart rate. It is responsible for the body's fight-or-flight response and is active when we are faced with a stressful situation. Sympathetic nerves travel from the spine to all parts of the body and stimulate the body's organs to respond to a stressful situation by increasing heart rate, releasing stress hormones, and increasing adrenaline in the system. This is the gas pedal. Chronic activation shortens life and health spans. It is counterbalanced by the parasympathetic nervous system which is the brake and is associated with rest repair and health.

T score: A T score is a type of standardized score that is calculated by converting raw scores into a standard scale with a mean of 50 and a standard deviation of 10. T scores are often used in bone density testing to provide an easy way to compare scores across populations and to give you information on how you compare to your peers.

T3: T3 is a type of thyroid hormone that is minimally produced by the thyroid gland but is made in the blood and tissues by converting T4 to T3 by the removal of one iodine atom. It is one of the two hormones produced by the thyroid, the other being the predominatT4. T3 enters the nucleus of the cell and modulates the expression of hundreds of genes. It is responsible for regulating a variety of metabolic processes, including growth and development, metabolism, and body temperature.

T4: T4 (thyroxine) is a thyroid hormone that helps regulate the body's metabolism. It is the primary thyroid hormone produced in the thyroid gland and is the precursor to active T3. T4 works by binding to receptors on cells throughout the body, stimulating them to produce proteins, carbohydrates, and fats. This helps the body maintain a healthy metabolism and helps regulate body temperature.

TSH: TSH stands for thyroid stimulating hormone. It is a hormone produced by the pituitary gland in response to the brain that helps regulate the production of hormones in the thyroid gland. It is used as one measure of thyroid function, aids in the diagnosis of thyroid disorders, and monitors the effectiveness of treatment. It is not as reliable as a resting metabolic rate for diagnosing hypo or hyper-thyroid states.

TTAGGG: TTAGGG is a unique DNA sequence that is used in telomere analysis. It is also known as the telomere repeat sequence. Telomeres are made up of nucleic acids like the rest of the DNA and are found on the ends of chromosomes.

Telomerase: Telomerase is an enzyme that helps maintain the length of telomeres, which are segments of DNA at the end of chromosomes. Telomerase adds repeating sequences of nucleotides to the ends of telomeres, which helps them to remain stable and prevents them from becoming too short. Because telomeres shorten over time, telomerase helps to counteract this process, allowing cells to stay alive for longer periods.

Telomere: A telomere is a region of repetitive nucleotide sequences at each end of a chromosome, which protects the end of the chromosome from deterioration or from fusion with neighboring chromosomes. Telomeres are essential for proper cell division and are thus critical for maintaining the integrity of the genetic information within a cell.

Testosterone: Testosterone is a hormone produced by the human body. It is primarily responsible for the development of male characteristics and sex drive. It is also responsible for the production of red blood cells, muscle mass, and bone density. Testosterone levels peak during adolescence and early adulthood and decrease with age. Low testosterone levels can lead to a variety of health problems, including decreased libido, erectile dysfunction, depression, and lack of ability to cope with stress.

Thymus gland: The thymus is a small organ located in the upper part of the chest, behind the breastbone. It is part of the lymphatic system, which helps the body fight infection and other diseases. The thymus produces two types of lymphocytes (white blood cells): T cells and B cells. These cells help the body recognize and fight off foreign invaders, such as bacteria and viruses. The thymus gland involutes and is replaced in part with fat cells at a rate of 3% per year until age 35-40. At this point, it has very little activity left. One Hallmark of Aging, Immunosenescence, is thought to be addressable by rebooting the Thymus gland with Growth hormone or with peptides and stem cells.

Transcriptomics: Transcriptomics is the study of the transcriptome, which is the set of all RNA molecules, including mRNA, rRNA, tRNA, and other non-coding RNAs, produced by the transcription of genes in a cell. Transcriptomics is a field of molecular biology that studies the expression of genes and the regulation of gene expression. It is used to understand how different genes are expressed in different tissues and under different conditions including aging, as well as how gene expression is altered in response to interventions designed to slow or reverse aging. Transcriptomics is also used in cancer to better understand the vulnerabilities of cancer cells.

Tricyclic: Tricyclic is a type of antidepressant drug that was developed in the 1950s to treat depression. It works by blocking the reuptake of norepinephrine and serotonin in the brain, which increases the levels of these neurotransmitters in the brain, leading to improved mood. Tricyclic antidepressants are generally used to treat moderate to severe depression but are also used to treat anxiety and other mental health disorders. They can be associated with a dry mouth dizziness constipation and weight gain.

Triglycerides: Triglycerides are a type of fat found in the blood. They are made up of three separate molecules of fatty acids that are bound together by a glycerol molecule. High levels of triglycerides in the blood can increase the risk of heart disease, stroke, and other health problems.

VO2-max: VO2 max stands for maximal oxygen uptake and is a measure of the maximum amount of oxygen that an individual can utilize during intense exercise. Cardiac output is a surrogate marker for VO2 max. It is one of the most important indicators of aerobic fitness and is a measure of the body's ability to transport and use oxygen during exercise. A high VO2 max is associated with a longer life and fewer disease of aging such as heart disease, dementia, and cancer.

Xenobiotics: Xenobiotics are chemical compounds that are foreign to an organism's natural biochemistry. Examples of xenobiotics include pharmaceuticals, pesticides, industrial chemicals, and pollutants. Xenobiotics can have both natural and man-made origins. They represent a burden for the bodied detox systems.

Zombie cells: Zombie cells is a slang term for senescent cells.

Z score: A Z score is a statistical tool that allows you to compare yourself to a healthy 30-year-old. It is used in reporting bone mineral density as a compliment to a T score which compares you to your age-matched peers.

Acknowledgments

I wish to thank my family, friends, mentors, and collaborators who have encouraged and supported me in my life journey and medical career. They have all left an indelible impact on this book.

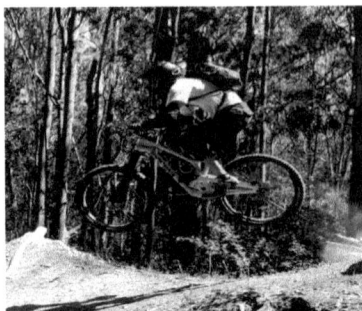
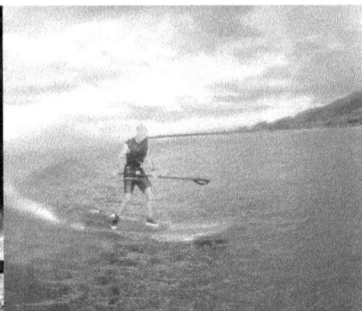
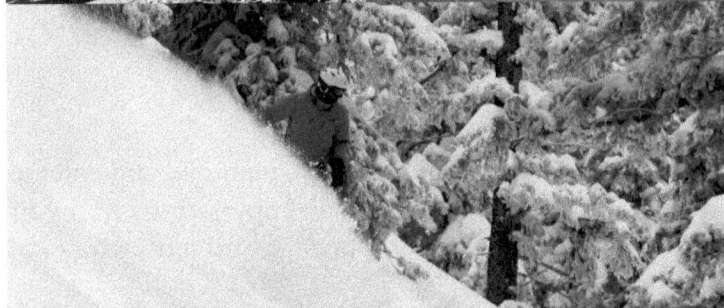
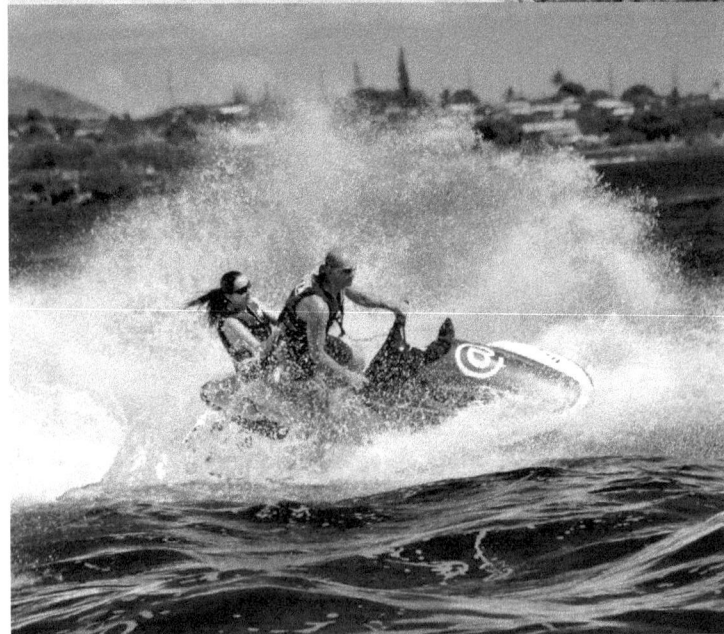

About Dr. Jeffrey Gladden

Dr. Jeffrey Gladden, chronologically 69 in 2023, has a mosaic of biological ages ranging as low as his mid-20s, with the majority in his 30s and 40s. Some would call it a miracle, but he calls it Playing the Symphony of Longevity to Live Young for a Lifetime. The Symphony is composed of a truly exponential plan for the exponential problem of aging. We don't age in a linear way. Aging accelerates exponentially, and virtually all plans that simply focus on eating better, exercise, sleep, stress reduction, hormone replacement, and supplements are a linear strategy to an exponential problem.

From a young age, Jeff saw what aging did to those he loved. At a crucial moment in his life, he can still hear his grandmother telling him, *"Jeff, don't ever get old … it's hell to get old."* Her words were more than a warning, it was a plea for him not to grow old the same way she had.

As a true trailblazer in Life Energy, Longevity, Health, and Human Performance Optimization Science, Dr. Gladden's groundbreaking work applies the best science, deepest insights, and the greatest technologies to unlock the secrets to longevity at his clinic, Gladden Longevity.

Being a leading cardiologist for over 25 years, Dr. Gladden regularly brought the latest cutting-edge technologies to his patients. During that time, he co-founded the Heart Hospital Baylor Scott & White, was the founder and CEO of a cardiology group with 10 offices and 12 doctors, and created cardiac catheterization labs, rapid response heart attack programs, heart arrhythmia programs, and congestive heart failure programs for outlying communities and hospitals. In addition, he became involved in several medical device startups and, as of this writing, sits on the board of two of them. He discovered that he could always get a better result for his patients by having a deeper understanding of them and the problems they faced enabling him to create precise solutions for them. He brings that same mindset to his work at Gladden Longevity.

In his early 50s, despite his successes, he started to feel rundown, was putting on weight, had less energy, and when stressed, started to feel depressed, struggling to do things that used to be easy.

When he went in for medical testing, he was told that "everything checks out ok for your age. You're just getting older... why don't we start you on an antidepressant."

Jeff knew his doctors were not addressing the underlying issues, they were asking the wrong questions, so he went deeper, much deeper, to ask better ones. He extensively trained and got new certifications in functional and age management medicine. His hard work paid off, and after two and half years, he reversed all of his symptoms and started feeling better than ever.

He then began to wonder, "How good can I be? How fit, how strong, mentally sharp, how spiritually aligned, how relationally replete."

This empowering question led him to leave the sick care world and focus all his energies on longevity, health, performance, and life energy optimization.

"How good can you be?" became the genesis for Gladden Longevity, and he's never looked back. Having a mindset of only being married to his questions, not his current answers, Dr. Gladden continues to make massive strides in the fields of longevity, health, human performance, and life energy. Gladden Longevity is running IRB-approved trials to safely bring the most cutting-edge technologies to his clients, and he wants to share them with you.

Dr. Gladden is confident that we can function like a 30-year-old when we are 100. His work and research now include three additional questions:

- **How Good Can We Be?**
- **How Do We Make 100 The New 30?**
- **How Do We Live Well Beyond 120?**
- **How Do We Live Young for a Lifetime?**

Today, as the founder of Gladden Longevity, he and his longevity staff create Truly cutting-edge, exponentially impactful individualized health rejuvenation, performance longevity, and life energy plans for each and every client, helping them navigate and resolve their issues and teaching them how to play their personal symphony of longevity to maximize their vitality, quality of life, and impact.

When he's not at work, he enjoys his athleticism, artistic, and spiritual sides. He has a super active life: surfing, mountain biking, hiking, snowboarding, playing the guitar, spiritual growth and enlightenment, and spending time with his loved ones. His goal is to follow his trajectory for greatness and make his greatest impact on the planet by having the transcendence and wisdom of a 300-year-old mind in a 30-year-old body. His grandmother is smiling, he's not growing old, he is growing stronger, mentally sharper, more athletically capable, and spiritually wiser while loving every moment of the journey.

Connect with Dr. Gladden at GladdenLongevity.com

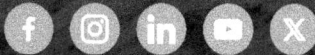

GLADDEN
LONGEVITY
Live Young

CONNECT WITH

Dr. Gladden

Follow him on your favorite
social media platform.

www.gladdenlongevity.com

About Gladden Longevity

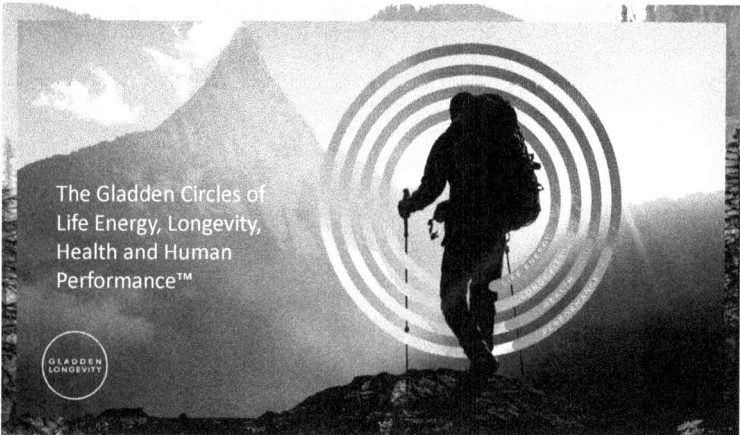

The Gladden Circles of Life Energy, Longevity, Health and Human Performance™

GLADDEN LONGEVITY

Discover a new path to vitality, rejuvenation, and a youthful life at the Gladden Longevity Clinic and Advanced Performance Center. Our mission is crystal clear: to revolutionize aging through the fusion of deep understanding of our clients, innovative personalized care, and the use of cutting-edge technologies. With unwavering dedication, we strive to unlock the keys to living your best life with peak health, human performance, and optimal longevity.

Together, we'll architect and implement tailored health plans, harnessing advanced diagnostics and regenerative therapies to empower you with boundless energy, mental clarity, equanimity, and physical resilience.

Join us on this transformative journey and embrace this opportunity to "Live Young for a Lifetime."

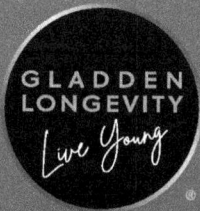

GLADDEN
LONGEVITY
Live Young

LIFE-RAFT
Life Energy, Resilience, Anti-Fragility Trail

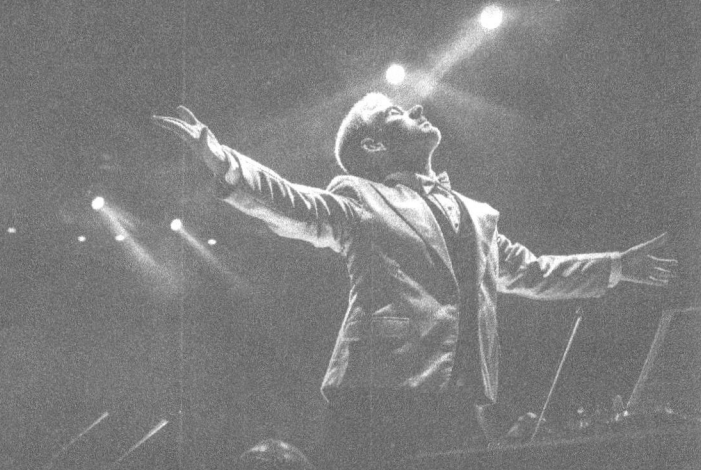

Playing the "Symphony" of Longevity

Interested in joining this exclusive
IRB approved study?

www.gladenlongevity.com/Life-RaftStudy

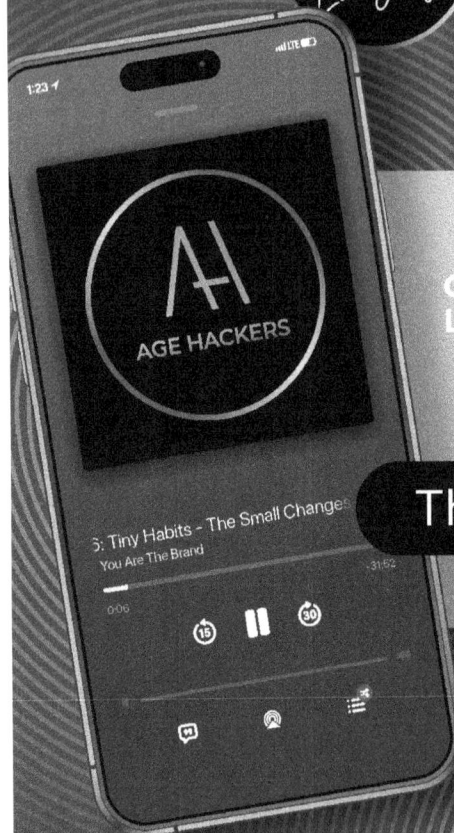

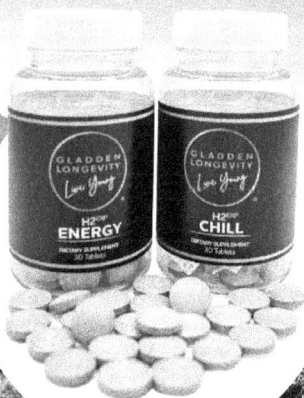

GLADDEN LONGEVITY
Live Young

ENERGY

CHILL

Supplement Shop

Explore a wide array of supplements recommended for a healthy approach to longevity

www.gladdenlongevityshop.com

THIS BOOK IS PROTECTED INTELLECTUAL PROPERTY

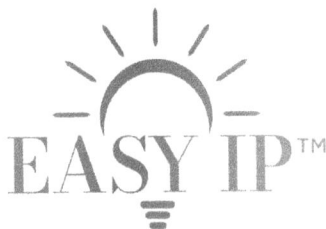

EASY IP™

The author of this book values Intellectual Property. The book you just read is protected by Easy IP™, a proprietary process, which integrates blockchain technology giving Intellectual Property "Global Protection." By creating a "Time-Stamped" smart contract that can never be tampered with or changed, we establish "First Use" that tracks back to the author.

Easy IP™ functions much like a Pre-Patent™ since it provides an immutable "First Use" of the Intellectual Property. This is achieved through our proprietary process of leveraging blockchain technology and smart contracts. As a result, proving "First Use" is simple through a global and verifiable smart contract. By protecting intellectual property with blockchain technology and smart contracts, we establish a "First to File" event.

Powered By Easy IP™

LEARN MORE AT EASYIP.TODAY